A New and Untried Course

A New and Untried Course

Woman's Medical College and Medical College of Pennsylvania, 1850–1998

Steven J. Peitzman

RUTGERS UNIVERSITY PRESS
New Brunswick, New Jersey, and London

Library of Congress Cataloging-in-Publication Data

Peitzman, Steven J. (Steven Jay), 1945–
    A new and untried course : Woman's Medical College and Medical College
of Pennsylvania, 1850–1998 / Steven J. Peitzman.
        p. cm.
    Includes bibliographical references and index.
    ISBN 0–8135–2815–1 (cloth : alk. paper) — ISBN 0–8135–2816–X (pbk. :
alk. paper)
        1. Medical College of Pennsylvania—History. 2. Medical
colleges—Pennsylvania—Philadelphia—History. 3. Women physicians—
Study and teaching—Pennsylvania—Philadelphia—History. I. Title

R747.M48 P45 2000
610'.71'174811—dc21   99–045850

British Cataloging-in-Publication data for this book is available from the British
Library

Manufactured in the United States of America

*In memory of Ida Draeger, B.S. in L.S.,
and Harry Gottlieb, M.D.*

Contents

Illustrations

Preface and Acknowledgments

In 1996, leaders of the Allegheny University of the Health Sciences, which included the MCP Hahnemann School of Medicine, commissioned new sesquicentennial histories of the two medical colleges that in 1993 entered into merger under Allegheny: Medical College of Pennsylvania (MCP, the former Woman's Medical College of Pennsylvania, founded in 1850) and Hahnemann University, the former Hahnemann Medical College (founded in 1848).[1] In writing this history of Woman's Medical College and MCP, I have tried to both offer a full portrait which will appeal to alumnae/i, faculty, and students and to provide a "contextualized" and interpretive account that historians might find useful. In due time, I will no doubt learn from both intended audiences how successful I have been. Regrettably, space has not allowed inclusion of the history of the College's School of Nursing.

I have, of course, many acknowledgments and thanks to offer. For the first, I choose a woman and her (first) book: Regina Morantz-Sanchez and her *Sympathy and Science: Women Physicians in American Medicine*, published by Oxford University Press in 1985 and the landmark work on its subject. Since it would prove tiresome to cite Professor Morantz-Sanchez in every tenth note, my general reliance on her scholarship must be clearly stated here, and I am grateful for her generosity in reading my draft chapters.

Other historians who either read chapter drafts or in other ways offered assistance include Edward Atwater, Vanessa Northington Gamble, Jennifer Gunn, Robert Kaiser, Kenneth Ludmerer, Joan Lynaugh, Russell C. Maulitz, Edward Morman (who shared his research on Frances Emily White), Ellen More, Janet Tighe, and Susan Wells.

Kristin Bunin, while a medical student at MCP Hahnemann, served ably as a research assistant and collaborated in the development of chapter 11. The salutary influence of Maria Trumpler, Toby Appel, and Kristin's other mentors at Yale University shows clearly.

Virtually all the primary resources for this book are held by the Archives and Special Collections on Women in Medicine of MCP Hahnemann University (the present name of the former Allegheny University of the Health Sciences). I am especially indebted to the help and friendship of current archivists Barbara Williams and Joanne Grossman and former staff Sandra Chaff, Margaret Jerrido, and Jill Gates Smith. Within a few weeks of herself first exploring the WMC/MCP collections, Barbara Williams presented me with unexpected gems. Former archives assistant Peggy Morris was unfailingly kind and eager to assist. Courteous help was also provided at the Quaker Collections of Haverford College, the Friends Historical Library at Swarthmore College, the Historical Society of Pennsylvania, the Van Pelt Library of the University of Pennsylvania, the Library of the College of Physicians of Philadelphia, and the Urban Archives of Temple University.

All photographs used in this work are courtesy of the Archives and Special Collections on Women in Medicine.

At the then Allegheny University of the Health Sciences, the vice president for development Michael O'Mahoney and Chancellor D. Walter Cohen helped arrange a sabbatical leave from my clinical and teaching duties to work on the book, and have been supportive in many other ways. Also helpful were their assistants, Jackie Adamczyk, Murielle Telemaque, and Regina Bernhardt. The Sesquicentennial Book Committee provided encouragement and advice, and I acknowledge Carol Hansen Montgomery's supervision of that group's work. I am also grateful for the help of Marlie Wasserman and her staff at Rutgers University Press and for the gentle but careful attention of copyeditor Debbie Self. I was fortunate to enlist the indexing skills and knowledge of longtime friend and mentor Lisabeth Holloway.

A number of Woman's Medical College/Medical College of Pennsylvania alumnae/i, faculty, and officers have offered information and opinions both in formal interviews and more casual conversations: Doris Bartuska, Lawrence Byrd, Angie Connor, Lourdes Corman, Jean Forest, Deborah Goldstein, Mary Ellen Hartman, Virginia Hedrick, Lila

Stein Kroser, Phyllis Marciano, Rachel Pape, Charles Puglia, Jay Roberts, Lillian Seitsiv, Alton Sutnick, Doris Willig, Margaret Gray Wood, and others I may be forgetting.

During my sabbatical year, Zia Ahmed and Jean Lee in the Division of Nephrology of MCP Hahnemann School of Medicine assumed additional work.

Financial sponsorship of this book was generously provided by the alumnae/i of Woman's Medical College and Medical College of Pennsylvania; Jonathan Gomberg spent many hours effecting the alumnae/i rescue following the Allegheny collapse. The Barra Foundation also provided critical help in achieving the goals of both sesquicentennial histories.

I am grateful for the friendship, stories, tolerance, and counsel of June Klinghoffer, internist, teacher, and resident spirit of Woman's Med dwelling in MCP. She would probably have preferred that all warts be excised from this book. Unwilling dermatologist, I have left some in, but suspect that the story nonetheless will help explain why she and many others look back with profound respect and affection for this unique medical College and its people.

A New and Untried Course

Introduction

Ladies, in welcoming you here today, let me extend to
you the warm hand of sisterly sympathy. I know the
heart of a woman, and especially that of one entering
upon a new and untried course, like that before you.

Ann Preston, *Introductory Lecture to the Course*
of Instruction in the Female Medical College
of Pennsylvania for the Session 1855–56

O̶f the three old professions of law, medicine, and the clergy, medicine was the first in modern times that women entered in large numbers. This social movement began in mid-nineteenth-century America, and the Woman's Medical College of Pennsylvania (WMC) in Philadelphia played an instrumental role. Founded as the Female Medical College of Pennsylvania in 1850, it was the first school anywhere established to train women in medicine and offer them the M.D. Just as "firsts" are common in the city of Benjamin Franklin, so is institutional durability: WMC was also the longest surviving of the several women's medical schools that arose in the United States. Following a decision in 1969 to admit men to its medical classes the school became the Medical College of Pennsylvania (MCP) in 1970: now, enrolling *men* became the "untried course."

This book is an account of Woman's Medical College and its coeducational continuation. It comprises several accounts, because there are many parallel stories to tell; for this reason, most chapters do not form neat chronological or thematic narratives. What one might call the "*political*" history of WMC forms a tale of numerous crises, mostly financial, overcome by dedicated leaders, faculty, and particularly alumnae. Generating loyalty and motivating the will to carry on was the development of a College "saga" (using the phrase of the educational sociologist Burton Clark), a compilation of historical sensibility, hagiography, and a belief in shared purpose. Certainly an understandable self-interest of women faculty and administrators also defended the school over the long period when most American medical schools offered women few such opportunities. In the decades following World War II, new expectations and opportunities coupled to federal funding drove American medical schools to become complex "academic centers" of research and sophisticated medical care. This new context and the civil rights movement of the 1960s challenged both the original purpose of teaching only women and the unwritten policy of maintaining a largely female faculty. "Woman's Medical" yielded to Medical College of Pennsylvania and the latter confronted a need to both preserve and reinvent identity.

The *curricular* history of WMC and MCP as told here will stress the College's early efforts to emulate (or even surpass) the offerings of the strongest "male" medical schools, so that opponents of the medical women's movement would not be able to equate women's medical education with irregular or inferior training. Influenced by notions of what a woman physician would most likely do in her career, either by choice or restriction, WMC long excelled in the teaching of obstetrics/gynecology and preventive medicine. Owing to lack of funds and perhaps paucity of imagination, however, no major new provisions for training the woman physician arose in the later twentieth century to help justify the school's continuation and to attract students.

The *students* have their story, and stories, to tell, and they did so perhaps most vividly in those early decades of the College history when the young "hen medics" knew themselves to be unconventional beings, even adventuresses in a foreign realm. But well into the years of the coeducational MCP, its students have shared a camaraderie and cohesiveness which helped perpetuate the College saga and its durability. The voice of the students must be part of a full collegiate history. Only addressed episodically, owing to lack of space, are the careers of the graduates, the patterns of which of course varied over time. Available information for nineteenth-century alumnae in particular reveals a surprising diversity and success in the practice of medicine. The College evolved a tradition of training medical missionaries, whose medical and evangelical work in India or China tied together several elements of the nineteenth-century American woman's worldview. For most of its history as WMC, a majority of the school's women faculty and deans was alumnae; this led to continuity and helped sustain fealty at the expense at times of a limiting parochialism.

Other themes to be explored may be adumbrated here as a set of contrasts or even paradoxes, which necessarily add further complexity to the narrative. Although WMC won national and international significance as a training site for medical women, including missionaries, it thrived or struggled very much as a Philadelphia institution; its staunchest lay friends included local Quakers, patricians, and finally wealthy partisans of its neighborhood. An institution established for women and in good part led by women, WMC also serves as an early case study of male-female collaboration, particularly within the faculty. Oddly, it became most pervasively a women's institution in the 1920s and 1930s, by which time most American women studying medicine did so in other, coeducational schools.

WMC embodies the story of a women's institution whose feminist purposes empowered its triumph over early opposition and repeated adversity. At the same time, consequences of its gendered existence within American medicine and society, such as smallness, poverty, and low prestige, limited its standing in the medical world and bequested vulnerability to its second life as MCP. (Indeed, this book also represents one of the few careful studies of a "non-elite" medical school.) In the new and intensely competitive "medical marketplace" of the 1980s, this vulnerability led finally to takeover by a large hospital corporation centered in Pittsburgh—another "untried course," unknown at the time to any other American medical school. Initial optimism gave way within a few years to an unimagined calamitous outcome that will be noted in the Afterword but left for full accounting to a future historian.

To place some of the above themes and events in their proper setting, it has seemed desirable to periodically discuss throughout the book three contexts always influencing the College and its people. These contexts are the evolving practices and expectations of medical education, the changing social status and activities of American women, and (as already suggested) the local environment of Philadelphia. And to Locust Street in old Philadelphia we now turn to witness the commencement of "a new and untried course."

Chapter 1	"A New and Untried Course"

On 30 December 1851, Philadelphia—a city accustomed to "firsts"—witnessed a "novel and interesting occasion," in the understated words of one newspaper reporter.[1] The Female Medical College of Pennsylvania conducted its first commencement in the elegant Musical Fund Hall, usually the home of "concerts, balls, lectures, and singing-schools."[2] "The platform was occupied by the officers and patrons and patronesses, together with the pupils of the College. The graduating class were seated upon a front settee to the left of the speakers' stand. Their names were called by Professor Moseley, the Dean, when the President conferred upon them severally the degree of Doctor of Medicine."[3] The president was William J. Mullen (1805–1882), an unlikely combination of watchmaker, dentist, businessman, philanthropist, women's rights advocate, and future prison reformer. A few American women had previously been awarded the M.D., but never eight together on one platform and never before from a medical school established specifically for women.

Joseph S. Longshore, a founder and the professor of obstetrics and the diseases of women and children, gave the valedictory address; he was a radical Quaker physician, antislavery and pro-temperance. Not given to muted expression, he told the graduates that "this day forms an eventful epoch in the history of your lives, in the history of woman, in the history of the race. This day *society* assigns to woman an exalted position, one never before conferred upon her by general legislative sanction."[4] Later, he offered some general and professional advice: "In your practice, avoid routine. . . . Never prescribe without a reason for your prescription . . . remove causes rather than treat names; aim to *assist* nature . . . continue to study, to think, to reason. . . . In your intercourse with your patients, be frank, candid and truthful. Avoid all deception and prevarication."

He also advised the women never, because they are women, to "consent to receive less for the same duties than is demanded by the profession generally."[5] Prayers had opened and would close the ceremonies, and "an efficient orchestra . . . discoursed excellent music."[6]

Despite the conventional prayers, oratory, and music, the controversial occurrence had not escaped some critical notice:

> There was a numerous attendance of the young men belonging to the different schools of medicine in our city, a very small minority of whom evinced a slight disposition to indulge in merriment and ridicule at the expense of the ladies present, but they were soon shamed into propriety by the good sense of an overwhelming majority. A few were inclined to be boisterous, but they were prevented from annoying the assemblage by the presence of a detail of the Marshall's police, under Lieut. Watkins.[7]

In later accounts of the first commencement, two thousand persons are said to have filled the hall, of whom five hundred were male medical students. A squadron of fifty police supposedly had been summoned in expectation of a riot by the young men.[8] Though the actual event may have been less dramatic (two thousand attending a graduation of eight?), the first commencement became one of the defining legends of the earliest medical school for women, one of the stories of quiet triumph over opposition that helped form the College's distinctive and motivating institutional saga, a notion to be developed later in this work.

Background to a New Reform

It was no accident that a medical college for women arose in 1850, and in Philadelphia, both the "Quaker City" and the "City of Medicine." Many members of the Society of Friends ardently joined the interlinked reform movements that transformed the United States in the decades before the Civil War. These decades have been aptly termed the period of "Freedom's Ferment," an age of "romantic reform."[9] The United States seemed intoxicated with ideas and energy. Among the causes urgently championed were peace, temperance, betterment of health and diet, and perhaps above all, abolition and the "Woman Movement," the term for that early phase of American feminism. Many persons, particularly Quakers, both opposed slavery and supported woman's rights on secular or religious grounds: these linked campaigns rejected the subjugation of human beings, God's children. The abolition movement also provided for women an opportunity to exert agency outside the sphere of home or farm—even to lead and speak in public.[10]

American women in the early nineteenth century with few exceptions could not vote, owned few civil or legal rights as individuals, could not control property when married, and found themselves almost entirely excluded from professions other than teaching. In the 1840s women began to reject this status. The first Woman's Rights Convention was held in July 1848 in Seneca Falls, New York, and others followed. The Woman Movement claimed, with gradual success, correction of some of the civil and legal inequities.

American women also demanded entry into schools of higher learning and into exclusively male occupations and professions—such as medical schools and the formal practice of medicine. Two of a handful of American women who managed to earn medical degrees before the founding of women's medical schools found encouragement but ultimate disappointment in Philadelphia.[11] Sarah Adamson Dolley (1829–1909) apprenticed to her uncle, Hiram Corson (1804–1896), a practitioner in Montgomery County outside Philadelphia and a lifelong advocate for women physicians. Refused admission to Philadelphia's schools, Dolley succeeded in enrolling at the Eclectic Central Medical College in Rochester, New York, from which she graduated in 1851. "Eclectic medicine" was one of several therapeutic sects of the nineteenth century; some of these accepted women more readily than did "regular" medicine.

The other early woman medical graduate with Philadelphia connections was Elizabeth Blackwell (1821–1910), who came to the city in 1847 to seek, unsuccessfully, entry into a medical school. She was befriended by the Quaker physician and author William Elder, who later would serve on the Woman's Medical College board of corporators.[12] Blackwell found acceptance (an isolated experiment) at the regular Geneva Medical College in western New York State, from which she graduated in 1849. Elizabeth and her sister Emily Blackwell would in 1857 found the renowned New York Infirmary for Women and Children and later its Woman's Medical College.

Why did women of the 1840s and 1850s want to train as physicians? Obviously, many simply wished to (and did) enter a profession and earn an independent living by practicing medicine. But other motivations have been identified by historians such as Regina Morantz-Sanchez.[13] Many women were eager to improve women's health by learning and teaching the workings of the body and hygiene. A demand clearly existed: wives and mothers attended "ladies' physiologic institutes," which arose in large cities for this purpose, or lectures on health presented by early female medical graduates. Some early women physicians were motivated by knowledge that norms of modesty and "delicacy" made many women shun treatment by male doctors, especially for gynecologic symptoms. Other women who sought medical education had acquired a fondness for science, as then understood. Hannah Longshore (1819–1901), a graduate of the first class of the Female Medical College, "had for years been an interested reader and student of the natural sciences." Though she did not study for the degree, another early matriculant was Graceanna Lewis of Chester County, Pennsylvania, also a Friend, who became one of the most acclaimed women scientists of nineteenth-century America.[14]

What of the *opposition* to the idea of women as physicians?[15] Why did almost all regular medical schools refuse to accept female applicants, thus making necessary new, separate schools for women? The Victorian mind saw woman as morally superior to men, but inferior in strength, resolve, and intelligence. Thus she would be unable to manage the arduous work of medical education and practice or to tolerate the gore and blood necessarily encountered. Indeed, the use of purgatives, emetics, and blood letting and the frequent resort to amputation characterized early nineteenth-century practice. Furthermore, detractors argued, even if successful, women would be "de-sexed" by medical work—robbed of their unique feminine delicacy and grace.

Male American medical students of the early and mid–nineteenth century acquired a reputation as a "coarse and uneducated lot . . . regarded with suspicion by all respectable boarding-house ladies of the town." Rowdy behavior not infrequently disrupted lectures or dissection. Opponents of female medical education, and probably parents as well, feared exposing women to such companions.[16] Women soon pointed out that "medical literature and medical feeling, it is all too obvious, need the refining and ennobling influences that the purity, and peculiar endowments of the true woman are calculated to give."[17] Historian of American medical women Regina Morantz-Sanchez showed that the leaders of the woman's medical movement often embraced, at least publicly, the prevalent assumptions about women's attributes, then found ways to use them in advocating their cause.[18]

In retrospect the arguments against medical work for women seem patently specious. Women, after all, had long been strong enough to raise children, run a household, and share in farm work and were sufficiently indifferent to blood and pain to nurse family members or serve as midwives. Some male physicians certainly opposed women's entry into the profession because they rightly feared competition, knowing that many women would prefer a woman doctor.[19] Finally, and perhaps least easily documented, the Western cultural worldview largely accepted by men and women saw the genders in separate spheres, a plan seemingly ratified by time, nature, and the Bible. It did not fit in the order of things for woman to serve as doctor, soldier, or railway engineman. "It is much to be regretted," wrote a leading American medical journal in 1849, "that she has been . . . led to aspire to honors and duties which by the order of nature and common consent of the world devolve upon men."[20] As we have already seen, some dissident thinkers disagreed.

The Founding of the Woman's Medical College of Pennsylvania

Decades after its doors first opened, those writing about the early years of the Woman's Medical College of Pennsylvania recounted the events in different ways, championing one or another "founder" and founding story.[21] This confusing disparity indicates that the College came to mean much to those who participated in its early struggles and growth. Clara Marshall (1847–1931), graduate of WMC and dean from 1888 until 1917—the period when most women's medical colleges expired—preferred to see the founder as Bartholomew Fussell, M.D., like her a Friend from Chester County, Pennsylvania. Fussell was a battling abolitionist and successful practitioner in his community. He much respected his sister Esther Fussell Lewis, a woman of competence and intelligence who in his mind would have made a fine physician. (In fact *her* work was no less demanding: widowed early, she raised five daughters, for a time taught school, ran a farm and home, initiated iron-ore mining on her property, and maintained a rich correspondence with friends and relatives.)

Sometime in the 1840s, Bartholomew Fussell concluded that a woman's medical college was needed; this became a deeply felt "concern" much in the Friends' tradition. In 1846, he gathered at his house several physicians who he thought would prove sympathetic to the odd notion, including his nephew Edwin Fussell (1813–1882). His niece Graceanna Lewis, mentioned above for her later attainment in science, while visiting Bartholomew Fussell's home that day registered the event in her memory, and recalled it many years afterward in a letter, now lost, to Marshall. "In general terms I know that the project was approved by those present and that each was counseled to look about him for the best persons to carry out the enterprise."[22] Bartholomew Fussell then dropped out of the picture, seemingly playing no practical role in creating the College.[23] His nephew Edwin would, however, become a crucial early faculty member, and the Chester County Quaker communities would later contribute Ann Preston (1813–1872) and Clara Marshall, both faculty members and deans of the school.

Another physician of Quaker origins, Joseph S. Longshore, a graduate of the University of Pennsylvania School of Medicine, like Fussell fervidly upheld the causes of abolition, temperance, and the access of women to medicine; he became a founding faculty member of the Female Medical College (as the school was known until 1867). Both his sister Anna Longshore and his brother Thomas's wife, Hannah Longshore, would enter the first class. Hannah became one of Philadelphia's first successful women physicians. Joseph Longshore and others sympathetic to the undertaking also set up the "American Female Medical

Education Society" to "sustain the Female Medical College of Pennsylvania, and the cause of Female Medical Education in general."[24]

Joining Longshore was William J. Mullen. Born in Lancaster County, Pennsylvania, Mullen became a jeweler's apprentice at age sixteen, attended medical lectures at the Medical Department of Pennsylvania College (one of Philadelphia's extinct medical schools), engaged in dentistry (jewelers sometimes crafted false teeth at the time), and apparently made his fortune through the invention of a new process for making gold watch dials. From 1840 he lived in Philadelphia, devoting much of his energy and income to philanthropy. For the poor of his neighborhood of south Philadelphia he helped establish the "House of Industry," which offered food, shelter, education, and a dose of temperance lecturing. His other concerns included women's emancipation and prison reform. In 1854 he helped invent a new occupation—"Prison Agent"—at which he remained for thirty years. This work entailed visiting prisoners at Philadelphia's Moyamensing Prison, aiding their families, helping those discharged find lodging and employment, and, most dramatically, seeing to the release of countless victims of false or unjustified incarcerations. These included women falsely charged by drunken husbands, a nine-year-old boy accused of "larceny of an egg," even a woman who had attempted suicide on learning of the deaths of her husband and sons. Mullen made no small contribution to easing the wretchedness of slums and prisons, even if (as some later accounts suggest), he too much enjoyed the commendations his work attracted.[25]

Mullen took the chair as president at the first recorded meeting of the board of corporators of the Female Medical College, held at Philadelphia's stately Merchants' Exchange on 4 January 1850. Joseph Longshore was appointed secretary. The small group expressed their "sentiments in relation to the project" and discussed "the preliminary measures necessary to be adopted." The Pennsylvania Assembly passed an act incorporating the Female Medical College of Pennsylvania on 11 March 1850, for "the purpose of instructing females in the science and art of medicine."[26]

Longshore and Mullen set about finding a few faculty and rooms—all that was needed for a medical school in 1850, when instruction consisted almost entirely of lectures. In August, space was rented in a small

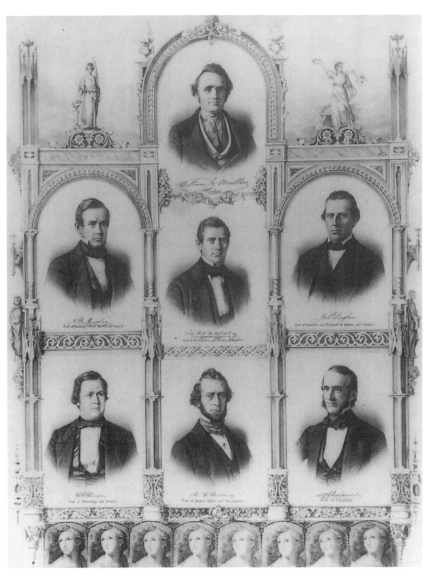

Figure 1. William J. Mullen, first president of the College (at the top), and the initial faculty, some of whom were also corporators.

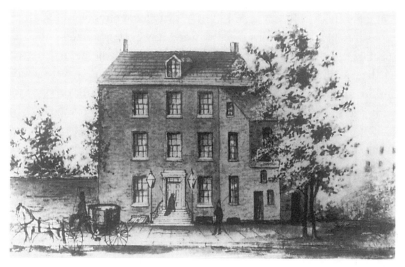

Figure 2. A drawing which first appeared in the 1920s purports to show the building in the rear of 627 Arch Street, Philadelphia, which first housed the Female Medical College of Pennsylvania.

building at the rear of 229 Arch Street (627 Arch after Philadelphia renumbered streets in 1858), and rooms were fitted up at a cost of $1,504.72, promptly creating the institution's first debt (which Mullen paid), since contributions were scant. In fact, raising funds to run a creditable school proved a vexing and ceaseless chore from the start and virtually ever after. The early minutes of the board of corporators and faculty reveal numerous fiscal disappointments and strategies for raising money.[27]

The Early Faculty

Finding suitable faculty presented a greater challenge than renting rooms. Few established male physicians in the 1850s chanced to associate with the highly unorthodox undertaking of training women in medicine. In that era students in medical colleges bought tickets for each professor's lectures, typically at ten to fifteen dollars each, and these fees provided the speaker's reimbursement. The prospects for garnering much income at the small Female Medical College probably seemed doubtful (though men like Longshore and Edwin Fussell saw the College as a cause, not a source of revenue).[28] In the early years, faculty members chaotically came and went, mostly local physicians for whom no historical trace remains. Several were, however, graduates of the respectable University of Pennsylvania School of Medicine or Jefferson Medical College.[29] Scant information suggests that most were young and inexperienced as medical teachers. One professor was dropped for failing to show up for lectures, another when it was discovered that he lacked a medical degree.[30] Nonetheless, as a student in the first class, Ann Preston found reason to praise: "There is a considerable and increasing apparatus and the Professors seem enthusiastic and to have their hearts in their business."[31] The "apparatus" referred to included anatomical preparations, papier-mâché models, samples of materia medica, charts, and other aids gathered by the instructors.

A wrenching event of these tumultuous embryonic years was the eviction in 1853 of Joseph Longshore, founder and faithful friend to the cause.[32] Longshore, and at least one other early professor, Abraham Livezy, stood tainted with controversial sectarian leanings. Longshore embraced eclecticism, one of the less extreme of the alternative systems, but still heresy to regular medicine.[33] According to his brother, he also favored mesmerism, spiritualism, and "nerve theories in occult sciences." Mullen and others leading the new school intended that the already suspect activity of teaching medicine to women not lose further credibility with the established medical community, thus the purge of "irregular" faculty members.

The high-spirited Longshore fought back, eventually with a lawsuit.[34] He, Livezy, and Nathaniel Moseley (another member of the initial faculty) promptly founded the Penn Medical University, a progressive eclectic school that taught both men and women in separate sessions. It became a competitor to the tenuous Female Medical College. None of this was unusual: in the nineteenth century medical school professors frequently engaged in "bitter controversies and disputations," threats, and lawsuits. Often a faction seceded and started its own medical school down the road.[35]

In 1852 Hannah Longshore, a graduate of the first class of the Female Medical College, was appointed "demonstrator in anatomy"; owing to prevalent anxiety about exposing breasts or genitalia in mixed company, the College leadership wanted the demonstrator to be always a woman.[36] On 25 February 1853 the board of corporators resolved that "the president of the College be requested to ascertain by the next meeting of the Corporation if there are any Female Physicians who would be suitable and who would accept chairs in this College."[37] While this may have reflected the difficulty of finding acceptable male teachers, more likely it meant that the early leaders (mostly Quakers) had in mind creating a "Female Medical College" that would be largely staffed and eventually run by women—as indeed occurred. Martha Mowry of Providence, Rhode Island, was appointed professor of obstetrics (after being awarded an honorary M.D.) on 10 May 1853 and served during the 1853 term. Mowry was one of the scattered successful women physicians of the pre-1850 period who had apprenticed to physicians but had no way of obtaining a degree.[38] At this same board meeting of 10 May 1853 a letter was read from Ann Preston "accepting the chair of Physiology and Medical Institutes." As professor and first woman dean, she would soon become the central figure in strengthening the College.

Furthering their wish to involve women in the affairs of the school, the board of corporators (then all men) in 1858 appointed "a board of lady managers to aid in the supervision of the interests of the College."[39]

The Curriculum during the First Decade

Throughout most of the nineteenth century, American medical schools provided lectures, some dissection, and little else—practical work with patients hardly existed.[40] Students obtained the clinical part of their training through an apprenticeship or, as the Female Medical College required, two years of supervision by "a respectable practitioner." Of course, the quality of the apprenticeship varied with the ability and generosity of the preceptor. During the 1850s the students of the Female Medical College seeking the M.D. typically sat in lectures from nine to five, over a term of four or five months commencing in October, and did so again the following or a subsequent year, hearing the same subjects. This plan matched exactly that of other schools. The subjects were anatomy, theory and practice of medicine, obstetrics and diseases of women and children, surgery, materia medica and therapeutics, and chemistry.

In medical education some habits defy change: early in the inaugural term one professor moved at a faculty meeting that "each member of this faculty cease lecturing as soon as he finishes the sentence after the first bell." In 1857 another resolution acknowledged the "too great crowding of lectures and the inability of the students generally to master so much in a little time without injury to their health."[41] Some lectures were enhanced with drawings, anatomical specimens, and models of wax or papier-mâché. According to an 1852 Philadelphia guidebook, the College's museum was "amply, and, considering its age, we should say richly, supplied. It contains an extensive collection of wet and dry preparations . . . together with a large proportion of French models and wax preparations."[42] Like their male counterparts, students at the women's school also worked on the cadaver; their College's yearly announcement for many years claimed "abundant material for dissection."

The American medical school of the 1850s provided little or no clinical training. The faculty of the Female Medical College, however, did set up a small dispensary or clinic practice for practical instruction. Selected patients were demonstrated and discussed before a group of pupils. An extant clinic notebook from 1856 to 1858 suggests that the classes were grouped into sections for this activity, each attending for several weeks. Students observed the history taking, physical examination, and treatment of patients with coughs, scrofula (tuberculosis of the lymphatic system), dyspepsia, abdominal pains, headache, conjunctivitis, dropsy (edema), tonsillitis, menstrual disorders, and a variety of other problems. The faculty relied on the popular remedies of the time prescribed in combination, but not infrequently a recommendation for exercise, fresh air, or the outdoors precedes the prescription. The notes also reveal several dental extractions, minor operations, and at least one treatment with electrical shock for a stubborn abdominal pain of "obscure" origin. The patients' names suggest that many belonged to the increasing number of Irish immigrants settling in Philadelphia. Recognizing that their pupils would eventually care for mostly women patients, the early faculty also tried to arrange for some "lying-in" (obstetrical experience), though one cannot know how successful they were.[43]

In 1859, the faculty, after voting on each candidate for the M.D., resolved "to recommend to the graduates the propriety of spending some time in the New York Infirmary or some other place where they may obtain a fuller practical knowledge of pharmacy and disease."[44] Elizabeth Blackwell had recently founded the New York Infirmary for

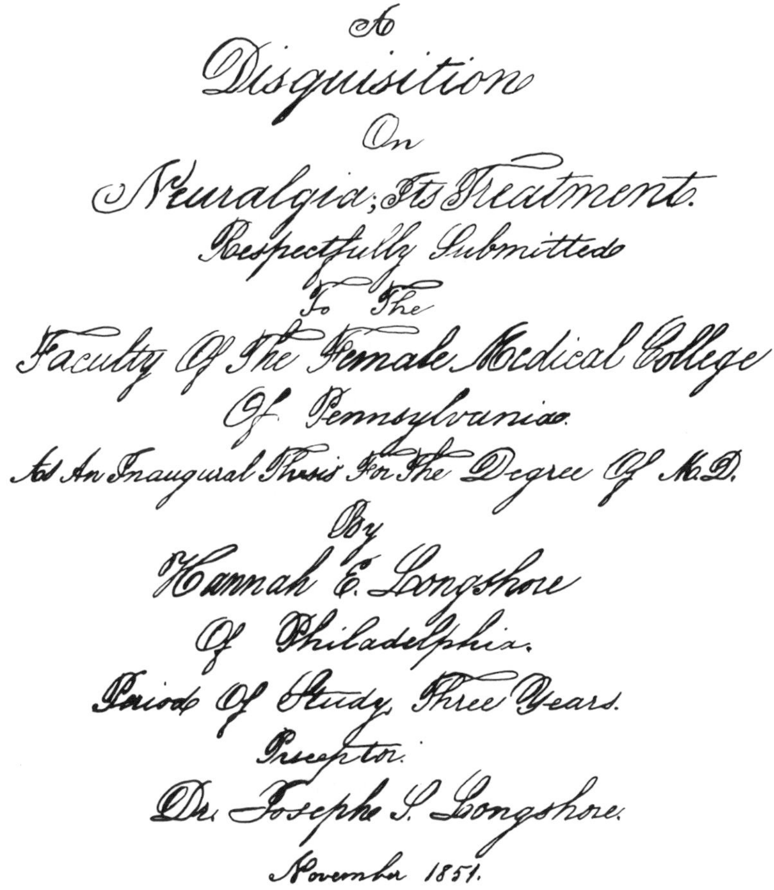

A

Disquisition

On

Neuralgia; Its Treatment.

Respectfully Submitted

To The

Faculty Of The Female Medical College

Of Pennsylvania.

As An Inaugural Thesis For The Degree Of M.D.

By

Hannah E. Longshore

Of Philadelphia.

Period Of Study, Three Years.

Preceptor:

Dr. Joseph S. Longshore.

November 1851.

Figure 3. Handwritten title page from Hannah Longshore's graduation thesis on "Neuralgia and Its Treatments." Longshore became one of Philadelphia's first successful women physicians.

Women and Children in 1857 for clinical education of women physicians, and several Female Medical College students had already worked there during the summer.[45] The Female Medical College probably offered no less than the typical male medical school and appears to have strived to do more. But the faculty recognized the limits of their program and urged students to make use of the only teaching hospital then available to women.

Students were required to write a thesis from the beginning of the College to as late as 1942; again, the early faculty adhered to customary practice. These theses presented reviews of a topic, not products of actual research. Most students chose clinical subjects of the day: from the first class (dated 1851), Frances G. Mitchell wrote "A Disquisition on Chlorosis," Margaret Richardson chose "Phthisis," Ann Preston "General Diagnosis," and Martha Sawin "Anaemia." Others chose more wide-ranging topics, such as Angenette Hunt on "The True Physician" (1851), Augusta Montgomery on "The Medical Education of Woman" (1852), Mary Smith on "Thoughts that Would Strike Out All Order from the Universe" (1855), and Elise Pfeiffer Stone on "The True Position of Woman" (1867). Faculty minutes recorded each professor's comments, mostly indicating general and literary rather than scientific judgments (e.g., from 1857: "very well written," "tolerably fair," "very respectable," "badly spelled and ungrammatical").[46]

To complete requirements for graduation, students underwent an oral examination, after which faculty voted to pass them or not, for some years using the traditional device of tossing white or black balls into a bowl.

The First Students

The ultimate fate of the new College depended upon the future proficiency and reputation of its early students. Fortunately, many proved capable and determined; clearly they were bold enough to take themselves to a wholly unproved school to pursue an uncharted course for women. Who were they?

Biographical materials in their alumna folders provide information only for some of the first decade's students, and obviously those who practiced medicine and made a name for themselves are more likely to have left paper traces. From these few clippings, yellowed obituaries, and other fugitive shards, we can form some tentative portrait.[47] Most came from Pennsylvania or New York, with a scattering from New England and other states, and one each from Canada and England. Several were the daughters or sisters of doctors, and when they married they sometimes wed physicians. The early students at the Female Medical College obtained preliminary education, often quite sound, at the proliferating female "academies," local Friends' schools, or the "seminaries" newly available to middle-class girls beginning in the 1820s. Orie

Moon-Andrews (class of 1857) in fact went to the famous Troy Seminary in New York, founded by educational reformer Emma Willard, which became a prototype for many similar schools. At least one student, the brilliant Emeline Horton Cleveland (1855), attended Oberlin College in Ohio, among the first U.S. institutions of higher learning to enroll women.

The early students commonly taught school before choosing a medical career.[48] After graduating, a few managed further clinical education, then most entered practice, sometimes relocating several times in search of a post (a pattern equally common for recently fledged medical men). Predictably, many early graduates, and not just of the first decade, turned out to be the first women M.D.'s in their town, county, territory, or state. Several either established or worked for institutions such as water-cure resorts or other sorts of sanitariums, occasionally combining medical and entrepreneurial careers.[49] Ann Preston, Anna Longshore-Potts, and Samantha Nivison engaged in public lecturing on matters of health, aimed at a female audience. In this way, they fulfilled the ideal of using their training to provide needed information to women, and they also gained some income. Attending lectures of all sorts was a popular activity in the early nineteenth century.[50]

One would like to know something of the thoughts and hopes of these young women, but the historical record for the earliest period offers only minimal help. In a fine letter of 4 January 1851, the most famous Female Medical College graduate of the first decade, Ann Preston, told a friend of "the joy of exploring a new field of knowledge, the rest from accustomed pursuits and cares, the stimulus of competition, the novelty of a new kind of life, are all mine, and for the time possess a charm. And then, I am restful in spirit and well satisfied that I came."[51] These few words express through one person's invigorating experiences the awakening expansion of women's opportunities in the United States of the 1850s. Ann Preston relinquished domestic drudgery in favor of challenge and competition.

Students probably lived mostly in boardinghouses near the College and reached it by foot or horse-drawn omnibus. Lectures occupied much of the day, with clinical demonstrations on Wednesday and Saturday mornings. Medical students of the time took notes during lectures, sometimes using a form of shorthand, then created lengthy synopses of the lectures in the evening.[52] They also devoted at least several hours a week to dissection. We can assume safely that the early students of the Female Medical College enjoyed little leisure time, but did find their way to church or meeting on Sundays, and perhaps at times went to hear a traveling political or literary lecturer or a musical performance. Old or new friendships and, where practical, visits with family no doubt helped sustain spirit and well-being.

Events of the First Decade

The next meeting of the faculty after the first commencement took place, oddly enough, in Boston, on 3 March 1852. The previous year, an attempt arose to form an alliance between the Female Medical College of Pennsylvania and the recently launched New England Female Medical College, the outgrowth of a school for midwifery founded by Samuel Gregory, a non-physician lecturer on physiology and advocate of women practitioners for women patients. The two M.D.s on the Boston school's faculty in 1851, Enoch C. Rolfe and William Cornell, obtained Female Medical College appointments, while most of the Female Medical College faculty apparently joined in a course of medical lectures in Boston beginning in February of 1852, following the fall term in Philadelphia. Surprisingly, in March of 1856 the board opened discussions about merger with Longshore's Penn Medical University. No such arrangement ensued.[53] These early brushes with merger, like many others that would follow throughout the school's history, arose almost surely out of pecuniary desperation and—for the first decade—inability to secure permanent faculty.

Indeed the first decade tried the resolve of the early supporters and faculty. Whereas eight women won degrees in 1852 (technically, December 1851) and nine in 1853, only four did so in 1854, six in 1855, four in 1856, seven in 1857 but then four again in 1858, six in 1859 but only one in 1860. Faculty desertions continued, and by 1856 those attending the faculty meeting represented the true nucleus of loyal teachers and leaders: Ann Preston, Emeline Horton Cleveland, Edwin Fussell, Elwood Harvey, and for a time Sylvester Birdsell. In 1857 Fussell and Birdsell took on the lectures of two resigned faculty members in addition to their own. Even as it grew the College would always remain small: we will see how smallness became its sustaining strength but its economic weakness.

The year 1857 saw one of the periodic financial panics of the nineteenth century, which would have lessened contributions. Despite the presence of well-known abolitionists, Philadelphia in the 1850s enjoyed many ties with the South and was not widely sympathetic to abolition or blacks. The fervid antislavery position of some of the Female Medical College's Quaker progenitors and leaders probably attracted animosity, not donations.[54] In 1858 the faculty recommended to the corporators the "appointment of lecturing and financial agents—to travel throughout the country lecturing upon the cause of female medical education and endeavor to collect students and funds for the college." In 1859, the board of corporators decided to "draft a memorial to the legislature [of Pennsylvania] asking for pecuniary assistance."[55]

Confederate forces attacked Fort Sumter on 12 April 1861, thrusting the nation into war. Customary social and business dealings deteriorated. Medical men went off to military service in the field or at the temporary Civil War hospitals; several of these functioned in Philadelphia. In July of 1861 the board of corporators of the Female Medical College felt "compelled by the general prostration of all business to give up and vacate the buildings now rented."[56] On 10 October 1861 the tiny faculty confronted a resignation from Sylvester Birdsell, called to "imperative duties elsewhere." The small band of Female Medical College faithful, mostly Friends, suffered the compound sadness of seeing their hopes for peaceful abolition vanish, and possibly their local cause as well. On 17 October 1861 "after much consultation on the probable number of students, it was moved by Dr. [Mark] Kerr that owing to the embarrassed state of the times the sessions of 1861–2 be omitted." A vote was taken and the motion passed, though Dr. Cleveland opposed it, and "a letter was read from A. Preston," no doubt also urging continuation of operations.[57] One can only imagine the grievous disappointment felt by the small group, and particularly by Ann Preston, a product and now a leader of the College. A week earlier, with poignancy and eloquence that still touch her unintended reader, she had written in her diary: "I have been sad for my country, because it is so slow to learn the wisdom which would bring prosperity; sad for my disabled mother and desolate home; sad in the prospects of the Institution to which I have given so much of my time and strength, for there now seems no possibility of success; and I fear that, after all these years of toil, we may be doomed to succumb to the weight of opposition." But, she went on, "Tonight the inward encouragement is, do thy best; work where the work opens; applauded or condemned, speak and write thy grandest inspiration, thy noblest idea, and sing hosanna, for thy work has been no failure, and the Everlasting will preserve it, and attest it forever."[58]

In fact, owing in good part to Dr. Preston's earlier initiatives, hope rekindled quickly, and the work found an opening. Soon after giving up 229 Arch Street, the board arranged to rent rooms for the College at the Woman's Hospital of Philadelphia on North College Avenue in Philadelphia, near Girard College, and by February of 1862 resolved to resume lectures "the coming winter." Ann Preston had originated the Woman's Hospital to provide the College's students with clinical experience; unintentionally, she had also provided for the school's temporary home.

Building Within, Opposition Without

Chapter 2

In rooms rented from the Woman's Hospital of Philadelphia, the Female Medical College of Pennsylvania reopened in October of 1862 to instruct a discouragingly small group of pupils. By October of 1875, a respectable number of students, professors of wide reputation, and a loyal board of corporators gathered to officially inaugurate the College's first real home, a handsome and spacious building designed to accommodate a progressively expanded curriculum. Within fifteen years, a remarkable step upward had occurred.

In broad strokes, the period from 1862 to 1875 must be seen not just as an interval of shoring up facilities, faculty, and course work, but the beginning of a transformation driven by internal insistence on doing the best, and external influences from the world of medicine and science. The transformation began to reduce the stress on "Woman's"— albeit only slightly and imperceptibly—and focus more on the changing imperatives of "Medical College." What should a medical school *be*? How might a faculty define the requisite knowledge base to be taught? Who ought the teachers be: might any holder of the M.D. teach any subject in the curriculum, or does one need experts among experts? What place in the school should be claimed by laboratory science, flourishing in the German and French medical academy? How might faculty be paid, especially any whose work or background precludes earnings from practice? What sorts of building design and equipment does medical education require? What clinical work could be offered, and where? WMC began to deal seriously with these and related questions during the 1860s and 1870s: this period saw progress in what one might term the "professionalization" of the medical school.

Not coincidentally, also in the 1860s and 1870s the women of the College sought broader entry into the existing organized medical profession, which in Philadelphia tended to glacial conservatism. Though the College was able to attract several valuable male allies with standing in the larger profession, efforts to join it more fully met with opposition. So various aspects of professionalization form the thematic suturing for this chapter, which comprises an array of practically and symbolically meaningful events.[1]

The Woman's Hospital of Philadelphia

In large part to provide clinical experience for WMC students, a group of Quaker women founded the Woman's Hospital of Philadelphia in 1861. Ann Preston headed the effort: to her efforts "more than to all other influences may be traced its very origin." "I went to every one who I thought would give me either money or influence," she later said.[2] Two large row houses were purchased near the beautiful campus of Girard College in Philadelphia's Twenty-ninth Ward, a district to the northwest of the old downtown newly popular with Quakers seeking residence in a less bustling neighborhood.[3] When the College resumed classes in 1862, having given up its quarters at 627 Arch Street, the hospital rented space to the school on favorable terms.[4] Eventually in its own building, WMC would call North College Avenue home until 1930.

The purposes of the hospital as incorporated in 1861 were to "establish in the City of Philadelphia a Hospital for the treatment of diseases of women and children, and for obstetrical cases; furnishing at the same time facilities for clinical instruction to women engaged in the study of medicine, and for the practical training of nurses; the chief resident physician to be a woman."[5] This statement encompassed several forward-looking needs. Philadelphia women needing hospitalization who might wish to do so could now receive care from women physicians and surgeons. Second, WMC students would obtain practical instruction rare in American medical schools of 1861, few of which could claim an affiliated hospital. Male students and graduates could more easily than women find clinical experiences through a hospital internship or attendance at the several "private" or supplementary medical schools conducted for profit in large cities.[6] Though most medical care in the nineteenth century occurred at home or in a practitioner's office, the "teaching hospital" could provide, as "clinical material," many patients gathered in one place for some time, who could be examined while the course of their diseases was observed. The tension between the needs of patients and interests of students often led to discord between hospital and medical school, as we will later see arose between WMC and the Woman's Hospital.

The Woman's Hospital would also undertake the "practical training of nurses." The development of nursing as a skilled profession claimed attention as another new pathway to expanded spheres for women. No doubt to the surprise of Dr. Preston and her colleagues, the educational needs of medical students and nursing students eventually showed signs of conflict.[7]

Finally, the charter provided that "the chief resident physician [is] to be a woman." This policy symbolized another critical function of WMC, the Woman's Hospital of Philadelphia, and similar institutions in New York City, Boston, and elsewhere: not only to provide training to students, but to provide opportunity for some of those students later to enjoy full professional expression as doctors—to teach, manage, investigate, perform surgery. The existing institutions, controlled by men, would be infuriatingly slow to welcome women.

Ann Preston and her friends were astute in founding the hospital for another reason. Transformed by the discoveries of anesthetics in the 1840s and Joseph Lister's antisepsis in the 1860s, surgery, especialy gynecologic surgery, boldly expanded its scope and power in the late nineteenth century. Once routinely done at home, surgery soon required a hospital equipped for the technical needs. Woman's Hospital allowed for the development of surgical careers for WMC faculty and graduates in Philadelphia.[8]

Woman's Hospital accepted its first patient, to the "Lying In Department (maternity)," on 16 December 1861. By April of 1862 twelve patients occupied beds.[9] A dispensary and "outdoor" practice soon opened. The Woman's Hospital grew steadily; by 1875 it housed thirty-seven beds, treated nearly two thousand patients at their homes (this carried out largely by students), and saw over three thousand visitors in its dispensary.[10] Women and children were admitted "without regard to their religious belief, nationality or color," but unwed maternity cases found little welcome, despite the pleas of at least one woman staff physician who recognized that sometimes "sympathizing care" could do more to change a life than moralistic rejection.[11]

Emeline Horton Cleveland

As an integral part of establishing the hospital, Emeline Horton Cleveland (1829–1878), a Female Medical College graduate of 1855, was sent for further clinical training to Paris in order to serve as the first resident physician of the new institution. During her seven months abroad, she acquired the French language, advanced knowledge and techniques, the diploma of the school of the Maternité Hospital, and five prizes, two of them firsts. She was already professor of anatomy at WMC since 1856, but took the more suitable chair of obstetrics in 1862. She then combined a career of teaching, administration, and private practice until illness forced her reluctantly to retire shortly before her death. For two years Horton Cleveland served as dean, following the death of Ann Preston. She was one of the first women surgeons in the United States to perform major gynecological procedures.

A published case report from 1875, after describing a successful ovariotomy by Cleveland, made the political claim that woman *can* perform surgery. Both the medical and sociopolitical contents of this case report are striking. It is noteworthy that it appeared in a somewhat obscure regional journal produced in Cincinnati: presumably, no Philadelphia medical periodical would take the paper, or the writers chose not to try. Cincinnati was known at the time as a liberal, tolerant city. Dr. Cleveland's patient suffered wretchedly from a cystic ovarian tumor that induced an enormous deposition of fluid in her abdominal cavity, only briefly relieved by drainage procedures. The article's writer (not Cleveland herself) carefully reviewed the patient's history, operation, and postoperative period. She noted that three weeks after the operation the patient "had regained a healthy appearance, having a good color, and looking many years younger than before the operation." Several concluding passages reveal the second agenda of the publication: "there have been seven cases of ovariotomy in all, at the Woman's Hospital [of Philadelphia], four of which have recovered, which is certainly a fair proportion for a hospital. . . . The rapid advances that will be made in this direction in the next few years, will go far towards dispelling the doubts of those who consider the point still unsettled, as to whether or not women can make good surgeons."[12]

Perfected during the nineteenth century, the ovariotomy was a surgical landmark, one of the few permissible operations requiring entry into the abdominal cavity. A young surgeon, or woman surgeon, especially one declaring expertise in gynecology, could not have been fully credited by peers without successfully taking on the "big" operations. In another report, Cleveland modestly recounted her inventiveness that allowed the correction of a particularly difficult gynecologic disorder, vesico-vaginal fistula. This work, along with teaching and deaning for several years, she combined with motherhood and marriage to a man invalided at an early age!

Probably the most brilliant of America's nineteenth-century women physicians, Mary Putnam Jacobi (1842–1906), an 1864 graduate of Female Medical College, called Horton Cleveland "a woman of real ability [who] would have done justice to a much larger sphere than that to which fate condemned her." She was "possessed of much personal beauty, and grace of manner." Another graduate recalled the "tall, graceful figure . . . as she came upon the platform, laid her handkerchief on the desk, took her seat (for she never lectured standing) and stroking her hair with both hands began her lecture with an easy, fluent speech which was both clear and elegant."[13]

Virtually everyone who wrote about Cleveland commented upon her "womanliness" and her natural lack of pretension or self-assertion. This was the esteemed model for the woman physician in the nineteenth century, acceptable to those of both genders who welcomed female doctors at all. Above everything, medical competence and even leadership must *not* make a woman into a man: that would too much upset the dictates of God or Nature—and threaten the established advantages of males. The woman physician, even surgeon, might still marry and become a mother and exude the feminine qualities. Thus, supporters of medical women could rejoice in this masterful surgeon and teacher, whose gracefulness and charm validated the cherished ideal. Emeline Horton Cleveland represented a powerful image for her students and a persuasive claim for credibility outside the College walls.

Early death deprived the College and Woman's Hospital of this able worker. On one wall in the current home of the descendant medical school hangs her portrait, which yet commends to its viewers unmistakable intelligence and beauty.

A New Name

In 1867, the College legally changed its name from "Female" to "Woman's" Medical College of Pennsylvania. The *Annual Announcement* for the 1867–1868 session explained the name change as "a simple recognition of the growing purity of our English tongue, which demands that terms shall be distinctive in their signification; and of an increasing regard for the dignity of woman—the co-worker with man, and his companion in the noblest thoughts and pursuits."[14]

Sarah Josepha Hale (1788–1879), Philadelphia author and editor of *Godey's Lady's Book*, since the mid-1850s had campaigned with unrelenting zeal for the eradication of the term "female" when applied to women. She believed it vulgar, ungrammatical, and discordant with the Bible, Shakespeare, and all of Anglo-Saxon usage. Much of her verbal bombardment fell on Matthew Vassar and other men at Vassar Female College, as it was first known (she entirely supported the school but not its name). In one sharp letter to the inoffensive founder, she asked: "Female! What female do you mean? Not a female donkey?"[15] Hale prevailed in 1866, when Vassar dropped female from its name. It can be no coincidence that the Female Medical College, in Sarah Josepha Hale's own city, traded "Female" for "Woman's" the next year.[16]

As the years and decades would go by, the former Female Medical College grew into a comfortable local familiarity as the "Woman's Medical College," or most amiably, "Woman's Med."

New Faculty and Their Significance

Ann Preston succeeded Edwin Fussell as dean in 1865. Almost certainly, she had much to do with the improvements and faculty appointments over the next five or six years.[17] On 14 October 1865, the board appointed a small committee to "confer with Dr. Preston" regarding filling vacant chairs for the coming course of lectures, due to begin in two days.[18] In December the board approved Rachel Bodley (1831–1888) as professor of chemistry and toxicology. The board and the faculty may not have entirely comprehended the significance of this appointment. First, Bodley was *not* a physician; rather, her training and experience were those of a scientist and teacher of science, so far, at least, as understood in mid-nineteenth-century America. Second, she came from another city and state to accept a position at the College. Third, since she could not earn a living by practice, she necessarily received a salary from the College—she was a paid, professional teacher. She would also become an effective dean of the school and something of a precocious medical sociologist.

Bodley, born in Cincinnati, attended its Wesleyan Female Seminary then taught there until 1860. During 1859 and 1860 she was the first woman to attend the Polytechnic College of the State of Pennsylvania, in Philadelphia, an early school which taught chemistry, natural science, engineering, and especially principles of mining.[19] She took the chemistry course. On return to her native city she taught natural sciences at the Cincinnati Female Seminary and classified a large botanical collection.[20] She became known to WMC in 1856 through a chance meeting with board member Isaac Barton.[21]

Bodley's education in science was unusual for the 1850s and 1860s; it comprised a mixture of what she acquired in the "seminary" she attended (some of these were quite strong), self-learning, and—more remarkable—her attendance at an early science school. Despite her training in chemistry and membership for some years (the sole woman!) in the American Chemical Society, she seems to have favored botany. In the early nineteenth century, botany (or "botanizing" in the field) attracted many middle- and upper-class women and became the most "feminized" of sciences.[22] Bodley fulfilled other expectations that allowed her to fit in and serve WMC well: she was a devout Christian and had been well bred to a "suave and courtly manner."[23] The standing lent by her knowledge of science and her social abilities both counted when in 1874 she was appointed dean.

During the later 1860s, faculty continued to come and go, though not so chaotically as in the 1850s. Three men who joined merit special attention: Charles Hermon Thomas (1839–1921), appointed in 1867; Henry Hartshorne (1823–1897), appointed in 1868; and J. Gibbons Hunt (1826–1893), a member of the board, appointed as faculty in 1870. All were or would become Fellows of the prestigious College of Physicians of Philadelphia, and Hartshorne claimed a wide reputation well outside the city.

Thomas combined capability in general and gynecologic surgery with expertise in ophthalmology, but joined the College as professor of materia medica: chairs needed to be filled and rigid specialization did not exist in the 1860s. Though doing some practice, Henry Hartshorne earned his living and reputation largely as professional teacher and scholar of medicine. He earlier had taught at the medical school of the University of Pennsylvania, Haverford College, and Philadelphia's Central High School.[24] Hartshorne wrote numerous articles and several widely used medical textbooks.[25] A prominent Philadelphia surgeon of this period believed that authorship of textbooks by faculty did more than anything else to spread notice of a medical school, and Hartshorne did list WMC on the title pages of his later editions.[26] He also wrote poetry and essays and edited the *Friends Review*.

The authors of the *Standard History of the Medical Profession of Philadelphia*, published in 1897, state that Thomas and Hartshorne "were the most successful of any up to that time in winning respect for the college among the profession at large."[27] According to the historian of Philadelphia medicine Whitfield Bell, "men who were graduates of the University of Pennsylvania, were on the staff of the Pennsylvania Hospital, were Fellows of the College of Physicians of Philadelphia, and were authors of a text or treatise, were widely regarded . . . as at the top of the profession."[28]

No assertion is intended that Thomas and Hartshorne were superior in intellect to Emeline Horton Cleveland or Ann Preston. But they did represent an expansion of teaching within the school, credibility with the male profession at a time when "character" mattered, and a trustworthy intermediary between the College and the larger medical world. Hartshorne and Thomas represented WMC at meetings of the American Medical Association in 1870 and 1871.[29]

If Hartshorne represented the medical gentleman, J[ohn] Gibbons

Hunt, like Rachel Bodley, brought valuable new expertise to a medical school trying to stay current in 1870. On 25 November 1870 the board recorded this resolution from the faculty: "Resolved that as the exhibition of organic tissues by the steriopticon and gas microscope belongs to the advanced modes of teaching and has already been introduced into the Jefferson Medical College and the University of Pennsylvania we would respectfully ask the Corporators to secure the same advantages to our students by employing Dr. J. G. Hunt to give a few of these exhibitions at our College."[30]

The next *Annual Announcement*, for the 1871–1872 session, reported that Dr. Hunt's demonstrations during the previous year had proved "a new and interesting feature in the Winter's exercises." Hunt, already a member of the board of corporators and a staff physician at the Woman's Hospital, was one of Philadelphia's most skillful microscopists, adept at techniques of preparation and staining.[31]

In March of 1872, Hunt initiated a totally new secondary chair, professor of microscopy and histology, with a salary of $250.[32] The new title and the payment both speak for the ambition and alertness of those leading the school. The microscope, simply put, *stood for science*, and steadily gained privilege in the better American medical schools. The microscope had produced the cell theory and the categorization of disease at the histologic level. A well-educated physician should have some experience with this symbol of the scientific foundation of medicine; and the microscope, it was argued, offered practical diagnostic aid, such as examination of urinary sediment. Soon after 1872, the microscope would help give rise to the new science of bacteriology.

Seeking to Enter the Male Medical World: The Medical Societies

The women physicians in Philadelphia during the 1850s and 1860s deferred attempts to move beyond their own practices, schools, and hospitals, but they could not totally ignore the actions of medical organizations.[33] The state societies sometimes influenced legislative decisions about licensing. The American Medical Association (AMA), founded in 1847 but hardly commanding until much later, concerned itself especially with reform of medical education. Meetings of county societies provided opportunity to discuss cases and professional affairs, and, in cities, to establish "networks" and referral patterns. Together, the various societies sought to define "regular" medicine and distinguish it from sectarianism and quackery. Though of limited power, they represented the closest thing to a governance of medicine in the United States. The societies also attempted to codify and enforce medical ethics, which in the nineteenth century referred more to how physicians behaved with one another than with patients: the protocol for consultation, dealing (or rather, *not* dealing), with irregular practitioners, and—particularly irksome—advertising.

Far from accepting the city's new medical women onto its rolls, in November of 1858 the Philadelphia County Medical Society's Board of Censors effectively forbade its members to "consult or hold professional medical intercourse with their professors or alumnae," referring to the Female Medical College. The Pennsylvania State Medical Society endorsed this odious injunction in 1859 and again in 1860, supposedly on the grounds that "some of its professors are irregular practitioners."[34] Thus the women and men of the College found themselves set outside the walls of an increasingly self-demarcated profession.

Dr. Hiram Corson, mentioned in chapter 1 as the practitioner in Whitemarsh (northwest of Philadelphia) who championed medical women, led yearly attempts to rescind the state society's rulings, almost succeeding in 1866 and 1867. A setback occurred in 1867, however, when at a meeting of the Philadelphia County Medical Society a member produced a circular touting a "Compound Asiatic Balsam," which was "prepared only and sold wholesale and retail by Dr. M. G. KERR, physician and chemist."[35] The advertiser was Mark Kerr, professor of materia medica at WMC. Here was an instance of the most detestable sort of medical advertising—pitching a secret remedy. The board of the College requested and received Kerr's resignation, then communicated to the county society that it knew nothing of the offending advertisement.[36] Poor Kerr, whatever his failings, had served loyally on the faculty since 1854, even contributing a particularly bland valedictory address in 1866.

In March of 1867, following the Kerr debacle, the Philadelphia County Medical Society issued a lengthy "Preamble and Resolution" that rejected the idea of women physicians with familiar arguments about woman's incapacity for the work, and the threat to modesty, marriage, and family. It concluded with a resolution that "the members of this Society cannot encourage women to become practitioners of medicine, nor, on these grounds, can they consent to meet in consultation such practitioners."[37]

This manifesto prompted Dean Ann Preston's acerbic and eloquent response, described in the next chapter. One might speculate that the vehemence of this 1867 proclamation by the Philadelphia society arose not *despite* the now proved accomplishment of medical women in the city, but in fact *because of it*—the social outrage declared itself unmistakably and the threat of competition promised only to sharpen.

Not coincidentally, also in 1867, and more than one thousand miles to the west, women and a few male allies undertook another, more momentous, political campaign. Feminists Lucy Stone, Olympia Brown, Elizabeth Cady Stanton, and Susan B. Anthony braved frontier conditions to travel throughout Kansas, urging a favorable vote in the state referendum on women's suffrage. They suffered defeat in this first of fifty-six such referendums.[38] The bellwether campaign in Kansas and the Philadelphia medical women's struggle with the county and state societies aimed at the same radical demand: enfranchisement, the full and rightful exercise of citizenship, in a nation or profession.[39]

Not until 1871 did the Pennsylvania State Medical Society rescind its resolution prohibiting professional dealings with women physicians and faculty of female medical schools. And not until 1888, after several attempts, did a woman first gain membership in the Philadelphia County Medical Society. She was Mary Willits, a Friend from rural Pennsylvania, and—not surprisingly—an 1881 honors graduate of WMC.[40]

Blackguardism at the Nation's First Hospital

While engaged in the medical society battles, the increasingly self-assured Philadelphia medical women also saw the time as ripe to apply for entry into a majestic home of high-caste Philadelphia medicine, the Pennsylvania Hospital. Opened in 1752 mainly to serve the poor, this first general hospital in the United States became a center of clinical education. It offered lecture-demonstrations ("clinics") attended by male medical students from all the city's schools. These clinical lectures, at which selected patients were presented and discussed, and even operated upon, were taught by renowned faculty members of the University of Pennsylvania and Jefferson Medical College, who also held prestigious staff positions at the hospital.

In September of 1869, the Quaker managers (trustees) of Pennsylvania Hospital gave permission to their friends on the WMC board for the College's students to attend the hospital's clinical lectures. On 6 November 1869, about thirty to thirty-five WMC students presented the tickets they had purchased from the hospital steward and took seats in the new octagonal amphitheater. Though accounts vary, what occurred shocked the women and when broadcast in the Philadelphia newspapers and beyond amazed and outraged the larger community. The *Philadelphia Bulletin* said that when the women first entered the amphitheater, several hundred male medical students greeted the newcomers with "yells, hisses, 'caterwauling,' mock applause, offensive remarks upon personal appearance, etc."[41] Other newspaper accounts stated, however, that the rooms remained calm during much of the first hour of clinical presentation ("Malaria, sunstroke, and dropsy, illustrated by their victims, claimed the general ear").[42]

During the second part of the instruction, surgical cases were demonstrated, including an unfortunate man with a poorly healing fracture of the femur. The discussion of his situation required, according to some journalistic accounts, a momentary "exposure" (presumably, of the thigh or groin area), which proved "the signal for an explosion among the students—mock applause, clapping, stamping, and shouts of laughter, mingled with hisses and jeers, in one wild uproar."[43] Other accounts fail to include this seeming nadir of a wretched affair. All accounts agreed that upon the conclusion of the Saturday clinic, the WMC students were harassed as they left the clinic hall through the Pennsylvania Hospital grounds. "After the lectures the [male] students took possession of the walk leading through the yard from the Hospital, thus compelling the objects of their audacity to take the carriage way to the street. Reaching the street, the students followed them some distance, greatly to their annoyance, uttering various uncouth noises and indecent comments, and making other manifestations peculiar to this class of 'gentleman.'"[44] Another account referred to the "jeers, hisses and other distinctive traits of rowdyism, from the future M.D.s of the country!"[45] With few exceptions, the press condemned the male students and supported the reality and idea of women doctors.[46]

For weeks, articles, interviews, and editorials flowed through the pages of the *Philadelphia Bulletin*, *Ledger*, *Post*, and other newspapers, a huge mass of words set in the minuscule type then so popular. These words in turn multiplied along telegraph wires, so that the entire country read about the Philadelphia male students' "blackguardism" (a favorite word at the time). The women who attended documented the event in notebooks and scrapbooks, and of course recalled it later. Sarah Hibbard, who received her M.D. in 1870, wrote of enduring for two hours the "groans and hisses of as *ungentlemanly* a set of fellows as one would care to meet," in order to learn.[47] Elizabeth Keller, who also received her M.D. in 1870, remembered in 1906 how "We entered in a body amidst jeers and groanings, whistling and stamping of feet, by the men students, who had determined to make it so unpleasant for us that, from choice, we would not care to attend another. On leaving the hospital we were actually stoned by those so-called gentlemen."[48]

Graduate of 1871 and future faculty member Anna Broomall (1847–1931) in 1926 recollected for a newspaper writer that "the [male] students rushed in pell-mell, stood up in the seats, hooted, called us names and threw spitballs, trying in vain to dislodge us."[49] The stately minutes of the board of managers of the Pennsylvania Hospital refer to the "serious disturbance" in which "a number of the male students in attendance behaved in a very indecorous manner."[50]

Calm and decorum ruled the clinic on the next Saturday, though only a small fraction of the male students came.[51] Eventually, the contention and verbiage receded, and mixed clinical lectures resumed as a routine component of Philadelphia's medical life.[52]

What underlay this extraordinary event in which a mass of young men, indeed future doctors, violated the most sacrosanct Victorian standards for treating the opposite sex? For one thing, coeducation of any sort within higher education met with overwhelming opposition in nineteenth-century America.[53] In the concise phrase of the historian Carroll Smith-Rosenberg, "coeducation threatened the very principle of gender polarity."[54] But surely more was at stake on Philadelphia's Pine Street in 1869.

For any man with even a pretense of breeding to jeer, mock, perhaps even stone and spit upon women could hardly be imagined in mid-nineteenth-century America. And therein lies one piece of explanation: by coming to the Pennsylvania Hospital in order to look upon exposed skin and flesh in the presence of men, which true ladies could never do, the WMC students—in the judgment of the male students—had already de-sexed themselves, and abrogated their right to customary gender-based deference and respect. In a vicious letter published in the *New Republic*, "R.W.M.," a University of Pennsylvania student present on 6 November, with phrases fed by some black lode of misogyny assailed the "shameless herd of sexless beings who dishonor the garb of ladies—this beardless set of non-blushers."[55] In his nineteenth-century male worldview, these students, despite their long hair and dark dresses, were *not* in fact true women, and need not be so treated. Consciously or not, this assumption must have unleashed the behavior of the men students.

Beyond condemnation of indelicate women who would attend mixed medical classes, the men no doubt themselves felt discomfort at witnessing, or wondering if they would witness, exposure of male genitalia in the presence of women—to the Victorian mind, the idea was appalling. In opposing medical co-education on this basis, a Chicago physician, who did not oppose women becoming doctors, in 1878 referred to "the universal feeling of the sexes toward each other—a feeling with which from childhood up we are indoctrinated by the civilization of our time."[56] If true, as some of the newspaper accounts told it, that upon the brief uncovering of the fractured man's thigh and pelvis, the male students at once burst into a new height of uproar, one may be justified in positing some sort of acute sexual anxiety linked to nineteenth-century prudery and the emotional immaturity of the young men. Some of them were young men indeed, really older boys, among themselves and away from home. Historian E. Anthony Rotundo refers to a "boy culture," which exuded (along with admirable values like mastery and skill) impulsiveness, rowdyism, violence, and aggressiveness.[57] Even adult men when together in groups had traditionally indulged in drinking, smoking, profanity, and sometimes violence: among other purposes, such behavior served to exclude women.[58]

Although the men may have perceived the newcomers as "de-sexed" by their mere presence in the teaching theater, the WMC contingent was still sufficiently female to represent an intolerable invasion of what had been an all-male temple—the privileged halls of Pennsylvania Hospital. The group from WMC chose to "infest the rights of four hundred regular medical students who have sustained the clinics from their foundation," wrote R.W.M., who also referred to "our citadel in possession of this neuter thirty-four."[59]

Throughout the nineteenth century, all-male "secret societies," such as the Masons and Odd Fellows, attracted huge memberships in the United States. At their meetings, these societies offered rituals built of arcane language and signs, in which inductees or members moving up by degrees enacted contrived myths and stories; sometimes these involved partial stripping.[60] Is it too fanciful to suggest a loose analogy with the all-male weekly clinical lecture? It was closed to the non-initiated and all women, and offered—along with undeniably valuable instruction—a sort of fellowship, educational ritual, esoteric medical patois, and the display of partial nudity. For established medical men, the county societies amounted to another form of all-male environment. At least it is plausible to suggest that men's opposition to women physicians in the nineteenth century revealed not only their entrenched notions of what it meant to be feminine, but also cultural aspects of masculinity.

For the thirty-four or -five women who endured the jeers at the amphitheater, it was a true rite of passage. The event prefigured the countless smaller acts of insult and disapproval that women medical students would encounter for many decades to come. The notorious Pennsylvania Hospital incident became one of the defining stories of Woman's Medical College: a very real and vicious event which grew into legend.[61] A graduate of 1889 in her autobiography wrote that "one of our most cherished traditions when I was a student there was the story of Dr. Ann Preston, the first dean of the College, leading a small group of women medical students in forced march down the middle of Chestnut Street protected by the police from a mob of male medical students who had hooted them out of a clinic which the women had been given permission to attend." This alumna remembered not the event, but the institutional *memory* of the event as propagated forward in time, a now canonized part of the College's saga.[62]

The Pennsylvania Hospital fracas surely belongs to that class of stories, personalities, and myths which helps create the living identity of a school and helps pupils and faculty cleave to it and feel part of something long-lasting, heroic, and distinctive. It is tempting to believe that the oppressive events of 1867 and 1869 helped instill in the women leaders of the College of those years and for decades to come a persistent sense that, however attitudes might progress, caution prescribed the sustenance, at least in some one place, of a medical education environment reserved for women. The Pennsylvania Hospital "jeering episode" occurred in 1869; Woman's Medical College would not admit male students until exactly one hundred years later.

Firming Up the Course: Curricular Reforms of the 1870s

This passage newly appeared in the *Annual Announcement* for 1869–1870: "A demand has for a long time existed, both in Europe and in this country, for a system of progressive medical education. The plan now prevalent involved the great evil of "cramming" too many branches at once. . . . With this view, we propose to offer to our students the option of adopting a progressive course."[63] The two-year lecture curriculum (the same lectures both years) seemed to some inherently absurd and too demanding on the students, who then as now struggled to fix the mass of facts into their heads, or at least lodge it there until exams. The new three-year "progressive" option allowed students to complete the "fundamental branches" (anatomy, physiology, hygiene, chemistry) during the first year, and the "immediately practical" subjects (therapeutics, practices of medicine, surgery, etc.) in years two and three. The *Announcement* also promised for the third year "instruction upon ophthalmology, auscultation and percussion, and such other special teaching as the resources of the College and Hospital may afford."[64] WMC numbered among the earliest American medical schools to offer the progressive course (which did not really entail much more faculty work), and though it was not mandatory until 1881, its introduction antedated similar plans at the University of Pennsylvania and Harvard.[65] By 1872, twelve of thirty-three new students elected the progressive course.[66]

In 1871, the board authorized the faculty to undertake a spring term, "so long as it can be done at no expense to the College."[67] Again, WMC stood progressively among the first schools to adopt this addition.[68] Topics covered in the ten-week spring course for 1872 included practical chemistry, regional anatomy, practical anatomy, botany, dental physiology and pathology, auscultation and percussion, bandaging, and diseases of the eye. The catalog promised that much of the instruction would be practical. The program also included clinics in diseases of women and children, surgery, and ophthalmology, as well as dispensary service at the Woman's Hospital, and quiz (review) sessions on primary courses of the winter term.[69]

Probably not every bit of this actually occurred; college catalogs tend to proffer more than their authors can deliver.[70] Still, the spring semester (and the three-year course) indicate clear recognition by the faculty that medical knowledge was expanding and being categorized into specialties. Also, the faculty and dean no doubt realized the need to instruct in "practical" ways that went beyond the customary lecturing, even though doing so would increase demands on faculty time, budgets, and space. The later nineteenth century would see medical schools, at least the stronger ones, accept the notion of "learning by doing," and begin to implement it through greater reliance on teaching in the laboratory, and eventually, by invention of the clinical clerkship.[71]

Like most medical schools of the 1870s, WMC for a time lacked the resolve to require the spring session, probably fearing that doing so would overtax resources and might discourage applicants with lesser ambition, or who needed to work part of the year.[72] By 1870, there were five other women's medical schools in the country, so competition for women students had increased.[73]

The College's First Real Home

New programs would require more space, yet the Woman's Hospital found its own work expanding and hoped to see its tenant College vacate. As early as 1871, some signs of disharmony arose, even though, as we have seen, the governance bodies of the two institutions were interwoven. In April of 1871, the hospital's "House Committee" suggested, "as there are more nurses than usual on duty, that the number of house [medical] students be lessened or altogether dispensed with; and if need be secure the services of a paid apothecary in the place of students."[74]

It is unknown to what extent the College responded to this ominous misconception of the role of medical students in a teaching hospital.[75] Between 1871 and 1874, Woman's Hospital sent increasingly pressing requests that WMC vacate its rented space.[76] Fortunately, by 1874 the College was able to begin construction of its own building, thanks to an earlier bequest of a faithful Quaker corporator named Isaac Barton, a shy and diligent merchant and advocate for women's rights.[77] In 1873 the College had purchased a lot adjoining Woman's Hospital on North College Avenue; it was eager to maintain its then uncommon pedagogic access to teaching beds.[78] The board solicited plans from several architects and, after an exasperating period of review, awarded the contract to Addison Hutton, a well-known Friend and designer of houses, schools, and institutional buildings.[79]

Construction began in August of 1874.[80] At the cornerstone ceremony held on 1 October, the president of the board, T. Morris Perot, indulged in some prematurely optimistic comments:

> Now, however, everything looks bright; the prejudice has
> almost entirely disappeared, and popularity has taken its place,
> while the profession has been forced by public opinion to
> concede the right of woman to practice medicine. Under these
> favorable circumstances it is my pleasurable duty to lay this
> corner-stone, which I here do, *in the name of woman, and for her
> advancement in the science and practice of medicine.*[81]

Other speeches followed.

On 8 March 1875 the College formerly took possession from the builder, and the janitor moved into his apartment. The official opening was held on 11 March, the twenty-fifth anniversary of the founding and also commencement day, when "a large company assembled and spent the early evening in promenading through the brilliantly-lighted halls, and inspecting the spacious building in every part."[82] Then came the requisite speeches in the west lecture room, followed by a "bounteous collation."

Rachel Bodley, recently elected dean of the faculty, delivered the central address, containing these words: "When and where in the world's history before to-night, have the feet of women trodden halls reared solely for the professional education of women? The Woman's Medical

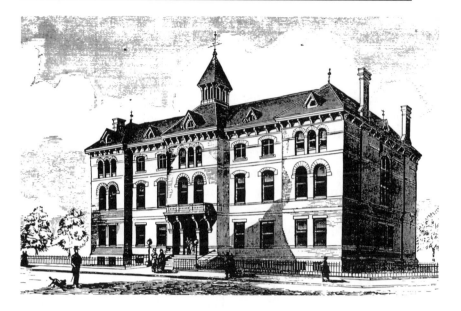

Figure 4. Opened in 1875, this was the first building the College constructed for its own use. It was designed by well-known Philadelphia Quaker architect Addison Hutton.

College enters a home, *her own home*, and you are witnesses of her joy."[83]

Indeed, it is hard to underestimate the exhilaration felt by the gathered faculty, corporators, and alumnae. A student wrote to a friend that the new structure was "a fine one, very completely arranged, and fitted up, and the professors, both gentlemen and ladies, who have been working under great disadvantages for so many years, are very justly proud of it."[84] The College family found itself, as if through the deed of some deft and beneficent conjurer, suddenly in the halls of its own solid and up-to-date building. The three-story edifice in a subdued Italianate style contained a large dissecting room; a library; a museum; laboratories for microscopy, pharmacy, and chemistry; a recitation ("quiz") room; two lecture halls each able to seat 250 persons; and other assigned spaces.

The two large lecture halls consumed vast space on both the second and third floors: their presence attested to the faith in the lecture method and wildly optimistic expectations for future enrollment. The dissection room occupied space on the third floor in the front, well-lit by skylights and dormer windows; students called it the "sky parlor." The building had no elevators and only one, grand, central stairwell. It is not known how the cadavers reached the sky parlor.[85]

In 1876, the year after the North College Avenue building opened, Philadelphia proudly hosted the great Centennial Exhibition in Fairmount Park, not too far from WMC. Mrs. Elizabeth Duane Gillespie, on behalf of the committee overseeing the Woman's Pavilion, invited Woman's Medical College to mount a display. The faculty selected pharmaceuticals, which students made in the new pharmacy laboratory. Mrs. Gillespie stated approvingly in a letter that the "exhibit of the pharmaceutical department of the Woman's Medical College could not be dispensed with," creating with this phrase a new department and a perfect pun.[86]

The "bright and clear tinctures" and "perfect form and finish" of the pills fashioned by the WMC students made for an impressive display at the Centennial. Of course, hand-fashioning medications, though still a potentially useful skill for physicians of the 1870s, hardly typified the real work of the woman medical student or physician: the display represented not intellectual capabilities, but a sort of traditional feminine handiwork extended to a medical craft. The Centennial Exhibition *was*, however, an exhibition, and needed *things*.[87] In any case, the presentation afforded the young medical school a unique opportunity for making itself known to American women while assuming a place at a major Philadelphia event.

It was the new building itself, not the display from its laboratory, that symbolized the progress and status of the College and of Philadelphia's medical women. The large brick structure proclaimed that women's medical education was no transient or trifling fancy. Yet, in her dedicatory remarks, Bodley muted her enthusiasm long enough to disclose her "single fear . . . a vision of a lecture-room capable of seating two hundred and fifty persons, containing a handful of fifty or sixty students."[88] Bodley had reason for concern. During the previous four years, the number of yearly matriculants ranged from fifty-seven to seventy four (in 1872–73), but it dropped to under fifty for the 1874–75 session.[89] In an 1874 letter to a friend and supporter of the College, Emeline Horton Cleveland suggested the basis for this alarming decline:

Several causes have probably operated to make the numbers so small among which the stringency of the money market has probably not been the least. The classes in the other schools are smaller than usual this year & we could not hope that we should not suffer out of measure with other schools from this cause. One or two new schools have become opened to women during the year in addition to the half dozen or more previously existing. . . . I have no doubt that another winter will find our class fuller when it shall be known that our new building is completed. Some have always gone to Ann Arbor in preference to coming here because of more comfortable lecture & dissecting rooms & better laboratory accommodations. When we shall be able to rival Ann Arbor in these I trust our superior clinical facilities will attract numbers here who would otherwise go there.[90]

The economic collapse Cleveland referred to, the financial panic of 1873, resulted in part from the railroad-building mania of the nineteenth century. Savings vanished and money became tight. Potential women students would have encountered difficulty financing their schooling; some would need to work rather than attend school. Cleveland was correct in assessing the competition offered by the University of Michigan ("Ann Arbor"): in 1870, it became the first major American university to open its medical division, unquestionably one of the country's best, to women.

So indeed an enormous amount depended upon the new building of 1875, the faculty within it, and the ability to implement instructional advances promised in the catalog. Despite the rejection by the medical societies and the rebuff at Pennsylvania Hospital, gains exceeded setbacks during the 1860s and 1870s, and the women and men of the board and faculty, mostly Quaker, remained steadfast in their commitment. The early deaths of Ann Preston and Emeline Horton Cleveland deprived the school of their continued example and guidance, but provided heroines to help begin adducing a distinct and usable history around which old and new members of the College community could rally. Woman's Medical College would never see a class size of 250: smallness would always be an attribute of the school, one which allowed a special emotional ambience but contributed to financial insecurity. Still, a growing number of students *would* come to the school in the 1880s and 1890s to find a remarkably strong enterprise offering women a solid medical education as then understood. An already historic sense of purpose animated the College, and—amounting to a remarkable nineteenth-century social experiment—in it progressive women and men worked together, knowing what needed to be done.

Chapter 3 Ann Preston, M.D.

An Excursus

Though not herself a founder, Ann Preston more than anyone else personifies the formative years of the Woman's Medical College. It is generally agreed that her inspiration and leadership carried the school from its tremulous beginnings to its first years of stable credibility. Having left conventional domestic responsibilities and country schoolteaching at the age of thirty-eight to enter the first class of the first women's medical school, Preston embodied the extension of woman's sphere through the act of bold, individual choice. She also prefigured what came to be known as the nontraditional student in medical school, generally someone older than most students, leaving one career or way of life for a new path. As the first of the lineage of women deans of the Woman's Medical College of Pennsylvania, a succession that stretched over one hundred years, she exemplified woman as leader, adept at managing complex affairs and motivating colleagues. Nothing has appeared in the College's promotional literature more often than one of the familiar few images of Preston—stiff early photographs showing her refined and regular features, into which the viewer imaginatively reads strength and resolve.

Ann Preston, in addition to serving as a doctor, was both moral and political reformer, visionary, fund-raiser, and institution builder. She was a fighting Quaker, her weapons being moral suasion, active example, and—not least of these—the forceful written word.[1] It was often with

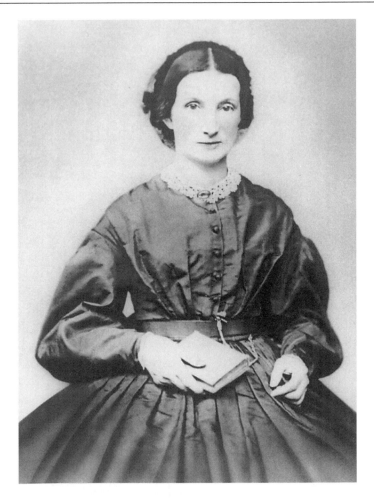

Figure 5. Ann Preston, graduate of the first class, abolitionist, teacher of hygiene and physiology, medical practitioner, poet, rhetorician, institution builder, Friend.

words that she influenced others while alive, and it is mainly writings that she left behind after death. This excursus on Ann Preston will recall her particularly as craftswoman of the pen, with the aim of allowing her words to supply the portrait.

When reading memoirs and writings about Ann Preston, one is struck by the unfailing reference to her small size and fragility: she is described as "little," "petite," "tiny," and, endlessly, as "frail." One newspaper report from 1870 told how "this delicate *petit* person in black silk and velvet" was so small that she had to "stand upon a bench while addressing students."[2] Yet coupled with her name repeatedly is also this word: *indomitable*. Contemporaries referred to her shortness and delicacy because these characteristics, if marking her as acceptably "feminine," contrasted so strikingly with, and thus highlighted, her tenacity and accomplishment. Though never untrue to her Quaker birthright, she yielded quietness and reticence in order to publicly speak, write, teach, and lead, as her causes demanded. But she was never aggressive or "masculine": hers was a "cheerful, lady like persistence." That indeed she did periodically suffer from ill health only rarely interrupted her work.

Ann Preston was born in West Grove, Chester County, Pennsylvania, in 1813, daughter of Amos and Margaret Smith Preston. Amos, a prosperous farmer, landowner, and Quaker preacher, embraced the Hicksite movement early on, and fervidly supported abolition, as did Ann and at least two of her brothers. They grew up in a comfortable home alive with intellect and concern for one's relation with God and with other human beings. Ann Preston studied at a local Quaker school and briefly at a boarding school in nearby Chester, Pennsylvania. She enjoyed both literature, as a member of the local lyceum, and the book of nature, gloriously accessible throughout Chester County's hills and fields. Since her mother experienced chronically subdued health, Ann assumed much responsibility for the household and the supervision of her six brothers and one sister.

As a young woman she joined the local antislavery society, in which her growing skill with words found ample exercise. At least once she went well beyond persuasion: a much-told story relates how she hid an escaped slave, astray from the nearby Underground Railroad, then disguised her as an elderly Quaker woman (bonnet and veils). With courage and forethought, she conveyed her camouflaged charge by carriage *in* the direction of pursuing slave catchers, safely reaching a house they had already searched. Ann Preston also supported temperance, and, of course, women's rights. For some years she also taught school locally and found time to write, including a published book of verse for children, *Cousin Ann's Stories*.

While these activities that centered on family, meeting, and community might have sufficed, for the future Dr. Preston they did not: her life was to be distinctly divided into two phases—West Grove in Chester County, then Woman's Medical College in Philadelphia. The shift typified nineteenth-century trends—from farm to city, and, for a few women at first, from home to public place. At the age of thirty-eight, she left her beloved (though at times demanding) home and family to enter the heaped uncertainties of studying medicine as a member of the first class of the Female Medical College and was gratified to feel "the joy of exploring a new field of knowledge, the rest from accustomed pursuits and cares, the stimulus of competition, the novelty of a new kind of life."[3] Throughout her career, however, she cherished family visits and an annual vacation at home.

After graduation, Dr. Preston stayed at the College to hear the lectures again (not an unusual decision at the time) and soon found herself invited to join the faculty as professor of physiology, a title expanded to "physiology and hygiene" in 1858. Physiology held some of the same meaning it does now—functions of the organs and the body—but it also encompassed principles of hygiene and the sustenance of health. Motivated to aid the well-being of their sisters at a time when American culture saw women as almost intrinsically sickly, early female physicians embraced the teaching of hygiene. The New York Infirmary's Woman's Medical College and the Philadelphia school added this subject to their curricula in advance of male medical schools. It could include reproductive and sexual functions, so mid-nineteenth century attitudes demanded a female instructor for women students.

Ann Preston urged the value of preserving health and offered ways to accomplish it. In her valedictory address to the 1864 graduates, she told them of "the necessity of guarding your own health, by all prudent and right precautions. This is a part of your capital, and an instrument essential to full success."[4]

Other WMC faculty made similar recommendations in their addresses throughout the nineteenth century, and the notion could not have been limited to the College. Elsewhere Preston asserted that sometimes "by diet and regimen you may turn a man inside out."[5] Preston believed in the value of proper diet, exercise, fresh air, avoidance of overwork, and—aided by these—the "healing power of nature." She did not, however, deny the value of intelligently prescribed medication nor of surgery when needed, and expressed no tolerance for "every absurd

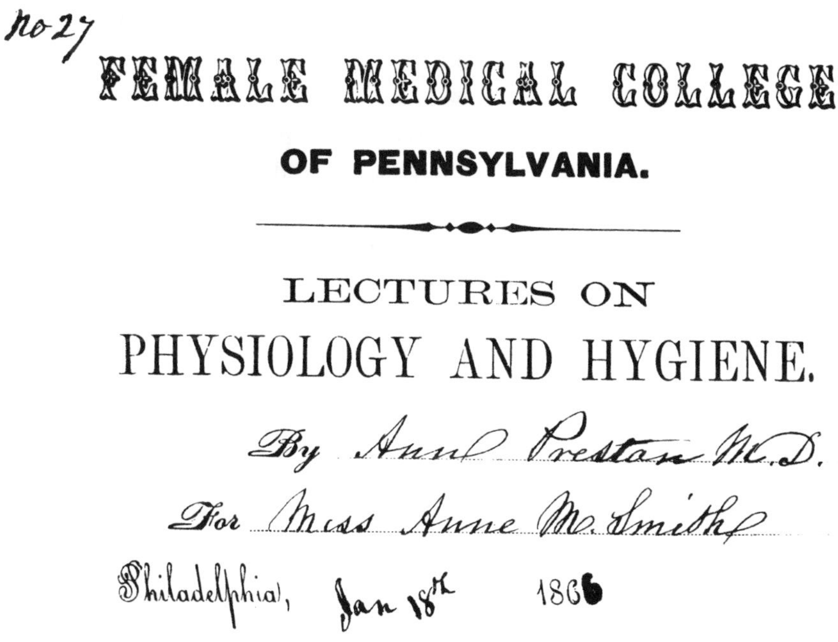

no 27

FEMALE MEDICAL COLLEGE

OF PENNSYLVANIA.

LECTURES ON
PHYSIOLOGY AND HYGIENE.

By Ann Preston M.D.

For Miss Anne M. Smith

Philadelphia,   Jan 18th   1866

Figure 6. In the nineteenth-century American medical school, students purchased tickets to each professor's lectures, such as this one for Ann Preston's course on physiology and hygiene.

new theory," "narrow creeds and partial schools," or "rushing blindly from one extreme of medication to its opposite, like trees tossed to and fro in a gale."[6] Though herself not a scientist, she endorsed the ways of orthodox medicine and science and steered this course during her watch as dean of the Woman's Medical College.

As we have seen, soon after joining the faculty Preston became an institution builder: even before becoming dean, she undertook the daunting task of establishing Woman's Hospital of Philadelphia both to provide clinical opportunities for the school's students and graduates, and medical services for women that would be carried out *by* women. She moved into deanship of the Female Medical College in 1865 and, despite periodic crises, guided it into a welcome period of growth and security. The mere accounting of events cannot convey the immense amount of work and unyielding persistence demanded. Dr. Preston drew from her singular spirit and conviction, and—like similar women of the times—possibly from organizational experience gained in the abolition and temperance campaigns.

Her accomplishments belied her imperfect health, for early in 1862 she had suffered another bout of what was probably rheumatic fever, followed by "complete prostration, mental and physical, [which] terminated in brief intellectual aberration."[7] This followed soon after the opening of the Woman's Hospital, a prolonged illness of Ann Preston's mother, and above all the College's suspension of classes: her collapse paralleled that of her beloved school. Stress, overwork, and perhaps her rheumatic disease (or its treatment) probably brought on Preston's illness. Whatever the cause, the physician necessarily became patient: she spent several months in the Pennsylvania Hospital for the Insane, under the care of Thomas S. Kirkbride, a renowned leader in the rational and humane treatment of mental disorder. He was also a Friend. In a grim irony, this pause in Ann Preston's productive life fit the rhetorical predictions of male physicians who asserted that the female constitution could not stand the work and strain of professional life. In fact, Dr. Kirkbride's charges included many *male* physicians and businessmen.[8]

Ann Preston enjoyed a full recovery of her intellectual powers and later in 1862 went on to her most important period of shaping the future of the allied institutions, including, of course, the recovery of the WMC. She was not, however, a medical educator who did no medicine: the dean maintained a limited but satisfying practice and attended at the hospital.[9] She never married, but established a lively household, where "dear friends live with me in harmonious relations, and do much to make this an orderly home circle."[10] For some years the "friends" included several other single women, a mother and son, and a young married couple. Ann Preston died on 18 April 1872, to the unbelieving sorrow of her family, friends, colleagues, and (I will assume) patients. They lost a friend and steady comrade, while the cause of women in medicine lost "a force, a factor, which carried an influence worth a regiment of men."[11]

Much of the force of Ann Preston's being gained its effect through language spoken or in print: she was a fine writer. "From earliest childhood she possessed the ability to express her thoughts with grace and facility."[12] In her schooling, she would have used one of several widely popular (at least with the instructors) manuals of composition, perhaps an edition of Samuel Newman's *Practical System of Rhetoric, or the Principles and Rules of Style*. "Rhetoric" now owns an almost entirely derisive meaning; but in the nineteenth century it referred to the process of constructing, and sometimes delivering oratorically, a sound and pleasing argument or essay.[13] Certainly in Ann Preston's day many Americans sought to win others to their point of view concerning slavery, whiskey, the Holy Trinity, tariffs, or dozens of other issues—so rhetorical skill mattered. A gender distinction did prevail, however, in the nineteenth-century teaching of rhetoric: girls were to learn a conversational, even sentimental style, boys a far more ordered and formal structure. Before the appearance of women activists for abolition and equal rights in the antebellum period, societal norms virtually prohibited a woman from speaking in public, except a few female ministers in the Society of Friends. Ann Preston was of the generation that *did* speak in public, and much of her recorded writing served that purpose. And, she chose and excelled in the more elaborated, "masculine" model.

The standard manuals stressed the form of the composition, the need for clear direction and crisp thinking, and several elements of style. These included "perspicuity," which mainly meant clarity; "vivacity" or "energy," a quality of forcefulness; and "elegance," the ability to delight the reader or listener's ear, with flow, melody, and harmony. The good writer chose words with precision and arranged them in lucid and energetic sentences, to enlighten and provide pleasure—and to persuade. A large part of Preston's work involved persuading skeptics and opponents that medicine suited women and that women physicians would suit certain needs of society.

Preston's prose often displays a craftsmanly selection of words and a skilled control of sentences (some of which are rather long, mortared with the then very popular semicolon). She consistently achieved a pleasing and seemingly natural cadence or rhythm that reveals her fondness for poetry, which she also wrote. Here is a simple admonition to graduates from her 1858 valedictory address: "Some of us have seen fearful mistakes, not so much because the disorder was obscure, as because pains were not taken to examine carefully, so as to separate the accidental from the essential, and detect, amid varying symptoms, the real seat and nature of the difficulty."[14]

The passage finds familiar but energetic words such as "fearful" and "obscure," nicely contrasts alternatives (accidental—essential), and concludes, in a kind of verbal release, with the strong phrase "real seat and nature of the difficulty." Such a sentence is referred to technically as "periodic." The content, incidentally, reflects the growing nineteenth-century interest in pathology (the local, organic "seat" of disease) which emerged from France and England in the first half of the nineteenth century.

In her 1864 farewell to graduates, she reminded them that their therapeutic agents included not only useful drugs, but that "all the common influences of daily life, and all the wide agents in nature which modify the condition of the body or mind are your legitimate instruments—the proper tools of your extended art."[15] Again she rings her sentence to conclusion with a brisk phrase that serves perfectly. Preston liked to choose adjectives carefully and favored this musical balance— "the *proper* tools of your *extended* art."

Ann Preston did not, of course, write always on professional subjects. Her few extant personal letters reveal charm and an inability to write English other than agreeably, despite a relaxation of punctuation:

> I must spend part of this most beautiful of autumn days in
> writing to my dear Hannah and notwithstanding her kind
> lecture on the advantage of taking pains with the "manner and
> matter which we discharge by way of letters," I fear alas I shall
> both scribble and pen my thoughts as they occur without much
> regard for perspicuity.
>
> I am sitting in my chamber with both windows open, have
> been surveying the beauty, fresh, variegated with the brightest
> colours, and watching various [?] animals of the human species
> whom the warm sun has enticed moving backwards and
> forwards and all appearing to enjoy themselves; I think after all
> this is rather a pleasant world to live in [;] it contains so much
> of the "spice of life."[16]

The writer was nineteen when she expressed these generous and youthful sentiments.

Ann Preston's student and friend Eliza Judson was charged with delivering a memorial address after the dean's death in 1872. In passing, Judson noted what later writers about Preston could not detect—her "innate love of the humorous."[17] Physicians love to tell clinical stories.

Here is an instructive case vignette from Dr. Preston's lecture on nursing the sick, delivered at the Woman's Hospital in May of 1863. The speaker argues that one should not discount the whims of patients, for sometimes nature speaks through such caprice:

> A lady related to me the case of her friend whose darling little girl was very ill, and grew weaker and weaker, until it was given up to die; a few weeks ago the lady met with this same little girl, plump and rosy, and on inquiring what miracle has so renewed that young life, was told that it was *raw oysters*; that the child had at first sucked a raw oyster and seemed eager for more; that it would awake in the night and cry for oysters, and still it grew stronger and stronger, as the mother, who read the wisdom of nature in the want of the child, fed it as it desired. It is by no means certain, however, that some other mother, hearing of this marvellous oyster cure, may not cram oysters down the revolting stomach of some little victim, to its serious injury; for thus people do.[18]

Here Dr. Preston makes her point with a lively tale whose strand of absurdity she tacitly and humorously acknowledges ("this marvellous oyster cure"). She appends a second caution (foolish mothers might wrongly generalize), phrased satirically; she both softens and underscores the message with the four words "for thus people do," a verbal sigh from the doctor who "has seen it all."

It was advocacy of medical women and the College that called forth what many consider her finest published essay of argument—the reply to the Philadelphia County Medical Society's manifesto forbidding its members to recognize women physicians, referred to in the previous chapter. In the almost classical tradition, she introduces her topic and summarizes the society's objections. She next develops her theme as she refutes each specious assertion of the Medical Society with a series of paragraphs whose language conveys her logic but never substitutes for it. Here is how she deals with the manifesto's familiar assertion that women cannot "bear up" under the strain of medical work:

> In regard to the first difficulty, few words need be expended. Pausing merely to allude to the fact, that in barbarous communities woman is pre-eminently the laborious drudge, and that in civilized society she is the nurse, keeping her unceasing vigils,

not only by the cradle of infancy, but by every bed of sickness and suffering, with a power of sustained endurance that man does not even claim to possess; that her life is as long, and her power of surmounting its painful vicissitudes not inferior to his, we come to the open, undeniable fact, that women *do* practice medicine, that they *are* able to "bear up under the bodily and mental strain" that this practice imposes, and that "natural obstacles" have not obstructed their way.[19]

Clearly, the dean of the Woman's Medical College has lost all patience with this particular cavil.

Lastly, Preston transcends the specific contentions to conclude with a stirring claim of rights for that righteous band her voice defends:

We regard this movement as belonging to the advancing civilization of the age, as the inevitable result of that progressive spirit which is unfolding human capabilities in many directions, and which has perceived that it is the condition of the highest health and happiness for woman, that she, also, should exercise the powers with which she has been endowed in accordance with her own convictions and feelings, and in harmony with her nature and organization.

That our position is womanly; that this work is established in the fitness of things and in the necessities of society, and that the movement belongs to the "revolutions which never go backward," we have no shadow of doubt.

For us it is the post of restful duty—the place assigned to us, as we believe, in the order of Providence, and we can do no other than maintain it.

But, on behalf of a little band of true-hearted young women who are just entering the profession, and from whose pathway we fain would see annoyance and impediments removed, we must protest, in the sacred name of our common humanity, against the injustice which places difficulties in our way, not because we are ignorant or pretentious or incompetent or unmindful of the code of medical or Christian ethics, but because we are women.

Truly yours,
Ann Preston, M.D.
Philadelphia, April 22, 1867.

Unfortunately, the response counted more as a literary than strategic success, for the recalcitrant Philadelphia medical men stood unready in 1867 to formally acknowledge their unwanted women colleagues. Eventually, of course, they would; the students Ann Preston taught and the institutions she helped build counted largely in securing respectability and reputation for Philadelphia's women physicians and surgeons.

Ann Preston can easily seem the remote and too-perfect heroine: a noble figure from very long ago, emanating from her tiny frame both unexpected energy and a faultless moral posture, always prepared to "work where the work opens" (this phrase apparently her personal motto) and wait or forgive when it remained closed. Some mystery surrounds her, centered particularly on the hospitalization at Pennsylvania Hospital. The personal journal she kept, quoted by her memorialist Eliza Judson, long has been lost, as are, oddly, the faculty minutes for most of her deanship—the only major gap in these holdings. We are thus hindered in knowing her as person and as professional. The few extant photographs help little. But her writing brings Ann Preston alive. The reply to the County Medical Society offers, through finely wrought prose, passion and anger, not patience or acceptance. Discovering in Dr. Ann Preston this union of righteous vehemence with force of language, one readily endorses those who have seen this half-known spiritual progenitor of WMC not only as healer, teacher, and reformer, but also as prophetess of a new idea.

Chapter 4

Deans Bodley and Marshall

Approaching a Golden Age

The period from the early 1880s to about 1910 can be considered a kind of golden age for WMC, and indeed for the women's medical movement in the United States. Enrollment of women in medical schools, both separate-sex and coeducational, reached a peak in this period. Strong medical schools for women operated not only in Philadelphia, but also in New York, Baltimore, and Chicago. Those choosing coeducation might win one of several places open to female applicants at Johns Hopkins, the University of Michigan, and some other first-rate university medical departments. Women also ran hospitals and made widespread gains in winning membership in medical societies. WMC by the late 1880s had developed into not merely an acceptable medical school, but in fact, by standards of the time, a superior one. Among the first American medical schools to require a four-year program, WMC by the late 1890s had grown into a complex institution, looking much more like the medical educational model of the next hundred years than the college of 1850. It claimed capable and dedicated faculty, responsible and attentive lay leadership, sufficient if not abundant physical resources, and an evolved ambience and spirit that fostered learning, loyalty, and a rich and formative social life among its students. This robust phase of the College story warrants full attention, for the mature institution had become a major participant in an extraordinary social phenomenon—the movement of women in now irrefutable numbers into a previously male profession. The present chapter will offer an overview of the development of the College from 1875, the year in which the new building opened, to the 1890s, and discuss the two deans who led the school into and through these years of strength. Subsequent chapters will expand on the attributes which made it so distinctive an institution in this period, including the unusual interplay of male and female faculty, the curriculum, and the lively and adventurous women students for whom the increasingly sophisticated institution existed.

Woman's Medical College always existed in a world of intellectual and social change, and the last decades of the nineteenth century proved no exception. To fully appreciate the College in this period, it will prove of value to look again at the three contexts traced in this work— the world of medicine and medical education, the evolving status of the American woman, and the local substrate of Philadelphia.

Medicine and Medical Education

Late nineteenth-century American medicine and medical education were marked by the ascent of the laboratory and science (especially bacteriology), the growth of clinical specialties, and the proliferation of hospitals. As use of the microscope spread, physicians, especially younger ones, began to comprehend disease in terms of specific causes at the level of cell or microbe, revealed only through the lens or laboratory. As the body of medical knowledge expanded enormously, many ambitious physicians, men and women, chose to cultivate a specialty such as dermatology, neurology, or otolaryngology. Such subjects eventually gained entry into the medical curriculum. The expansion of surgery under the safety of asepsis, and the large number of new immigrants who could not always obtain medical care in their crowded living quarters, drove the proliferation of urban hospitals and dispensaries. The number of general hospitals increased from about 170 in 1873 to over 700 by 1889.[1] For medical educators, the hospital offered "clinical material," meaning simply many ill patients gathered in one place.

The progressive medical schools sought to accommodate and prepare students for these transformations. A better school's faculty responsibly wanted to do a good job and to be part of a first-class institution;

they also competed for the better students. But setting up laboratories, paying for lectures in the specialties, and amplifying clinical instruction all demanded unprecedented faculty effort, and above all, money. Building or running a teaching hospital proved even more perilously expensive. Clearly, numerous marginal proprietary or even well-intentioned schools did not or could not upgrade, and many of these vanished in the first two decades of the twentieth century.[2]

The American Woman of the 1880s and 1890s

Throughout the 1880s and 1890s, most American women, even the growing number of college graduates, still largely accepted the role of mother and homemaker, though dissidents entered medicine, professional nursing, education, and—a very few—law. By the 1890s, about eight women's medical schools, some highly tenuous, operated at any one time, and by 1910 a notable 6 percent of all American doctors were female. This was a high point, and in fact the percentage diminished into the twentieth century.[3]

The movement for suffrage, having won regrettably few triumphs, reached a point of weariness by the middle of the 1890s. Many American women in fact opposed suffrage. But women continued to develop their individual and collective capabilities and their influence in other ways. The Women's Christian Temperance Union (WCTU) of the late nineteenth century, under the zealous command of Frances Willard, carried out work well beyond closing bars and spilling rum. It addressed, for example, child welfare and prison reform. Women's clubs also attracted massive numbers of members in the 1890s and early twentieth century. While many of these groups began with literary objectives, before long they became a force for urban reform. The club women extended traditional domestic concerns for health, well-being of children, and education, to an activist and effective force at municipal and national levels.[4] The educated and enterprising representative of this work and outlook in the 1890s has been called the "New Woman."

Philadelphia Near the Century's End

Finally, what of Philadelphia, home of WMC, in the late nineteenth century?[5] As the nation's third largest municipality in the 1880s and 1890s, it displayed all aspects of urban life. For example, Philadelphia's women engaged in reformist activities similar to those of their sisters elsewhere. They formed a branch of the WCTU, and some joined the Pennsylvania Suffrage Society, as well as one of the national groups. The pioneering New Century Club began in 1877, an outgrowth of Philadelphia women's participation in the 1876 Centennial Exhibition. It soon created its New Century Guild for working women, which provided a range of night classes, a gymnasium (in 1886), and other services. The equally meritorious Civic Club, which by varied routes strove for the betterment of Philadelphia, was founded in 1889, and the upper-class Acorn Club in 1894.[6] Some of Philadelphia's prominent medical women became active in one or more of these clubs.

Philadelphia's rapid growth and large working-class population provided ample opportunity for meliorist work by organizations and individuals. Increasingly larger factories produced textiles, carpets, shoes, sugar, cigars, furniture, steam locomotives, streetcars, steel, and nearly everything else. Working in the factories, service, and construction jobs, the large number of poor immigrants became the clientele of the free dispensaries, hospital wards, and clinics. As such, they became the human fuel of another of the city's characteristic industries—medical education. By the 1890s, four schools in addition to WMC (and all much larger) operated: the University of Pennsylvania School of Medicine, Jefferson Medical College, Hahnemann Medical College (homeopathic), and the extinct Medico-Chirurgical College. None admitted women or had women in major faculty positions. A postgraduate school, the liberal Philadelphia Polyclinic, did teach many women and shared some faculty members with WMC.

On the whole, Philadelphia of the 1890s moved along reasonably well: visitors remarked about its drabness, but also its modesty of scale, distaste for ostentation, and pleasing small-town ambience. To critics of its entrenched machine politics, the 1890s city was, at the same time, "corrupt and contented." Contented Philadelphians modeled snobbishness, with the "better people" looking down on first-generation money and on anyone dwelling "north of Market Street," where proper people did not live. Suitably located in this taboo zone, a novel group of mostly young women (and their male allies) on North College Avenue pursued not politics or social position, but rather their chosen work, the learning and teaching of medicine.

Growth and Constituencies

Into the lecture halls and laboratories of the new building came, in 1875, a total faculty of fourteen, comprising the full professors of the seven traditional courses and a secondary tier of instructors in the newer subjects. A total enrollment of seventy-two students chose either two or three years of work, which still depended heavily on lectures; the new subjects and practical work mostly filled the optional but popular spring course. A student could graduate if she passed oral examinations following two courses of the "Winter" lectures, completed dissection, wrote a brief thesis, and provided some documentation of a preceptorship.

Twenty years later, the 1895 *Annual Announcement* showed eight full professors and a corps of auxiliary teachers with a confusing array of titles—demonstrators, instructors and clinical instructors, adjunct and clinical professors, a prosector. Of the eight primary professorships (an endowed chair in gynecology having been added to the ancient seven), four were held by women, as were most of the junior titles. As in 1875, but more so, prominent Philadelphia male physicians taught at the school. The faculty and curriculum represented all the new specialties, even though some owned but a few hours in the roster.

The total enrollment in 1895 had reached 156. As of 1893, each student enrolling looked forward to a required course of four years that entailed the usual plethora of lectures, substantive laboratory work (including introduction to agar-agar and platinum loops, the exotic appliances of bacteriology), and as much or more clinical experience as most schools of the day provided. By the mid-1890s, WMC had acquired many of the recognizable attributes of the modern four-year medical school. Despite this growth in complexity, the management structure of WMC remained traditional: the dean oversaw most academic functions, but virtually every expense and most initiatives, no matter how minor, required approval by the board of corporators. The officers of the board decided what could be spent based on their judgment about the current state of the College's purse; no one drew up budgets, nor was there any organized fund-raising process. In 1896, the dean was allocated a part-time "sub-dean," but no secretary aided her work, and much business was transacted through handwritten letters and notes.

The board and the faculty for the most part worked together, but occasionally clashed sharply, particularly concerning the appointment or reappointment of faculty, and the willingness—or lack of it—to spend money. Gradually the students adduced a sense of group identity, complete with a "voice" that increasingly spoke up, or wrote down in the form of petitions. Thus, by the 1890s this third constituency believed it knew what the College needed. External influences arose as well, as the American Medical Association and the reborn Association of American Medical Colleges pressed for reform of medical education, and many states began to tighten their medical licensure systems.

In 1875, Emeline Horton Cleveland and Mary J. Scarlett-Dixon led in the founding of the Alumnae Association of the Woman's Medical College of Pennsylvania, one of the earliest women's medical societies. Its founding confirmed that WMC had become something worthy to think of and support as alma mater. By 1895, the association had about three hundred dues-paying members. The alumnae through the association assumed an enduring role in supporting the College and defending its founding purpose. It became another voice that could not be ignored, particularly after it repeatedly helped rescue WMC from successive crises in the twentieth century. Its annual meetings for many decades provided opportunity for graduates not only to remain in touch with the College and one another, but also to present and discuss papers; they easily proved that this element of medical life also could be carried out independently by women.[7]

The job of the dean became more laborious and diverse as the nineteenth century entered its last decades. She had to coordinate curricular changes and additions, represent the faculty to the board and to other institutions and agencies including alumnae, correspond with students and prospective students, read students' petitions and hear their complaints, record minutes of faculty meetings, and generally look after the daily running of the College. Considerable credit must go to Rachel Bodley (dean from 1874 to 1888) and Clara Marshall (dean from 1888

WOMAN'S
Medical College of Pennsylvania.

ALUMNÆ ASSOCIATION.

In response to an informal call, issued by Drs. Emeline H. Cleveland and Mary J. Scarlett-Dixon, to the Alumnæ of the Woman's Medical College of Pennsylvania, a meeting was held in the Foyer of Horticultural Hall, at Philadelphia, March 11th, 1875, to consider the feasibility of forming an organization for mutual benefit. The following named alumnæ were present:

Olive D. Aldrich,
Amy S. Barton,
Mary Branson,
Anna E. Broomall,
Mary Blehl,
Emily S. Brooke,
Harriet A. Bottsford,
Emeline H. Cleveland,
Rita B. Church,
Susan R. Cooper,
Mary J. Scarlett-Dixon,
Rachel A. Dickey,
Lucilla H. Green,
Mary A. D. Jones,
Elizabeth C. Keller,
Catharine M. Kennedy,

Anna Lukens,
Esther L. W. Marbourg,
Clara Marshall,
Sarah R. Munro,
Lizzie W. Needham,
Emma K. Ogden,
Charlotte A. Y. Olsen,
Mary Pratt,
Ermina H. Pollard,
Elizabeth C. W. Rockwood,
Arminta V. Scott,
Anita E. Tyng,
Mary E. Wilson,
Frances Emily White,
Ellen E. Zook,

Letters of regret at inability to be present, and expressive of interest in the object of the meeting, were received from the following named alumnæ:

Orie Moon Andrews,
A. C. Buckel,
Hannah B. Carter,
Mary Dubois,
Mary C. Putnam-Jacobi,

Lettie A. Smith,
Jenny K. G. Trout,
Odelia Blinn,
Amelia A. Christie.

Figure 7. A group of alumnae met to form an association on Founders' Day, 1875. Alumnae would become the most steadfast defenders of Woman's Medical College.

to 1917) for guiding and managing the school during these decades of growth.

Rachel Bodley, "The College Story," and Missionaries

We have already introduced Rachel Bodley in chapter 2 as the teacher and chemist-botanist who came to WMC in 1865. Poised and articulate, she evidently also possessed the sort of "breeding" and natural gifts that made her well able to perform an expanded public role. Bodley became dean when Emeline Horton stepped down owing to poor health.

During Bodley's watch, which ended with her sudden death in June of 1888, the College occupied its new building; several key faculty members came on board or rose to professorial rank; the curriculum expanded to a requisite three years and added new subjects; laboratory work was developed or expanded in physiology and chemistry. Although her duties as dean and professor of chemistry consumed most of her time, she managed to continue some botanical field work and lecturing. She also brought the College's name into nonmedical public spheres by serving on the Women's Committee of the Pennsylvania Board of Public Charities and on the school board of her district in Philadelphia.

Among her most interesting projects was the survey of alumnae she carried out for "The College Story," her valedictory address for 1881.[8] One historian of WMC, Gulielma Fell Alsop, aptly called attention to Rachel Bodley's own perception that her survey represented the same order of work as answering a chemical question with "test tube, reagent, and balance"—that is, actively gathering data, a component of science. She mailed "printed questions" to 244 living alumnae. A respectable 77 percent responded, many quite promptly (134 were back within two weeks). Bodley felt that the responses "have in a manner which is quite remarkable gathered these College Alumnae about me, and during the hours I have devoted to the preparation of this address, I have been among them and caught their spirit."[9]

Bodley's enriching experience while tabulating the results likely represented something more than just sentimentality. Though not herself a physician (her M.D. was honorary, from WMC), she had come to identify with a strengthening community of women whose individual and collegial activities formed a "cause." Through the College their cause became hers; and with *The College Story*, she validated the training of women doctors and helped assemble their history. The latter she nurtured as well through explanatory notes in the matriculation book and faculty minutes and by initiating a College collection of newspaper clippings which continued for over one hundred years.

The remarkable results of the survey refuted prejudicial assumptions about women physicians. Eighty-eight percent of the 189 respondents were "in active medical practice," and of those not, only 8 assigned the reason to "domestic duties," and six to "ill health."[10] Opponents to women entering medicine had asserted that women would drop practice when they married or would wither away due to the arduous demands of the work. Bodley showed that, as expected, the vast majority of their practices centered on obstetrics and gynecology, general practice, or some combination of these. Among the 76 women who answered the question about earnings, the mean annual income was $2,907.30, no small sum at the time.[11] About 40 percent of the alumnae attained membership in a county, state, or other local medical society.[12] Fifty-two of the 189 women had married, and Bodley rejoiced in finding that only 6 considered their work a "not entirely favorable" influence on their marriage and motherhood, and only one deemed it "unfavorable."[13] (It can be assumed that a couple with two incomes in the nineteenth century could easily afford servants.) Bodley never married, but like most advanced women of the nineteenth century did not challenge the "sacred" role of woman as wife and mother.[14] The dean included some frank comments from those who did find domestic and professional chores too much of a strain.

Bodley also called attention to the "small number of deaths" among the alumnae—only 32 over thirty years among 276 women, which she considered further evidence against the purported depleting effect that medical work would have on the supposedly more fragile female structure.[15] She then extracted some colorful and illustrative passages from the comments a number of her respondents added. Maria Minnis Homet, a member of the second graduating class (1853), recalled how she "bought a horse and saddle, also one hundred dollars' worth of medicine, and settled in a small village of Pennsylvania, with the Susquehanna River on one side, and mountains on the other. I often rode ten miles in the night as well as in the day. I made friends and my practice increased rapidly." Later, this early graduate married and also acquired a carriage; her supportive husband "never allowed me to harness my horse, and if I had a call in the night he always drove for me."[16] A graduate of 1875, also married and a mother, wrote from Nebraska: "During three weeks since the holidays I did not have a night's unbroken rest. We have had an unusually cold winter, with deep snows, and I have had to work to attend to my country practice."[17] One might easily imagine that such letters and the survey results as a whole would inspire the dean (and other faculty) as they tried to ensure as full and useful a medical education as resources would allow. "The College Story" formed almost a manifesto for the future.

A devout Christian, Rachel Bodley took a special, indeed evangelical, interest in the encouragement of women missionary doctors, thereby helping to create another lasting theme in the College saga. The foreign mission movement within American Protestantism reached full stride in the 1880s and 1890s, and women played a major role. Historians have referred to the "feminization of religion" in the United States during the nineteenth century.[18] As one outcome of women's reliance on religion and church work as a satisfying basis for extra-domestic accomplishment, they formed numerous female missionary societies, with membership reaching over three million by 1915.[19] The societies provided funds for the missions (mostly in China and India), and particularly supported medical services to women. The medical work in part served as an instrument of evangelism: while women waited outside the dispensary to see the female doctor, the "Bible woman" read scripture.[20] From a nineteenth-century Anglo-American viewpoint, certain aspects of the culturally determined status of Indian and Chinese women seemed to powerfully invite intervention. For example, even more than was the case in Western Victorian custom, the traditions of Hindu and Moslem women in India generally forbade examination by male physicians.

In 1851, Sarah Josepha Hale, Philadelphian and editor of the popular *Godey's Lady's Book*, had founded the Ladies Medical Missionary Society of Philadelphia to finance the medical education of women who would then go overseas. The first woman medical missionary sent to a "foreign field," aided by the Methodists, was Clara Swain, an 1869 graduate of WMC. Many graduates followed: some of the more notable early names include Mary Seelye, Sara Seward, Lucinda Coombs, Anna Kugler, Anna Fullerton, Elizabeth Reifsnyder, Mary Pauline Root, Mary Fulton, Rosetta Sherwood Hall. In 1975 Marion Fay, retired from the deanship and presidency of WMC and studying its history, estimated a total of 230 WMC graduates went to the field (and many more emerged from other medical schools).[21]

From a postcolonial perspective, we may well question the obvious theological and cultural imperialism so evident in nineteenth-century missionary work, along with unintended condescension. An 1888 account of the medical work of the Methodist missionary society reveals these now discredited attitudes: equating intelligence with ability in English, favoritism to the higher castes, assignment of Christian (Western) names to Indian orphans, above all the desire to combine cure and conversion.[22] Still, none can deny the heroism of these women, not a few of whom were buried young and far from home, dead of cholera or another hazard. Like many nineteenth-century women, many of the female physicians who went overseas indeed felt suffused with a profound sense of *mission*, comprehended as Christian charity alloyed with the highest meaning of the doctor's calling. The feminization of religion and the (partial) de-masculinization of medicine came perfectly together in the female, Christian, missionary physician.

It is worth pointing out here that many women physicians provided a secular form of missionary work in their own American cities by founding and staffing dispensaries in poor neighborhoods (sometimes within a settlement house), or by setting up night clinics for working women. One example of the former, the Alumnae Dispensary of WMC, will be discussed in a later chapter.[23]

Rachel Bodley, a contributor to missionary societies since childhood, urged students to become missionaries in her first introductory address at the opening of classes in 1875.[24] She took into her home Mrs. Anandibai Joshee, a young Indian woman who reversed the trajectory by coming to WMC to study medicine. Women from China, Korea, and other nations of the East would follow, lending to occasional classes an unexpected exotic quality. Bodley also established a friendship with Pundita Ramabai, an Indian poet and advocate for women. Gulielma Fell Alsop, herself for some years a practitioner in China, much admired the foreign mission work and its nurturing by Bodley, who, Alsop said, "used every means in her power to foster a Christian spirit in students and faculty."[25] With its pious Quaker roots and Bodleian influence, its active chapter of the Young Women's Christian Association, and the continuous presence of missionary students, the College in the nineteenth century manifested a strong Christian aura, entirely consistent with a product of feminine activism. By the mid-1890s, however, the variegated faculty included three adherents of "Ethical Culture," at least one a probable atheist.[26]

The missionary women won for WMC an international reputation at a time when few American medical schools were known outside their county. "It is often said that the name and fame of the College are better appreciated in foreign lands than in the quiet city of Philadelphia where the College originated and where it unostentatiously carries on its work from year to year," a College publication would assert in 1915.[27] It was not, of course, French or German scientists or specialists who recognized the school for clinical or scientific work, but rather educated Indians and Chinese, and British colonials, who knew it for its religiously based service by women, to women. Furthermore, the tales of the missionary women, Clara Swain and her followers, and the occasional woman who wore a sari or other ethnic costume to class, entered into the College's set of legends and attributes that filled out its identity and being.

As a lecturer and "quizzer" on chemistry, including the tiresome "old and new nomenclature," Bodley did not shine. But Kate Hurd-Mead, physician and historian from the class of 1888, recalled:

> There suddenly comes into my mind a picture of the same
> Rachel Bodley, no longer an inquisitor, but tactful, subtle and
> friendly, saying in a soft voice, "Ladies, you are invited to a
> reception . . . at my home to meet Ramabai, wisest of Indian
> women, and Mrs. Okami, your classmate, a pioneer from far
> Japan, and Mrs. Joshee, . . . and Susan LaFlesche, another of our
> students, a full-blooded American Indian from the great plains,
> and Sabat Islambooly, a Syrian from Damascus. . . . " She
> certainly was a good Dean, and we should not blame her for not
> teaching us what was not known until twenty years later.[28]

Bodley was known for her kindness to students, several of whom would live with her and her mother. She displayed considerable warmth in letters to Jane Addams, the famous activist and founder of Hull House in Chicago, who had been for one year a student at WMC. After thanking her for a gift (some sort of botanist's plant press), Bodley wrote in a letter, "I prize your love, and trust that it may long be mine! I reciprocate all you so generously lavish upon me. Do not wait until you come to Philadelphia again to say to me some of those things you 'saved to say.'"[29]

Rachel Bodley's bland and lifeless official portrait, made posthumously from a photograph, does little justice to a woman of intelligence, managerial capability, and no small amount of tempered exuberance.

Clara Marshall and Her Early Years as Dean

Clara Marshall, the fourth woman dean of WMC, served in that office from 1888 to 1917; this interval saw the pre- and post-Flexnerian transformation of American medical education (discussed further in chapter 7) and the closing of scores of schools that could not manage it. Also during the first decade of the twentieth century, the Woman's Hospital and WMC finally and bitterly severed their ties, just at the time when the new American Medical Association rating system for medical schools required for the highest designation that a school own or effectively control a hospital for teaching purposes. Under Marshall's leadership, the school succeeded in building a hospital and stayed open when all but one other women's medical school (a homeopathic college in New York City) shut down.

Marshall was born of Quaker parents in Chester County, Pennsylvania, not far from where Ann Preston lived.[30] She graduated from WMC in 1875, and took some course work at the Philadelphia College of Pharmacy in 1876. Before graduation from WMC, she was appointed auxiliary instructor in materia medica in 1874, then instructor in 1875, and professor of the same subject in 1876. The board appointed her to the professorship the day after Charles Hermon Thomas resigned as professor of materia medica and therapeutics; soon after, the faculty expressed its dismay and strong objection to this abrupt action.[31] Marshall may have known pharmacy, but she had little experience in

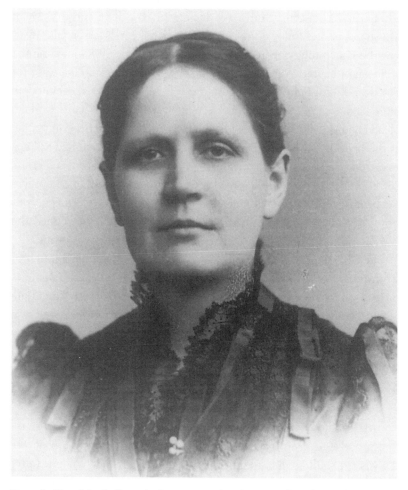

Figure 8. Clara Marshall taught "materia medica," practiced, and served effectively as dean from 1888 to 1917, the period of medical educational reform in the United States.

"therapeutics," and they predicted that she would not go into practice and gain it. (In this they proved wholly wrong: Dr. Marshall *did* practice and listed office hours in city directories as late as 1912.)[32] The faculty also believed that it should hold the privilege of selecting additions or replacements. It is possible that at this time the board was more concerned than the faculty with appointing women to the teaching corps, while the faculty felt it should determine its own membership as a professional privilege.[33]

During the 1890s and first decade of the next century, Dean Marshall's efforts followed the direction of her predecessor. She oversaw the continuing expansion of curriculum and faculty, including the addition of bacteriology. The mandatory four-year curriculum was proposed and adopted, and the building was modified to accommodate more laboratory work. As will be seen later, she and the faculty worked, pleaded, and negotiated to obtain more clinical instruction, including at the bedside, with some success. By 1895 Dean Marshall had to keep track of far more staff, students, teaching hours, hospitals, expenses, and correspondence than could have been imagined when she first entered the faculty. And she increasingly discovered that her job required a constant attention to money, as complexity and ambition multiplied the costs of running the College. She craved and begged for endowment.

Few of the graduates of the 1890s who penned autobiographies or reminiscences had much to say about Marshall as a teacher. Materia medica with its endless memorization held little potential to ingratiate medical students. Something of Marshall's personality is suggested by a letter she directed to the class of 1897, which had done exceptionally well in her materia medica examinations: "The papers in Materia Medica written April 25th, show evidence of such good work, and are so unusually free from silly blunders, that I think the students should be shown some evidence of appreciation on my part."

Marshall, no doubt well-meaning, chose this jolly reward: "I therefore propose to keep the examination papers until the session of 94–95, when I shall be glad to go over the paper with each student (after preparation on her part) so that she may not keep with her until her graduation year the mistakes of her paper in a crystallized form."[34] She was probably stern with students, and her enthusiasms more guarded than Bodley's or Preston's. Some of her writing and speeches do, however, reveal a sense of humor.

Like Bodley, she helped establish the official past of WMC through addresses, articles, and the first book-length history of the school, *Woman's Medical College of Pennsylvania: An Historical Outline*, which she published in 1897. A somewhat disjointed but useful work, it continued Ann Preston's idea of the "revolution that never goes back." Marshall recounted the beginnings, tribulations, and triumphs of the College and its graduates. She recounted their appointments as resident, assistant physician, or attending physician to a good variety of hospitals, and even municipalities (Frances C. Van Gasken became an assistant health inspector of Philadelphia in the 1890s, "on competitive examination"). Marshall herself in 1882 had been elected to attend at the obstetrical department of Blockley (Philadelphia Hospital), where she lectured to medical students from the several medical schools in the city. The dean concluded with a list of over five hundred publications by alumnae.[35] Such efforts by Bodley, Marshall, and their successors amounted to more than harmless antiquarianism: the established history and body of stories were meant to document a heroic past as a foundation for a future, to transcend the particulars of any individuals, buildings, or crises. Marshall's lists of firsts, society memberships, hospital appointments, and especially publications claimed further legitimacy for women doctors and for the Woman's Medical College by invoking these emerging standards and values of scholarly medical life. Bodley had hailed Christian missionaries as a means to spread the College's reputation; by 1897, Marshall preferred published case reports.

Marshall assumed the role of a public woman beyond her duties as dean: she won election to her district's school board in 1897 and joined two of Philadelphia's activist women's clubs, the New Century and the Civic.[36] She spoke to the annual meeting of the National American Woman Suffrage Association in 1898; and a local activist named Lida Stokes Adams ended a 1909 letter (aimed at setting up a presentation to WMC students) by saying to Marshall, "I know you are a true and loyal suffragist." Stokes Adams may have meant this as encouragement more than description, but Marshall was surely a "New Woman." As such, she tacitly taught her students something more than materia medica—the opening possibilities and responsibilities for the American woman.

And Rachel Bodley had done the same. The dean's job, as we have pointed out, grew immensely since the days of Ann Preston. Bodley and Marshall assumed leadership of a complex organization well before such opportunities commonly occurred in women's nonmedical higher education. So did Emily Blackwell, dean for thirty years at the Woman's Medical College of the New York Infirmary, another of the strong women's medical schools. It is clear that neither Bodley nor Marshall could win student acclaim as classroom teacher, nor could they claim national fame as practitioner of medicine or scientist. But, in the new setting of women's medical education, they and the other schools' female deans demonstrated the multifaceted capability of woman as manager in higher education and as managerial advocate of a cause. As Clara Marshall guided the College into the twentieth century and an awakening of medical educational reform, these tasks would approach the heroic.

Chapter 5

Curriculum, Clinics, and Coeducation in the Faculty

The 1880s and 1890s witnessed a profound expansion of the size and complexity of the medical curriculum in the United States. The better schools added more laboratory exercises, lectures in the new specialties, and some meaningful clinical experience—touching patients rather than gazing at them over the heads of several dozen intervening classmates. Yet even through the 1880s, neither government nor medical agencies promulgated much in the way of guidelines or requirements for medical schools. The Association of American Medical Colleges did reconstitute itself in 1890 and laid out a set of standards for its member schools. In 1891, a National Conference of State Medical Examining and Licensing Boards was founded, and it called for the three-year progressive course.[1] Pennsylvania's legislature created a "Medical Council" and boards of medical examiners which set standards for practitioners. Applicants for license in the Commonwealth would have to document four years of medical study as of 1 July 1895.[2]

Mostly, however, as pointed out by historian of American medical education Kenneth M. Ludmerer, advances in the educational quality of American medical schools in the nineteenth century can best be assigned to efforts of faculty working at their own schools.[3] The leaders of the most respected medical schools kept their eyes on one another, and on the approaching debut (in 1893) of something entirely new—the Johns Hopkins University School of Medicine and Hospital in

Baltimore, well endowed and set up to teach and carry out research in emulation of some practices of German universities.

Improving multiple components of medical education at the same time stretched most schools' financial capacity, including that of WMC.[4] By the 1890s the College could hardly be called poor if one looked at the sum of its investments: over $280,000 by 1897, probably more assets than most private medical schools could claim.[5] But much of it formed restricted funds rather than general endowment, and the chaotic financial milieu of the times often limited income. The frugal Quakers who raised the money used caution in spending it.

The following sections will not attempt to list every curricular modification and expansion during the period I have deemed the golden age of the early College. Rather, the focus will be primarily on adoption of the four-year course, the enhancement of laboratory work, the successful introduction of bacteriology, and the only partly successful search for clinical experience. I will also relate the failed attempts to establish a department of prevention, an objective that resonated with the feminist origins of the College.

The Four-Year Program

The direction seemed clear: before long no first-rate school could defer the required four-year course, which had been optional at WMC since 1882. Clara Marshall addressed inquiries concerning plans for the fourth year to the deans of University of Pennsylvania, Harvard, and the University of Michigan.[6] Each saw more bedside clinical work as its justification. Marshall also wrote to Emily Blackwell, dean of the Woman's Medical College of the New York Infirmary, the friendly competitor to WMC. If one but not both of these leading women's schools opted for a required fourth year, applications might for a time favor the more lenient college. But Blackwell replied that her faculty were "cordially in favor" of the reform.[7] Unlike the case with many other medical schools, in this case the women's colleges sought to cooperate toward progress.

Professor of surgery John B. Roberts proposed and the faculty moved to adopt the four-year course in 1891, though a faculty committee warned that "we have no clinical facilities under our immediate control" and that currently the Woman's Hospital allowed very little "bedside teaching." The faculty understood that a "profitable" fourth year would require the improvement in this lack of clinical opportunities, so common to nineteenth-century medical schools.[8] Requiring the extended course as of 1893–1894, WMC became one of only twelve schools (out of 136) to do so by 1894.[9] The four-year course remains the standard today.

Laboratory Work

An examination of sources leaves no doubt that the College did strenuously expand teaching in the laboratory, so that by 1893–1894 the first-year schedule shows more time spent in laboratory work than in the lecture halls.[10] The College building of 1875 had opened with laboratories for work in chemistry, "pharmaceuticals," and microscopy, mostly offered in the optional spring semester. Soon the practical work grew and entered the required curriculum. In 1881 the students themselves petitioned successfully for more time devoted to "practical work with the microscope." By 1898, the director of the histology and embryology laboratory reported that her course comprised nine hours of laboratory work over twenty weeks, with only one hour weekly given to a lecture or recitation. The class worked on sectioning specimens and also on embedding, staining, mounting, and, of course, studying the slides.[11]

No one pressed for laboratory teaching more ardently than professor of physiology Frances Emily White (1832–1903). Though never a published researcher, White believed profoundly in science, rejected traditional religion, and adhered to certain ideas of biological and social evolution. Suffice it to say that she saw learning physiology, especially in the laboratory, not merely as an underfitting of medical practice, but as a profound means of betterment, individually and for women. She also advocated physical improvement in the form of exercise classes for the students.[12] In 1879 she spent some time in Cambridge working with the renowned British physiologist Michael Foster, and—here another of the minor College legends—brought back with her a set of instruments.[13] Proudly listed in the *Annual Announcement*, with their alluringly arcane names capitalized, these included a "Pendulum Myograph, Revolving Kymograph, [and] a high resistance Galvanometer."[14]

White opened her laboratory as an optional addition to the spring

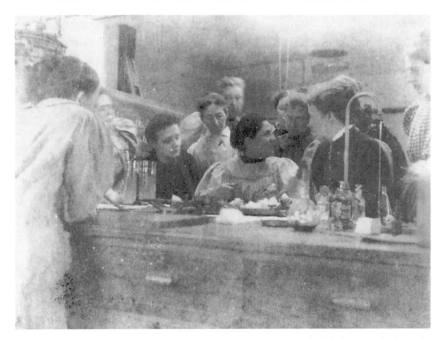

Figure 9. Russian-Jewish born Lydia Rabinowitsch, a pupil of Robert Koch, brought the new discipline of bacteriology to WMC in 1896; here she is surrounded by students, with whom she proved popular.

curriculum in 1881, and before long it claimed a sizeable number of obligatory hours and a special five-dollar surcharge. A student diarist of 1893 began her ten weeks of laboratory work on 24 February: "four hours of work in it today," which preceded three hours of afternoon classes and an anticipated two hours of dissection the same night ("nine hours of solid work is a good bit for one day beside study at home," she added).[15]

The culmination of laboratory work in this period came with the initiation of teaching in bacteriology, the newest medical science. In 1895 the board authorized five hundred dollars to appoint as instructor in bacteriology Lydia Rabinowitsch (1871–1935), an extremely promising young scientist who was born in Lithuania of Jewish parents. After receiving her Ph.D. at the University of Berne, she became an assistant to Robert Koch, the German doyen of bacteriology. With several publications to her credit, Rabinowitsch was already in Philadelphia in 1895, working at the University of Pennsylvania.[16]

A nearby row house was obtained and "fitted up as a laboratory."[17] In the laboratory, the students prepared cultures, learned plating techniques, stained slides, and of course studied and identified microbes under the microscope. One student in the first such class recalled the teacher's consternation when "someone dropped a culture of typhoid bacilli on the floor. It was much more impressive than the lectures."[18]

Rabinowitsch quickly became a well-liked faculty member and teacher ("one of the sweetest, prettiest, and smartest of women," wrote one student[19]), and would have brought to the College an entirely new capacity for research. Unfortunately, she left the faculty in 1898 when the board reluctantly denied her request to extend a period of summer work in Germany (she had also married there). Although the denial was defensible—she would not have been present for the beginning of fall classes, and had agreed in writing to a date of return—in retrospect her loss was a grievous mishap.[20]

Ironically, the board more than the faculty had recognized the potential importance of Rabinowitsch to the school: over faculty objections, they made her full professor and raised her salary to twelve hundred dollars (among the highest), to "secure [her] services . . . and have her best influence upon the school."[21] The faculty expressed some opposition to awarding such prominence to a non-physician practitioner of a novel branch of pathology, as some then considered bacteriology. The board in this case read the future better than the faculty, though it had to reluctantly enforce a reasonable written agreement.

Almost certainly, WMC of the 1880s and 1890s mounted more laboratory classes than all but a handful of American medical schools, an attainment largely overlooked because most of the history of medical education has focused on the elite schools. Clearly the school chose to emulate the advanced colleges, motivated by the need to declare that a women's medical school can be a scientific medical school, as symbolized by the laboratory. WMC would revise this message beginning in the 1930s with the inception of substantive faculty research.

The Search for Clinical Facilities

Providing good clinical instruction proved more difficult than firming up laboratory work, not just at WMC, but universally at American medical schools.[22] The late nineteenth-century rise of surgery, physical diagnosis, and clinical specialties hastened the demand for adequate practical experience. Students needed to extend the "learning by doing" of their physiology and bacteriology laboratories to clinical work, but in the 1890s few medical schools knew how to do this, even those that added the fourth year.

Medical colleges turned to hospitals in the community and generally received a tepid response. Hospital lay boards, even for those associated with a medical school, primarily wanted to ensure the efficient, least expensive, and paternalistically protective care of their charges, the sick but "worthy" poor. Those fortunate enough to house paying patients wanted to shelter them from bedside teaching. Hospitals strictly regulated when students could visit and what they could do. Medical school faculty pressed for more teaching privileges, both as worthy in itself and to compete for good students. Even Woman's Med won only limited clinical teaching from Woman's Hospital, its sister institution.

In the 1890s, the clinical presentation in an amphitheater continued, and where a school controlled a hospital (a rare situation) or managed some influence with one, the faculty initiated "ward walks" or "section teaching." In this transitional format, students in the third or fourth year formed sections of several to fifteen students, each of which in rotation spent assigned time in the affiliated hospital. Presumably they examined patients in small groups then reviewed findings with an instructor. Or the instructor may have literally walked from bed to bed, examining and commenting upon several patients. Students did not directly participate in the patients' care.

During most of the 1880s, clinical instruction at WMC relied mainly on the demonstration clinics at Woman's Hospital, Pennsylvania Hospital, Blockley, and the nearby German Hospital.[23] Clara Marshall made grateful mention in her 1897 history of the College of a member of the auxiliary faculty, Edward T. Bruen, who introduced "private classes of women students to the medical wards" at Blockley. This meant that during those months when Bruen served as attending physician at the city hospital, he arranged for small groups of WMC students to see patients with him on the wards. Such opportunity was as precious as it was scarce.

During the 1880s, relations with the Woman's Hospital remained cordial: the attending physicians were WMC faculty, and Dean Rachel Bodley served on the hospital's board of managers. Yet beyond the amphitheater clinics, neither did the College demand nor the hospital offer much clinical work to WMC students: the hospital's concerns seemed more the interns and the nursing school.[24] By the 1880s WMC students no longer could reside at the Woman's Hospital, eliminating an important if fragmentary opportunity for clinical learning.

In 1887, Anna Broomall, professor of obstetrics, announced a plan to establish a maternity outpatient service dedicated to student education in a poor area of south Philadelphia.[25] In its first year of operation, forty students had the opportunity to deliver babies; by 1895, many students cared for three or four deliveries.[26] They were assigned women "in their confinement" and visited them at home where they did pelvic measurements and urine examinations. Some babies were delivered there, others in the maternity hospital that later grew out of Broomall's department in south Philadelphia. Since Anna Broomall, unquestionably among the most able of the College's nineteenth-century faculty, combined the most current European techniques and ideas with a generous eagerness to teach, the WMC seniors enjoyed a valuable practical and intellectual experience, which as we will see formed a highlight in their memories.[27]

According to Lawrence Longo and Charlotte Borst, historians of obstetrics in the United States, before 1900 such practical maternity work occurred rarely in all-male American schools, from many of which it was possible to graduate without ever having delivered a baby. A few exceptions existed and home delivery programs eventually arose at many schools. Immigrant women, the typical patients of the student accoucheur, would have been accustomed to the midwife, so may have received the female medical students into their homes more confidently than young men. If so, the women's medical colleges had better opportunity to provide meaningful training in obstetrics, which they necessarily saw as a priority for their students, who would mostly look after women and children. The well-structured WMC program endured into the 1940s.[28]

But actual hands-on experience in other branches of practice at WMC remained scant through the 1880s, even if no worse than in the typical medical school. Wanting to do better but seeing little expectation from the Woman's Hospital, the faculty "earnestly" solicited the board of corporators to "take into consideration the feasibility of constructing and conducting a general hospital with general dispensary and outpatient department under the control of the College authorities."[29] This timorously phrased request may have been only symbolic: in any case, the board declined.[30]

In May of 1892 the faculty intensified its efforts to improve bedside instruction. Doctors Jacob S. Solis-Cohen at Blockley and Lawrence Wolff at the German Hospital (near WMC) agreed to take small classes of students into their hospitals. Some concessions were won from Woman's Hospital: in rotation, small groups of students (sections) could appear between seven and nine A.M. for instruction in the wards. Groups would receive dispensary teaching two days each week, and students would accompany each intern to her home deliveries.[31] Hospital physician Anna Fullerton (1853–1938; class of 1882) would supervise the teaching and conduct much of it herself. The students sent a note thanking the faculty for their efforts to amplify clinical experience. By the 1893–94 term, the plan was working reasonably well. But the arrangement required continuous monitoring, and by 1896 had deteriorated.

In 1895 Amy Barton, an 1874 graduate and clinical professor of ophthalmology, reported to the Alumnae Association her plan for a multi-clinic dispensary in the southeastern part of the city, not far from Broomall's obstetrical station. This region of South Philadelphia long had been Philadelphia's poorest, the same locale of slums and poverty where William Mullen helped build the House of Industry fifty years earlier. Barton and her friends (especially Drs. Ada Audenried and Gertrude Walker) had already raised some money and accomplished much of the preliminary work; now, they sought backing by the association. The founders chose the ample name "Hospital and Dispensary of the Alumnae of the Woman's Medical College of Pennsylvania," though they did not conceive of inpatient facilities at first. The dispensary's stated purposes would be to supply more "clinical material" for the College's demonstration clinics, to provide dispensary experience to recent graduates, and to offer free care by women to "poor women and children" of the district.[32] By 1897, some students had arranged to spend time as "assistants in the clinic, and . . . expressed themselves as delighted with the opportunity to do practical work under the friendly instructions of the chief clinicians," the latter being recent WMC graduates.[33]

The dispensary's founding and its lay support reflected the sense of collaboration and conviction so manifest within the WMC "community" of the 1890s, by which the causes of the charitable club woman and medical woman conjoined. Wrote Gertrude Walker: "This work of women for women is not only a blessed means of relieving the suffering poor, but also an important feature in the practical education of women physicians."[34] In this case the needy woman *patient*, object of sisterly sympathy, would become also the needed "clinical *material*," object of scientific scrutiny. So the charitable and professional impulses coincided, but also competed, even if not in the awareness of the well-meaning founders. The founding of the dispensary counts as among the first examples of the steadfast loyalty of many WMC alumnae to the College.

Preventive Medicine

One area of curriculum that WMC could not successfully establish in the late nineteenth century, despite evident interest, was preventive medicine. In the opinion of some historians, nineteenth-century women doctors taught hygiene and prevention more than most male physicians and saw as one of their tasks the elevation of female health.[35] In 1887, Lena Ingraham of the class of 1883 proposed at the annual meeting of the Alumnae Association that the society undertake to raise money for the endowment of a department and chair of preventive medicine at the College. Frances Emily White of the faculty endorsed such a plan, conceiving of a strong link between health, morality, and individual perfection.

The envisioned department would include the professorship, a gymnasium for students, and a "laboratory for illustrating sanitation."[36] Somehow, actual efforts aimed mainly at the gymnasium, which opened in a rented room at a nearby church in 1888.[37] This period was the peak of a wave of eagerness in the United States to "scientifically" elevate the state of health of sedentary businessmen, supposedly pampered women, and fat children: playgrounds and gyms sprung up widely. Women's colleges joined this movement: Vassar opened its gymnasium in 1889, Smith in 1892.[38]

Evidently tenuous in its infancy, the WMC gymnasium would require reinvention several times. At the 1891 Alumnae Association meeting, the president called for a report from the Committee on the Chair of Preventive Medicine, which she noted "seems to be rather a committee for the establishment of a gymnasium."[39] That year and the next, the alumnae discussed whether preventive medicine meant a gymnasium, linked to old ideas of self-discipline; or meant a bacteriology laboratory to help combat the spread of disease at a population level.[40] Given the confusion about what a preventive medicine department ought to be, and the difficulty of raising funds, no full-time chair would appear until well into the twentieth century.

In summary, the curriculum both on paper and in implementation grew enormously in substance and complexity, requiring much more effort by the dean to manage, the board to finance, the various levels of faculty to teach, and the students to learn. It progressed in a manner fully in keeping with trends in medicine and science, and—like the College building itself—looked little different from the programs of the better male or coeducational schools. Here was both a present strength yet possible risk for the future; for only the superior training in obstetrics marked the curricular content as meeting particular needs and interests of women physicians. Indicative was the failure to establish a chair and department of preventive medicine until decades after it was first proposed. When there came to WMC new periods of peril and struggle in the early twentieth century, actual embodiments of the central mission in the teaching programs might have benefited the school by better attracting students and financial support from affluent women.

The Faculty of the 1880s and 1890s

During this period, the WMC central faculty—the full professors of the major subjects—grew into a varied and accomplished crew. Medically and socially respectable, the faculty nonetheless included, fortunately, several indisputable "characters" and dissidents. No doubt the junior faculty and assistants, not discussed here, played an important role in the daily education of students. The friendship and egalitarian collegiality apparent in the dealings of the women and men form an unusual case study.

The major women professors of this period included Dean Marshall (also professor of materia medica), professor of obstetrics Anna Broomall, professor of gynecology Hannah Croasdale, and professor of physiology Frances Emily White. All were alumnae and all but White members of the Society of Friends.

Easily the best loved of the women faculty of the golden age of WMC, Anna Broomall has already appeared in this history several times. No reminiscence of the 1890s fails to recall Broomall, and never without affection and respect. One student called her a "soft voiced gentle creature," another recalled the "gentle, slender figure, in the simplest of black gowns, earnestly looking at her pupils through partly closed eyes as though her inner self dared not gaze openly at their dull faces."[41] One student enjoyed a moment of Broomall's kindness after feeling "set down on" by the dean; a graduate remembered a spontaneous offer of letters of introduction.[42]

But the self-effacing and generous Broomall allowed no laxity in her obstetrical work or teaching. She was a "firm believer in antisepsis," a "genius of a teacher" who could play the "strict martinet."[43] Before assuming her faculty work, she had ventured to the famous Vienna Frauenklinik, where she had learned the most advanced obstetrical techniques. Her student Anna Fullerton, like so many aspiring American doctors in the 1880s, also went to Vienna. She wrote back in 1884 that Broomall's teaching at WMC "is in every respect almost identical with that here."[44] Another student of the 1890s concisely summed up Broomall's charisma: a "very particular teacher yet full of fun."[45]

From 1880 (when the Quaker philanthropist Joseph Jeanes endowed a new chair for her) until 1902, Hannah T. Croasdale (1836–1912; WMC, 1870) served as professor of gynecology, yet little about her is known. Though a Quaker, she impressed students with the glories of her dress: a "trés grande dame," "a stylish figure in a fashionable gown of silk and velvet and lace." "When lecturing, she was absolutely uninspiring," but held the reputation as a fine surgeon with a delicate and sure "touch" who nonetheless also valued medical gynecology. To another student, Croasdale seemed the "ideal woman," probably denoting the synthesis of "womanly" attributes and surgical mastery, as remembered also in her predecessor, Emeline Horton Cleveland.[46] Also like Cleveland, Croasdale had married, and she became the mother of four children. She entered medical school after her husband died. She was, with Clara Marshall, a member of the New Century Club, and she supported suffrage.

Students remembered the physiologist Frances Emily White vividly, "an aristocratic lady with a Boston accent" (White was a New Englander though not from Boston) "clad in garnet velvet." But her socially conservative manner belied her advanced views concerning the nature of life and morals. "To do well in that subject [physiology]," wrote one alumna, "we had to learn to think, and with Dr. White we went through the throes not only of physiology but also of modern theology and materialism." Her lectures and laboratory work drew the best efforts from the students, and as with any such teacher, she terrified some, but came to be remembered with respect and affection by others.[47]

Certain board members must have recalled her as a different sort of challenge. She was her own woman and sometimes fostered controversy. Her initial lectures as the newly appointed professor of physiology in 1877 with their emphasis on evolution and the nature of life apparently mystified students, who preferred a more practical approach. White's lectures caused an unprecedented class protest (including a call for her removal) and a consequent series of painful problems for the dean, the faculty, and the board. In fact, this altercation may well have called the student voice into being, or at least provoked its first major deployment.[48]

Other noteworthy women faculty in the second tier included Mary Sherwood, who for some years commuted from Baltimore to give lectures in pathology. Unlike almost all other women instructors at WMC, Sherwood was not a graduate; she acquired her medical training in Zurich, whose university was an early haven for aspiring women doctors.[49] Russian-born Marie Formad (WMC, 1886) also taught pathology and became an admired surgeon at the Woman's Hospital of Philadelphia.[50]

More Men of Woman's Med

The men who taught at WMC in the 1880s and 1890s were also a proficient and colorful group. There were three successive generations of male faculty at the school during the nineteenth century: first, the founding and earliest faculty, a core of Quaker reformers of modest medical standing plus available marginalia of antebellum Philadelphia medicine; second, a group of liberal-minded, known, and respected medical men, Quakers or men of similar outlook; and third, as we will see, a set of mostly young, forward-looking practitioners, not Quakers, heavily involved in medical education and specialization. Here we will briefly describe only the most influential male faculty of this last group and seek to uncover their common characteristics: why did they wish to teach at Woman's Med?

Among the first of the new male faculty of the late nineteenth century was William Williams Keen (1837–1932), usually known as W. W. Keen, who served as professor of surgery from 1884 until 1889, when he accepted the same title at his alma mater, Jefferson Medical College. Before his WMC years, he had done postgraduate work in Europe and served under the illustrious Philadelphia physician, neurologist, and belletrist S. Weir Mitchell. After his days at WMC, Keen became nothing less than one of America's leading surgeons and surgical authors, with a special interest in what is now called neurosurgery. In 1893, Keen secretly operated on President Cleveland to remove a sarcoma of the jaw.

Kate Hurd-Mead referred to Keen as "one of the best friends the medical students ever had." His lectures "generally began before he reached the threshold of the hall with 'as I was saying last time' and his endings were often this injunction, 'After any operation the patient needs rest, REST, REST in BED.'"[51]

When Keen left for the position he no doubt coveted at Jefferson Medical College, the WMC faculty thanked him for his "unhesitating surrender of time in doing a generous share of faculty work" and added "warmest wishes for his success and happiness."[52] He long remained sympathetic toward WMC.

Professor of principles and practice of medicine from 1879 to 1892 James B. Walker (1846–1910) would never win the fame of Keen (or several of the other faculty), but proved a steady contributor and held the appropriate appointment to take students onto the floors at Philadelphia Hospital (Blockley). There he provided "invaluable bed-side instruction" without requiring a direct fee from students, as was customary. Hurd-Mead remembered his patience, parsimonious use of drugs, and advocacy of fresh air and sunshine in caring for the sick.[53] The faculty offered "best wishes for his continued prosperity and happiness" when he left in 1891.

Upon Walker's resignation occurred one of the few documented gender-based contests within the nineteenth-century faculty. The name proposed to take his place was Frederick Porteous (F. P.) Henry (1844–1919), a well-known, indeed weighty, figure in Philadelphia medicine. He represented another favorable and prestigious "catch" for the College, but the faculty minutes show that on 16 May 1891 "Profs. Broomall and Croasdale vote nay not from any personal or professional objection to Dr. Henry, but because they believe the chair should be filled by a woman physician, and they suggest the name of Dr. Ida E. Richardson and Dr. Alice Bennett."[54] Likely their vote voiced a gentle protest (Henry's appointment probably had been arranged already): within the senior clinical faculty, only the traditionally female subjects of obstetrics and gynecology were directed by women.

Catharine Macfarlane, an 1898 graduate and later distinguished gynecologist and WMC faculty member, recalled Henry as a "scholarly gentleman whose polished lectures were a delight to listen to."[55] Henry published two standard historical works on Philadelphia medicine in which WMC is well treated, a happy outcome of Henry's faculty position.[56]

Henry Leffmann (1847–1930), another of Philadelphia's idiosyncratic physician-intellects, served WMC as professor of chemistry from 1890 to 1917 (emeritus until 1923). He once wrote: "I would like my biography to begin as follows: 'Henry Leffmann was born on September 9, 1847, in Philadelphia. His ancestry on his father's side is partly Russian Jewish; on his mother side, partly Welsh Quaker. He was educated in the public schools, completing the course of B.A. at Central High School . . .' In these days of genetics and eugenics it is worth while to show that a mongrel may have some merit."[57]

Leffmann's merits included versatility. His national reputation rested

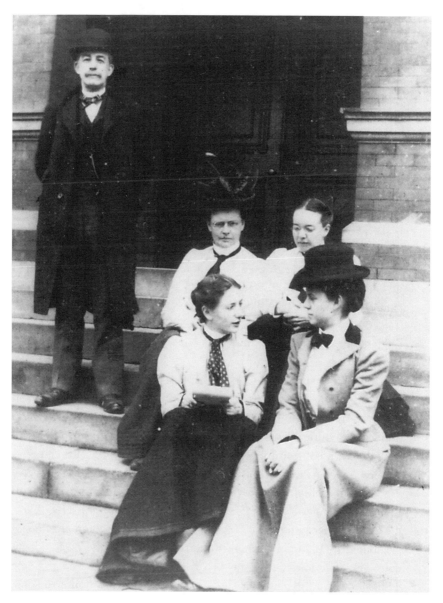

Figure 10. Many liberal male physicians taught at WMC, such as professor of chemistry and polymath Henry Leffmann, seen here on the College steps. Among the four students are future WMC president Ellen Culver Potter (upper right [WMC, 1903]) and future dean Martha Tracy (lower left [WMC, 1904]).

on his extensive work in analytic and consultative chemistry, but he also served as port physician. His hundreds of published papers ranged from technical topics to the works of Charles Dickens; his profound erudition and mighty memory astounded his friends and colleagues. One of these attested to Leffmann's "quaint quizzical humor" which made it "a joyous victory to be able to tell him a new story." Leffmann considered himself unconnected to any creed or "denominational church," and joined the Society for Ethical Culture, where he encountered WMC colleagues C. Newlin Peirce and Frances Emily White. Politically, he identified himself as "Democrat and Single Tax Advocate."

Diarist Mary Theodora McGavran said this about the popular professor of chemistry: "Our Dr. Leffmann likes the girls. He knows they are all earnest, working women and he is also aware of the fact that we all 'worship' him. I believe we are on more familiar terms with him than any other Prof. in school." She also recalled his attempt to ease the tension of final exams: "He didn't pay much attention to where we sat—Talked a good bit—Told a few stories &c &c. When Miss Clarke got too tired to stay in he said for her to get some one to stay with her & go off and rest."[58]

John Bingham Roberts (1852–1924) succeeded W. W. Keen to the chair of surgery in 1889 and served until 1910. Roberts, a Jefferson graduate, managed to combine public roles of scientific master-surgeon and serious political gadfly. Like Broomall, Croasdale, White, and Keen, he did additional training in Europe before commencing his career as surgeon, teacher, and author.

Undoubtedly a true progressive, Roberts sought improvement in himself, his profession and its educational process, and his city. A letter to Dean Marshall in 1897 (apologizing for missing commencement) originated in Baltimore, where Roberts was "taking the postgraduate course in bacteriology . . . I stay here four days each week and go home Thursday night." Roberts at the age of forty-five was going to some trouble to stay abreast of the most current science—and found himself sharing a laboratory table with several female Johns Hopkins medical students!

Angered by the notorious corruption and incompetence that pervaded Philadelphia politics in the 1890s and 1900s, he joined other reformers in leading the Committee of Seventy, founded to oppose election abuses and municipal mismanagement, and still in existence. Roberts later ran for city council on a reform ticket. At WMC, Roberts participated fully in attempts to develop clinical instruction and to maintain a high level of teaching.[59]

Other men on the faculty in the 1880s and 1890s included the longtime professor of anatomy William Parish (1845–1903); Arthur A. Stevens (1865–1944), who taught pathology and later therapeutics, pharmacology, and clinical medicine from 1892 to 1922; and Charles K. Mills (1845–1931), a leader in his field who lectured on neurology and medical jurisprudence. Stevens, like Henry Hartshorne before him, had written several popular textbooks and student manuals, and held a reputation as a skillful "quizmaster." "He really liked to teach and probably derived much personal satisfaction and pleasure out of his pedagogic life," according to his memorialist. In 1911, the senior class voted him one of their two favorite teachers.[60]

What might be said about the characteristics of the men who chose to attach themselves to WMC in the last decades of the nineteenth century? All but F. P. Henry were under forty years of age when they joined the faculty. Many would now be called specialists: Keen in neurological surgery, Leffmann in medical chemistry and toxicology, Mills in neurology, Stevens in pathology and drug therapeutics. Roberts, Mills, and Leffmann saw themselves as educational reformers: they established the Philadelphia Polyclinic and College for Graduates in Medicine, one of several "polyclinic" schools that arose in U.S. cities after 1880 to offer post-M.D. clinical experience and to teach the new specialties, mostly using the time-honored dispensary setting.[61] Few if any of the men under review could claim membership in old Philadelphia families or Philadelphia medical dynasties; Keen, Mills, Leffmann, and Stevens all had attended Philadelphia's Central High School, often referred to as "the Poor Man's College."[62] None, with the possible exception of Parish, was Quaker—a significant drift away from the College's roots, toward a broader basis in Philadelphia's medical community.

The men belonged to a new medical meritocracy of middle-class origins, confidently in tune with medical advance, but rarely destined to fill a sanctified major chair at Penn or Jefferson (Keen was an exception). Like many intellectually superior and ambitious young physicians, including their women colleagues, they sought teaching positions and

found a welcome at WMC, though they also built their own professorships at the Polyclinic. Leffmann and Roberts held progressive and even
nonconformist viewpoints and might have joined the women's medical school because of, rather than despite, its central feminist mission.

Coeducation at the Faculty Level

These men (and others before and since) chose to work as equals with
the College women in order to strengthen the institution in which they
believed and in which they had invested some important part of their
careers; the stakes totaled much more for the women, of course, who
had no hope of faculty appointment at the city's male medical schools.
The historiography of American women as written in the last thirty
years relied upon "separate spheres," the organizing idea that American women and men in the nineteenth century occupied distinct fields
of endeavor—women in the home, church, and temperance society;
men at work and in public life. Few case studies are available of women
and men working closely and harmoniously together in the nineteenth
century. Probably few examples indeed existed, but the dominant historical model of separate spheres may have impeded finding them.

The relationship between the men and women of WMC in the
nineteenth century can be seen as a rare model of fruitful and friendly
cooperation between the sexes. Since the years of Ann Preston, it stood
unquestioned that a woman would be dean. Each year at its annual
meeting, the faculty elected a "chairman" as well, largely an honorific
post to chair the meetings, who was always a man. The minutes amply
document that committee and curricular work was shared, and it certainly grew laborious with the major expansions of the 1890s. Clearly
the women and men strove together to improve ties with the Woman's
Hospital and amplify clinical opportunities. Isaac Comly, a professor of
the principles and practice of medicine during the 1870s, volunteered
to set up the museum after the move to the new building, and several
male faculty succeeded him in the time-consuming work of looking after it. Auxiliary faculty member Edward T. Bruen not only took students in small groups to Blockley, but offered to give "demonstrations
of morbid specimens to the class in Pathology" in small sections.[63]
When numerous male faculty departed to serve during World War I,

Leffmann and Henry, both slightly over seventy years of age, came out of retirement to rejoin their female colleagues at the College.[64]

Several times men and women professors agreed to assume additional lectures so that others could undertake overseas travel, as when Croasdale, Walker, and Marshall covered for Broomall in 1883.[65] Occasionally the faculty banded together in opposition to the board of corporators. For example, in March of 1882 the board declared its intent to not reappoint the professor of surgery, Benjamin Wilson; Rachel Bodley, with sympathetic anger, termed the board's act an "assault made upon him." In protest, the faculty demanded that charges be revealed and investigated. The following January, they defiantly elected Wilson their chairman, though this act did not deter his eventual removal by the board, after a protracted investigation.[66]

Plentiful evidence suggests that friendship, trust, and affection between the women and men on the faculty enhanced the sense of common purpose in the 1880s and 1890s. In an earlier period, professor of anatomy Mary Scarlett-Dixon confided as a friend in Edwin Fussell, who felt sympathetic interest in the College even after he endured an agonizing dispute with others on the faculty and left it.[67] Frances Emily White and Henry Hartshorne also shared their feelings and ambitions rather openly in letters; in one, Hartshorne gave avuncular advice about White's perplexing lectures.[68] Some of the resolutions passed by the faculty on the resignation or death of a colleague suggest more than just expected protocol, as when they expressed a "sense of personal loss in this severance of relations" with W. W. Keen, as noted above. Keen responded in a letter to Marshall that his "relations with the members of the faculty have been so absolutely agreeable that it was with the greatest regret that I resigned from a place so pleasant."[69] On the sudden death of Edward Bruen the faculty expressed "profound sorrow and regret" at the loss of a colleague who "was not possessed with a ready flow of language . . . [but showed] evident earnestness and honesty as a teacher . . . he made only friends among his colleagues and students."[70] When James B. Walker resigned in 1892 to attend to his enlarging practice, he sent a letter to the faculty in which he referred to attachments that he hoped would be "life long," and expressed a "keen sense of loss, personally and professionally, in severing myself from you in the interesting work which you are so successfully engaged."[71]

Other sorts of evidence support a high degree of good feeling be-tween the women and men co-workers. At a special memorial faculty meeting for Emeline Horton Cleveland, Benjamin Wilson, the profes-sor of surgery, spoke of her courage, indicating that he well knew it, being her physician.[72] Hannah Croasdale arrived late to a faculty meet-ing on 28 October 1882: she explained to Dean Bodley (who hated tar-diness) and the others that she had been visiting at the home of retired professor Isaac Comly, who had died that night after a long illness. Al-though it is doubtful that she attended him medically, probably Croasdale was a friend to the elderly Comly and his family. The meet-ing paused while some of the senior faculty recalled "our highly esteemed late professor."[73]

What fostered this high degree of male-female collegiality and friendship? Counting perhaps first would be individual attitudes and ex-periences that shaped these persons. Marshall, White, Broomall, and Croasdale, the women professors, had all graduated from WMC between 1870 and 1875: all had been taught by men and women and observed the involvement and interest of Comly, Hartshorne, Wilson, and Tho-mas. Three of the women professors grew up in the Society of Friends, whose tenets fostered a degree of gender equality and collaboration.

From a practical standpoint, the dean and senior women faculty members surely realized that certain male faculty could enhance the College's reputation. They could gain important sorts of political ac-cess and utilize professional privileges to take the students to the wards of hospitals for valuable bedside teaching. While the skilled women faculty must have felt daily indignation at not themselves gaining staff privileges at most Philadelphia hospitals, as a matter of expediency they welcomed opportunities for their students mediated by the male colleagues.

No doubt a prominent factor favoring the male-female alliance—perhaps the dominant one—was a jointly felt professional identity. The women and men of the faculty all held the M.D. (with the exceptions of Bodley and later Rabinowitsch) and worked in a world of medicine that increasingly demanded high levels of scientific and technical knowledge and thorough dedication for those who wished to excel. There was simply much more that intrinsically united the "Lady Pro-fessors" and "Gentlemen Professors" on North College Avenue than separated them. As one political component of this shared awareness, the women and men found need to stand together in conflicts with the board and with the Woman's Hospital, especially those that touched on professional authority.

A commonality of professional identity and expertise between women and men could occur in medicine—if only episodically—in the late nineteenth century in a way scarcely possible before in the United States, because women had not been allowed to enter other professions. For individuals such as Marshall, White, Broomall and Croasdale, and for Hartshorne, Leffmann, Keen, and Roberts, both a cause they supported, and their thorough self-identity as physicians and educators, transcended the inherited expectations of nineteenth-century gender separation and discrimination. So, paradoxically, WMC can be justly viewed as an institution run by women for women, *and* at the same time a locus of early and fruitful coeducation—at the faculty level. Thus it provided a secure female environment for its women students, while also allowing them familiarity with the ways of men physicians, with whom of course most WMC graduates would one day interact.

Some specifically gender-based disputes did arise at WMC and the Woman's Hospital. We saw that without objecting to Frederick P. Henry, two of the women faculty (but not two others) refused to vote for him, wishing to see a woman as the chair of medicine. Several times the call for more, or only, women faculty arose at meetings of the Alumnae Association.[74] As part of the first crisis with the Woman's Hospital, in 1896, accusations arose that men were expropriating surgical operations that ought be given to the women.[75] Almost certainly, however, the ability of the faculty women and men to work together and enjoy opportunities for harmony strengthened the College for its mission of training women in medicine and allowed it to successfully carry out the educational transformations of the 1880s, 1890s, and beyond.

Charlotte and C. Newlin Peirce

As an addendum to the history of male-female affiliation at WMC, we add the noble marriage of Cyrus Newlin ("C. N." or "C. Newlin") and Charlotte L. (Woodward) Peirce. For a remarkable span of over forty years (1867 to 1909), C. Newlin Peirce (1828–1909) toiled faithfully as a WMC corporator, much of that time carrying out the burdensome work of secretary. Born into the Society of Friends, and raised on his father's farm, as a young man he became an ardent abolitionist, and during his entire life promoted gender equality and women's rights. He became a dentist, dean of one of Philadelphia's early dental schools, and in addition to his service on the board taught "dental physiology and pathology" at WMC.[76] Unconventional in his viewpoints, he helped found the Philadelphia Society for Ethical Culture.

Charlotte Woodward had left a home overfilled with siblings at the age of fifteen to teach school, and found herself in Waterloo, New York, in 1848—in easy reach of the Seneca Falls Convention. She attended it and signed the Declaration of Sentiments. According to a friend of her later years, she returned from Seneca Falls to Waterloo in a wagon in which also rode Frederick Douglass, who had given a speech.[77] She remained an activist, suffragist, and clubwoman. After Pennsylvania's legislature ratified the Woman Suffrage Amendment, the then ninety-year-old feminist was asked if she expected to vote once the full national ratification process was complete. Charlotte Peirce (then her name) replied, "I'll vote if I have to be carried to the polls."[78] In fact she did vote in 1920 and is said to have been the only signer at Seneca Falls who survived to do so. In 1857 she had married C. Newlin Peirce, the right sort of man for such a woman. For some years she joined her husband on the board of WMC, but worked more actively for the Woman's Hospital of Philadelphia, serving on its board of managers and as the hospital's treasurer. Like her husband, Charlotte Peirce also actively participated in the Society for Ethical Culture.

Charlotte and C. Newlin Peirce may be thought of as an example of the American bourgeois radical couple, whose gift of a shared and healthy longevity carried them together from antebellum abolition and Seneca Falls, to the much more incremental and accommodating progressivism of the late nineteenth century. One wonders if WMC students of the 1880s and 1890s knew that such a pair of gentle revolutionaries dwelt among them.

Chapter 6

Student Life at the Mature "Woman's Med"

Through the 1890s and 1900s, enrollment at WMC ranged from 150 to about 190. As earlier, most students listed Philadelphia or other points in Pennsylvania as home; many came from New England and a scattering from every other region of the country, as well as a few from Canada. But there were some foreign matriculants, including young women from Turkey, India, and China, a set of sisters from Ecuador (Anita and Crucita Franco—it is tempting to suppose they were twins), and a series of Russians representing the enthusiasm for medical education among that nation's women. The vast majority of students were white and Protestant, but several African-Americans, Jews, and Catholics joined the classes (this diversity will be discussed later in the chapter). Of the Americans, about 10 percent came with college degrees, especially from Wellesley, Smith, and Swarthmore.[1]

Undoubtedly, as a group the WMC students represented a novel and lively addition to life in Philadelphia. Though relatively few in number, they were a presence in the city, which housed only one other women's college (the Philadelphia School of Design for Women); and Philadelphia necessarily became a part of them. The duration and intensity of medical education had changed markedly from the 1860s to the 1890s: before, a medical student might come to the city for two brief terms of four or five months of lectures in two different years, a small and transient investment of time. But by the mid-1890s, a WMC student attended medical school from October to May for each of four years. This constituted a sizable block of a young person's life, spent in one place, often away from home, among the same companions. The four-year span of full-time medical school allowed students not only to acquire a mass of knowledge and skills, but also to experience autonomy, build friendships, assemble or absorb traditions, even grapple with the vagaries and excitement of life itself.

At Work Day and Night

Two historical resources stand out as firsthand guides to student life at WMC in the 1890s: the diary of Mary Theodora McGavran, who graduated in 1895, and the unpublished autobiography of Edith Flower Wheeler, who received her M.D. in 1897.[2] Though she wrote her memoir fifty years after leaving WMC, Wheeler based her passages about school days on letters written at the time to her father.

For their experience of College work I will allow these and other participants to speak as much as possible for themselves. The sources suggest that students and later alumnae preferred to document the more colorful and distinctive aspects of their medical education. McGavran and Wheeler enjoyed using medical terms and slang to record events and thoughts which they knew to be esoteric or even shocking to non-medical persons; by doing so, they drew on language and experience to join themselves to medicine and to each other.

So they did not write much about lectures, the least interesting part of the curriculum, and pretty much a given. One student, as her mind drifted from the pathological topic itself, did capture the distracting mannerisms of one instructor: "She gasps and swallows a lump in her throat. . . . She is thoughtful. Horrors, there's a question. Who can answer it? She glances archly as we stumble over words. . . . She adjusts her sleeves more perfectly while she asks if we have seen specimens of 'nutmeg liver.'"[3]

Examinations brought anxiety and exertions to learn or at least "cram" the material. "This week has been one continued strain. We have an examination in physiology soon . . . and have been working hard at it," wrote McGavran in February of 1893. Several students came to her room: "We asked questions and volunteered opinions until ten o'clock. I think we benefited a great deal from it." Professor White's physiology examination did prove "long and hard—every one acknowledged it to be *exceedingly* trying." In April McGavran told her diary that the next day would bring an "anatomy Examination and it may be I should be studying for it now but I seem to be filled to overflowing with Gray. The next two weeks will be anxious ones for us. For a failure now means worrying for a year or at least until next fall."[4] Edith Flower Wheeler recalled a materia medica examination: "Medicines had to be recognized by their appearance, taste, and smell. Then this was followed by a written examination on dosage, use, etc." Wheeler and her friend did not feel "at all secure in their knowledge."[5]

Countless hours were spent in determined, solitary study, ever familiar to the medical student. The women toiled in the College's reading room or, more often, in their boardinghouses. A student's sister recorded this image: "At night she sat there and studied behind a screen. Once I tiptoed across the floor and looked over it. Helen, with a green shade over her eyes, and a big book open before her, was carefully examining what looked like a shin bone of beef. On the desk was a skull, and some osseosities for which I had no name. I tiptoed back to my seat, and after that the Bluebeard corner of the room knew me no more."[6]

Dissection of the cadaver, the early and transforming rite of passage into medicine, was seen by the public as a horrid practice, and particularly unsuited to the delicate sensitivities of women. Students' comments about anatomical work reveal their sense of accomplishment in overcoming feelings of aversion, as well as their eagerness to display medical sangfroid. Wheeler wrote: "Beginning dissection was rather a cross. The room in which this work was done did not smell like a rose garden. One also had to overcome the shrinking from touching a very cold dead body, as well as force herself to beat down the aversion to cutting flesh that had once been living, even as you or I, but it could be done, and, in time, the interest blotted out the shrinking."[7]

Anne Walter Fearn, an 1893 graduate, had done a year of medical school elsewhere, and while at WMC worked as a student-prosector: "It was very early morning at that hour just before the dawn . . . and I was all alone in the dissecting room, preparing a 'stiff' for the next day's demonstration. I was sleepy and anxious to finish my job and hurry

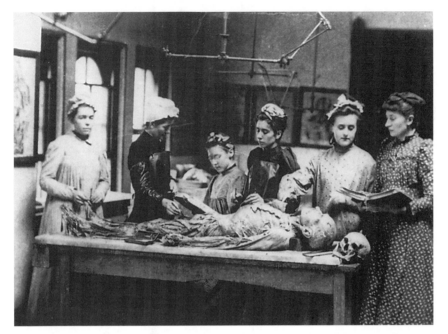

Figure 11. A WMC version of a medical school genre: a posed dissection scene from 1891.

home to bed. Impatiently I tugged at the tendon of the arm outstretched on a board. The arm jerked, clasped itself around my waist, and stayed there. This was too much for my 'hardened' nerves."[8]

McGavran reported on her anatomical work as follows: "To be sure the subject is rather odiferous: but lo me! what difference does that make to a med? The only trouble is we can only work a few hours at a time. If we overstay the proper time the effect is rather marked!"[9]

Having dissected, she is a "med"—a creature allowed strange privileges if one can endure them, as "meds" always have.

Almost a continuation of dissection into the later years of school, the course on "practical work in operative surgery" entailed "some practice in surgery on 'stiffs,' as they called them." Edith Flower Wheeler wrote to her family, probably in 1897: "I did a laparotomy on a patient today, a dead one. Had lots of fun. Succeeded in poking holes through everything that I ought not to. If my patient had not been dead to start with, she would have been deader'n a door nail by the time I got through. I sewed her up so she looked good on the outside, anyhow, no matter how badly disarranged her insides were."[10]

One strains to imagine parents' responses to reading such a letter, especially from a young woman. Delight in casual use of ghoulish humor appears also in Mary Theodora McGavran's quest for a brain: "Did I tell you [her diary] about getting or rather trying to get a fresh brain? Well I'll tell you. The girls wanted one and asked me if I couldn't get one thro Dr. Ross. Christy was rather anxious to have it and you know I'd have any head cut off for her if necessary."[11]

George Ross was a male resident at the German Hospital and a friend of McGavran. Despite her flirtations and irreverent phrases in the diary, McGavran was actually a conservative and devout woman, a missionary student who regularly attended church. But this sort of writing about acts and quests customarily deemed outrageous served several functions. It dissipated the terror and protected through identity— identity with the traditions and privileged expressions of medicine, and by extension with sisters in the chosen work.

Clinical work included demonstration clinics at the Woman's Hospital and elsewhere and some actual work with patients, infrequent as it was by later standards. Mary McGavran recorded several "clinics" in her diary: "To-day [11 November 1893] I went down to the Pennsylvania Hospital to hear Dr. DaCosta—He lectured on apoplexy and post typhoid fever. I like him very much only I must get used to his 'Gentlemen' in addressing a crowd of ladies and gentlemen—men and women, I should say. From there I came to the German and heard half of Dr. Wolfe's lectures on Medicine."

McGavran's reference to Jacob Mendez DaCosta's introduction indicates that women could still meet a tepid welcome at Pennsylvania Hospital twenty-five years after the great jeering episode of 1869. On another occasion McGavran described the fully conducted amphitheater clinic of the nineteenth century, in which even the surgical outcome becomes a public event: "Dr. Wolfe's lecture on the morphine habit was worthy of a clinic all to itself. Then he took up a case of obstruction making a diagnosis of the need of surgical measures. Dr. Deaver at once took the case up and proceeded to operate. It was very interesting and instructive altho the prognosis is yet doubtful. The woman was past middle age making matters worse."[12]

Edith Flower Wheeler during her stay at WMC wrote to her father that she would be expected to "attend clinics all over the city." She also remembered a clinic at Pennsylvania Hospital, given by one of its attending surgeons. A patient was wheeled into the amphitheater while the surgeon

> lectured to the class on the patient's ailment, which was
> tuberculosis with an abscess of the spine. The pus had worked
> its way down along the muscles of the thigh, producing quite a
> bulge. So, when all things were ready, the Doctor plunged his
> scalpel into the spot. The released pus shot upward in a large
> stream all over the Doctor's whiskers. . . . It made not a pause in
> his activity or talk. . . . The onlookers' stomachs turned slightly
> sideways but he was a shining example of self-control.[13]

And so, presumably, were the women students who joined their male colleagues in the Pennsylvania Hospital to witness this macabre performance—"what difference does it make to a med," and what difference makes the med's gender?

Possibly more than they counted educationally, these clinics constituted powerful socializing experiences. Our available witnesses chose to describe, either at the time or reflectively many years later, what must have been among the most dramatic of their clinical "lectures."[14]

The most extensive individual clinical work in the 1890s centered on obstetrics at Dr. Broomall's maternity service. For this and other practical work of medical education at the time, the working poor and indigent served as substrate, particularly impoverished African-Americans and recent immigrants from southern and eastern Europe. The students traveled to where the poor patients dwelled: the maternity practice on Washington Avenue in south Philadelphia lay nowhere near the school on North College Avenue. An 1897 graduate remembered the neighborhood around the maternity as a "confusion of streets and blind alleys" in which "Unpainted two-storied flats leaned their drab forms in unbroken, twisting double ranks, each house jostling its neighbor and spilling its occupants over worn thresholds."[15]

Immersion in the poorest reaches of the city revealed in the WMC students culturally entrenched assumptions and prejudices about class and ethnic origin. The young medical women were largely white, Protestant, middle class, and well washed; many no doubt encountered slums and the poor for the first time. The experience strained their ability to adhere to the traditional ideal of the physician's nonjudgmental benignity, and may well have tempered eagerness to embrace their women patients as sisters in need.

In previous years' course work, students had attended lectures in obstetrics, practiced on a manikin, and observed deliveries, all in preparation for their independent work as seniors. Edith Flower Wheeler recalled that "each student had to attend six cases on which she could give a complete detailed report. On the first case, a superior officer was with her, but the rest were taken care of alone." Revealing the development of her written medical facetiousness, and also typical class feelings, she wrote to her father:

> The first patient was a Jewess and, on examination, was found
> not to have been washed within the past nine months. . . . The
> Doctor, my superior, leaned up against the wall and went to
> sleep and I had plenty of time to observe my surroundings,
> interrupted at intervals by a curious moan like, oi, oi, oi,—
> . . . . I had lots of time to think over other and pleasanter places
> as well as to carefully go over all of my knowledge learned in
> books. . . . With very little preliminary warning, that stork
> dropped his burden suddenly, which was not what I had
> expected and I acted real commonplace by jumping. The job
> from then on I found to be practically and ordinarily speaking
> not all the most fastidious taste could desire but scientifically
> fascinating to the last degree. . . . I have been here a week and
> have to stay yet until I have three more cases. Those I have are
> all over the City. One way up in the northern part and one on
> the very last street in the southern part. When I get back to
> College I am going to ride my bike to see them.[16]

The importance of the outdoor maternity program will be discussed more in the next chapter.

Some students sought out clinical experience through a variety of initiatives. They might arrange to spend some time with an intern during her hours at one of the affiliated dispensaries, such as that founded by the alumnae (also in the poor area of south Philadelphia), or at the Woman's Hospital or West Philadelphia Hospital for Women. At the latter, Dr. Wheeler as a new intern "encountered, and mostly won over, measles, whooping cough, typhoid fever, tuberculosis, etc. She encountered a large number of puzzles, received much information and a few jolts. She found that patients do not always obey the doctor's orders or take their medicines as they are told."[17]

Rosalie Slaughter (later Morton), a classmate of Edith Wheeler, remembered the Alumnae Dispensary in her autobiography, probably romanticizing more than a little: "Here, daily, from nine till five, six women physicians from the Woman's Medical College came at scheduled hours to give gratuitous help to the poor. . . . Crowding into my office, they sat patiently while I extracted splinters, changed dressings, swabbed throats."[18] More seriously ill patients, often seen at home, suffered from cancers, bronchitis, diphtheria, Bright's Disease (nephritis), and typhoid.[19]

Mary Theodora McGavran demonstrated that a WMC student who made friends easily, including male friends, could obtain some bedside experience outside the prescribed curriculum. While visiting a friend hospitalized at nearby German Hospital with typhoid, McGavran received an invitation from a resident physician, Arthur Patek, to "see a case of typhoid in the ward—it was a very severe case—He allowed me to examine the patient and chart—I got several points." Patek went over several more patients with McGavran, whose diary records her pleasure at seeing patients "close-up" and gratitude to her resident friend: "guess he don't object to women doctors!"[20]

Managing Their Education

Well beyond such informal initiatives, the WMC students of the 1890s assumed that they had a responsibility and right to help shape their education and showed remarkable pluck (to use a word of their day) in doing so, mainly through their Student Association. The faculty minutes of the period show frequent requests for minor changes in quiz or examination schedules and occasional requests for more quiz sessions, including a series to help prepare for the new state board examinations.[21] At times the students requested a small expansion of the didactic program, as when they asked for "a short course of lectures on medical ethics" in 1891.[22] In general, the faculty agreed to these modest applications. But when larger issues arose, the students—unhindered by meekness and skilled in some organizational formalities—made their views known directly and forcefully to the board of corporators, and even once to the mayor of Philadelphia.

By 1896, much of the plan for enhanced clinical work at Woman's Hospital had fallen apart: that which the *Annual Announcement* promised did not occur. The Student Association sent to the faculty a detailed letter, formally structured with much display of "whereas" and "viz," listing the grievances and showing precisely which printed promises were violated. They also sent the letter to the Alumnae Association, and it was printed in the *Philadelphia Public Ledger*.[23] Suffice it to say here that the faculty responded with concern and the intent to remedy.[24]

On 16 November 1900, Dean Marshall read this startling letter "signed by almost every student of the College": "There is a house, No. 328 Federal St., which seems more suitable for the Maternity Hospital, now at 335 Washington Ave., than is its present house. It is owned by Mr. William Montgomery who holds it at $4500, and he is willing to hold a first mortgage of $2500."[25] In effect, the students had taken it upon themselves to identify a structure that they thought ought to be purchased to improve and secure the College's maternity program (and their comfort, of which the Washington Avenue house offered little); they had also made detailed inquiries concerning a mortgage. If they could manage to not shrink from cold dissections and bloody operations, why be daunted by transactions in real estate? They had opportunity, of course, to see that their women teachers looked upon all affairs, medical and managerial, as within their competence.

The Student Association in the 1890s also maintained a "Committee on Hospitals" or "Hospital Appointment Committee" which monitored the scarce availability of internships for women medical graduates. On one occasion, this committee sent a letter to Philadelphia's mayor protesting the absence of any WMC faculty member on the board that awarded internships at Philadelphia General Hospital.[26]

The Larger College Life

Despite the crushing amount of work, the WMC students managed to create a colorfully textured supplement to their academic schedules, much of it carried out through the class or Student Association. The

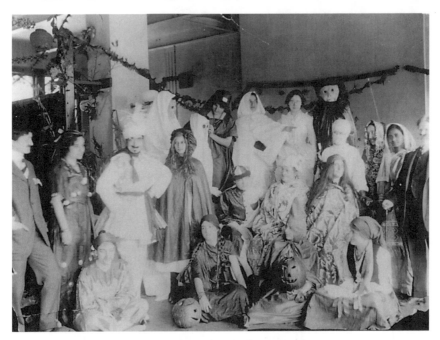

Figure 12. A long-standing tradition within the student culture at WMC was the annual Halloween party and dance attended by students and faculty, who enjoyed music, skits, and send-ups. This photograph is from about 1900.

sophomores traditionally provided a reception for the newly arrived freshmen, requiring the conveyance from boardinghouse rooms of pillows and rugs to a college quiz room or gymnasium.[27] An annual Halloween masquerade and party grew into a cherished tradition sustained deep into the twentieth century. The association also mediated the vexing dispute, inherited from earlier classes, over whether or not to adopt cap and gown for commencement. Eventually the costume was accepted in the late 1890s, probably first in 1897.[28]

At various times the Student Association arranged for a college pin (which required seeking permission from the board to use the College seal), and even the adoption of a "college cry."[29] The class of 1897 proceedings indicate a startling amount of energy given to the selection of a class color (green), then more to the shade of that color.[30] The association helped set up a basketball team, while groups of students also obtained permission to use a quiz room for fencing class. Others formed a glee club which gave concerts to benefit the maternity service and alumnae dispensary.[31]

Lacking in the minutes of the Student Association of this period, or in the reminiscences and diary, is much mention of women's rights or suffrage. Somehow, as a set of national, political questions, these issues did not often claim a place in the minds and schedules of the WMC students of the 1890s. Nor is there evidence of any prosuffrage persuasive endeavors among the faculty. Edith Wheeler admitted to not making her mind up about suffrage until much later.[32] One exception, 1889 graduate Lilian Welsh, remembered:

> The first suffrage meeting I even attended was when I was a student of medicine in Philadelphia in 1888, when the National Woman Suffrage Association held one of its annual meetings there. Strange to say, among the women medical students there was little or no sentiment on the subject at that time. Few of them were interested enough to attend any of the meetings. Several of us, however, went to an evening meeting and had no difficulty finding good seats.[33]

Before the turn of the century, evidence suggests that suffrage attracted little active interest or sympathy at the women's (nonmedical) colleges, where administrators sometimes discouraged discussion.[34]

A Bed, a Tub, and Typhoid Fever

Student activities included a committee to visit the sick and raising money to endow a student bed at Woman's Hospital. Though they hoped to kneel at the bedside, too frequently WMC students found themselves *in* bed as patients. Illness occurred with sufficient frequency to induce at least one class (1897) to maintain a "committee to visit sick members."[35] While colds and influenza must have annoyed the students, typhoid fever posed a serious and frequent threat. Both Mary McGavran and friend Ada McKee suffered long stretches of the illness while in College.[36] Catharine Macfarlane recalled that in 1899 or 1900, when she was a junior assistant in obstetrics, "there was a good deal of typhoid in the area near the waterfront," which was not far from the 335 Washington Avenue location of the College's maternity. "Three of us got typhoid fever. We were all patients in the Woman's Hospital at the same time. One student died. One very nearly died. I had a light attack."[37] Macfarlane remembered contriving in any way available to avoid the "tubbing"—cold baths every three or four hours—then thought essential for treating typhoid.[38]

Students, with support by the Alumnae Association and faculty, undertook a long-term project to raise enough money to endow a student's bed at the Woman's Hospital.[39] Professor of physiology Frances Emily White urged the Alumnae Association to help with the fund-raising, pointing out that when students became sick, usually they remained in their boardinghouses, where other students would "nurse their friends," a "serious draft on their time and strength."[40]

Catching typhoid fever, perhaps tuberculosis, or nursing an afflicted classmate made clear that the study and practice of medicine offered occasional dangers to health and even life. On the other hand, caring for each other in a boardinghouse or a hospital further brought the students together emotionally and helped them integrate the traditionally female role of caring with the therapeutic knowledge from their medical and surgical training. It can hardly be questioned that success in this self-realization must have aided in their development as physicians.

"A Book of College Tales"

At the Student Association meeting of 27 January 1896, the members discussed someone's idea for "a book of College tales" to introduce the College to the community; it would stress "college life particularly," more than medicine itself.[41] A committee solicited stories and essays, and, aided by the literary Henry Leffmann and alumna Gertrude Walker, saw to the preparation of illustrations and all other details for the book. On 18 February 1897 the class voted on the title: "Daughters of Aesculapius" thankfully won out over "Maids of Medical Mind" and "Women of the Evolution."

Daughters of Aesculapius can claim only modest literary merit; yet several of its "tales" and its few photographs offer a subtle charm to the reader, who looks fleetingly into the boardinghouse rooms and minds of these long-forgotten young women. Still oddities to many, they felt confirmed by their growing numbers, their friendships, their generally supportive College. The confidence and self-awareness—"life aware of itself"—of these intrepid *Daughters of Aesculapius* produced this printed token of their years as women medical students in the fin de siècle.[42]

Several of the stories, as well as McGavran's diary, confirm the importance and intensity of female friendships described by several feminist historians. Similar stories originating from the "seven sister" schools reveal an intent to document the formation of valued friendships, and perhaps an agenda to counter typical misogynic stereotypes of female jealousies and querulousness.[43] Medical women often maintained life-long friendships with their peers which originated in medical school.[44] No doubt some relationships included an erotic component, and many alumnae of the later twentieth century identify certain faculty alliances as lesbian or "Boston marriages." Certainly this element could contribute to the intensity of friendships among students or faculty and indirectly further foster cohesiveness and loyalty within the College. But among those in the larger medical community, which has been traditionally conservative, the suspicion or presumption of lesbianism at WMC could also serve as a silent source of derision or opposition, impossible to measure or even document.

At Home in Philadelphia

As noted several times, the students attending WMC mostly lived in boardinghouses not far from the College. Sometimes a few students would "keep house"—rent several rooms, or something like an apartment, and undertake all necessary cleaning and cooking. This choice might be made to save money, as in the case of "Alice" in the vignette called "Home life" in *Daughters of Aesculapius*, whose financial problems followed the "failure of the bank," probably during the 1893 fiscal panic. Alice and her two roommates did teaching and typewriting to support their college work.[45]

Many shared in this pecuniary plight, as had their predecessors. Few students came from rich families, and for some the financially perilous 1890s made it especially difficult to pay for their education, which was becoming more costly as expenses for new course work were passed down to matriculants. Edith Flower Wheeler's letters home to her father usually incorporated a plea for money.[46] Letters to the dean from women seeking information about the College's requirements often asked about expenses or included a phrase such as this from 1891: "I am the daughter of a clergyman and cannot expend but a certain sum on my education."[47] One of the African-American students from this period, Eliza Grier, in her letter of inquiry asked: "How much does it take to put one through a year in your school? Is there any possible chance to do any work that would not interfere with one's studies? Do you know of any possible way that might be provided for an emancipated slave to receive any help into so lofty a profession?"[48]

Grier did receive modest financial help from the College, managed somehow to pay the rest, and graduated in 1897.

Despite the demanding school work and lack of money (for some at least), WMC students used and explored their city, as natives or four-year visitors. Philadelphia has always been a city beloved of meanderers—full of odd byways, capricious little streets and alleys, nautical neighborhoods along the rivers, architectural curiosities aside buildings of dignity and elegance. And it boasted, and still does, of one of the largest and most beautiful city park systems, aligned along the Schuylkill River and Wissahickon Creek Valley.

In January of 1893 Mary McGavran and her friend Josie Moser

> took a walk up to the park—as we went to Horticultural Hall
> we came to a long steep path all covered with snow. Two small
> boys were there with sleds. We couldn't resist the temptation so
> we borrowed the sleds and had some old fashioned rides. It was
> so fine, first time I went down along there we tied the two sleds
> together and went down the slope and across the rustic bridge
> at the bottom together.[49]

McGavran also enjoyed taking walks around an elevated reservoir near the College, sometimes with one of her several beaus. With a classmate one February afternoon, she "lingered until the light began to fade, watching the rays shoot up and die away—and then walked slowly home, rested—ready for our nights work." She and classmates (and male friends) also used the park for croquet and tennis.[50] Following junior exams, McGavran joined a group of WMC students and a few friends in "the 'Rambler,' a Tallyho of the latest style, and set out for Indian

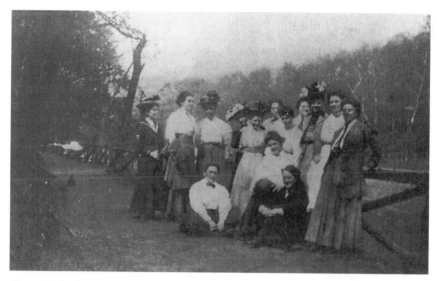

Figure 13. A class outing along the Wissahickon Creek in Philadelphia's Fairmount Park. *Scalpel*, 1911.

Rock." "The drive is grand beyond description. First up the Scuylkill [*sic*] & then up the Wissahickon creek. It took an hour to go out—an hour we spent in gathering flowers and ferns which grow in abundance. Then we started home. . . . We sang and talked and *enjoyed* ourselves *immensely* every minute. We reached the starting point at 7:30 P.M."[51]

McGavran attended church frequently, sampling from the immense number available in Philadelphia, and found time to volunteer at a Philadelphia mission.[52] Almost surely, many of the WMC women during the 1880s and 1890s attended church or Quaker meetings regularly or the services at their YMCA branch or at Woman's Hospital.

Edith Flower Wheeler, but probably not Mary McGavran, also went to theater, something young women could scarcely have done twenty years earlier. But the 1890s marked the beginning of a major movement toward greater social and sexual freedom for both genders that culminated in the 1920s. Wheeler took herself to see "The Black Crook," a notorious play in which the female characters wore "skin fitting black tights and . . . fancy short skirts"; these costumes succeeded in amazing her. She also saw tamer productions such as *Izoyl* (with Sarah Bernhardt), *The Little Minister*, and *Rip Van Winkle*. Wheeler heard

Paderewski play and Patti sing.[53] Mary McGavran and some friends attended concerts of the "German Symphony" and the Boston Symphony Orchestra.[54]

So at least some students utilized Philadelphia, made it part of their full lives, *perceived* it and found comfort in familiar and steady places. Wheeler said about herself: "She liked Philadelphia. It seemed very substantial, mature, and safe. The Medical College was situated directly across from Girard College, the main building of which was patterned after an old heathen temple, I believe. . . . and it was a never failing source of relief to the spirit, after contact with the ugly things of life, to look out on this building."[55]

Catharine Macfarlane wrote of her nights at the maternity practice in south Philadelphia, where students and the junior instructor slept in the building: "The long night vigils, the view of the shot tower against the rosy dawn, the gratitude of our simple patients, were the warp and woof of my initiation into the practice of medicine."[56]

Woman's Medical College as a Woman's College

Some facets of WMC student life vividly revealed by the authors of our diary, letters, and memoirs might seem at odds with sober expectations for what professional school ought to be. One can understand the impetus to communally address deficits of education and comfort and the need for friendships and recreation—but why school pins, colors, and cries, and years of debate over cap and gown? What of the successful but time-consuming effort to produce a book of college stories? Was there meaning beyond the obvious in the tallyho rides, fern picking, annual masquerade, canoeing, fencing, and a basketball league? What about the pyre of burning texts danced around the night before graduation, as described in a newspaper clipping?[57]

Virtually all aspects of the full life of the WMC student of the 1890s are comprehensible by seeing the experience as both a foundation for medical practice, and that broader foundation for life only recently open to women—college or university. In the nineteenth century only a minority of medical students had been four years at college or university. But "the life," student life outside the curriculum, had reached an alluring fullness particularly in the 1890s, and particularly at the women's schools. *So the women "meds" made medical school not only their professional training, but also their college experience.*

Most activities carried out by the classes at WMC matched counterparts at Vassar, Wellesley, Mt. Holyoke, and Bryn Mawr, as well as some coeducational universities and colleges.[58] Basketball and bicycling had become faddish on women's college campuses by the 1890s, and school cheers and colors owned a long history. The annual "gay masquerade" and dance at WMC approximated the popular girls-school theatrics: some women cross-dressed and played "chevaliers," while actual men were barred, except (if we believe a newspaper reporter) for several musicians, blindfolded and "chained to the floor" of an anteroom.

Students in women's colleges gained valuable organizational and managerial experience through their student associations, as also occurred at WMC. *Daughters of Aesculapius* is remarkable because it replicated in medical binding the volumes of college stories that had become popular around the turn of the century, such as *Harvard Stories* of 1893, *Princeton Stories* of 1895, *Yale Sketches* of 1895, *Cornell Stories* of 1898, *Vassar Studies* of 1899, *Vassar Stories* of 1900, *Wellesley Stories* of 1907, and others that preceded and followed these. The WMC collection actually preceded most of those from the other women's colleges. In sum, for students of this period, Woman's Medical College of Pennsylvania was not only their medical school, but also their college.[59]

In her brilliant book *Alma Mater*, Helen Lefkowitz Horowitz describes how student processions and various annual outdoor rituals at schools such as Smith, Wellesley, and Bryn Mawr "linked the students to the college landscape." Even "stretches of countryside beyond campus bounds became special places for important conversations or self-examination."[60] WMC and the neighboring Woman's Hospital obviously could provide no landscape of rolling hills, walking paths, cloisters, and ponds; so for the WMC students of the 1890s Philadelphia served as their campus, in multiple ways. Its Fairmount Park did, in fact, offer places to play tennis and croquet with friends, enjoy a year-end tallyho ride, engage in "important conversations or self-examination" along the pleasant walkway around the reservoir. The female "meds" refreshed in the parks and gained preparatory knowledge in their own classrooms and laboratories, but the particular work of this group of women students demanded that all of Philadelphia become their campus, as they found their way to scattered hospital amphitheaters, industrial sites to learn about ventilation and pasteurization, patients' homes to deliver babies, and other clinical work in the poorest areas of Philadelphia's south end. For such activities, the conventional women's colleges included no parallels.

And here lies the central phenomenon of four years at WMC in the 1890s: the whole experience wove together the increasingly valued features of women's collegiate life—including the formation of autonomy and friendships—with the powerful and intense tutelage in the ways and values of medicine. The "life" took place mainly in the company of women and fostered friendships and female identity; the medical education proceeded under the guidance of both genders and of course shaped professional identity. For at least some fortunate number of the young women, these long and daunting four years fostered a growing appreciation of life and friendship and made for a sustaining transition into their fuller adulthoods and professional roles. It is even plausible to claim that for a young American woman of the 1890s going to a women's medical school, at least one as fully developed as WMC, in a large and mature city like Philadelphia, was a rare adventure.

So it hardly surprises that commencement held much meaning, and to some extent borrowed from collegiate customs. By the end of the 1890s the students finally wore the much contested cap and gown as they marched in the Academy of Music.[61] To these formalities at least some classes added the nocturnal bonfire of hated texts, as reported in a newspaper article of 1898. The unknown reporter, seeing the event as collegiate, has found a "campus" for WMC where none really existed, and it is unclear exactly where this event occurred: "The campus was prettily lighted by strings of Chinese lanterns, but the mild radiance therefrom paled towards the close of the rites before the lurid glare from the burning pyre of books and other commodities, more or less mysterious, which were thrown to fuel the flames by the black gowned revelers who, separated by ropes from the spectators, moved in a circle around the fire, chanting original verses."[62]

The verses began as follows:

Where, oh where, are the lectures that vexed us,
Where, oh where, are the books that perplexed us,

Where, oh where, are the fears that oppressed us,
On May-day, so lately now flown?

And continued with reference to "drugs that we smelled at" and the
"soldiers that lived on quinine," but rather little else of medicine. And
they concluded poignantly:

Where, oh where, are the loving memories
Of all that has gladdened us here?
Laid away in our heart's deepest niches
To blossom for many a year.[63]

Clearly, despite its imperfections, WMC of the late nineteenth century managed to provide for its students not only a strong medical education, but also an experience of place and associations, and mostly—though
not exclusively—an experience of women together. This experience the
students largely created themselves, often with support from the faculty and board. Educational sociologist Burton Clark has referred to the
small liberal arts colleges of the nineteenth century as "intensive communities in which young people spent four critical years in places that
were highly conscious of their own struggle and achievement . . . [and]
that turned graduates into persons filled with fond memories and institutional devotion."[64] Surely this might apply as well to a small, four-
year medical college.

During the College's trying decades of the early twentieth century,
the Alumnae Association would become the single most insistent defender of the separate Woman's Med.[65] When in 1913 the College faced
grave obstacles, the president of the Alumnae Association sent a printed
note to other alumnae, imploring them to attend a special meeting "for
the sake of memories and associations of your student days."[66] In June
of 1921, financial failure made closure of the College seem inevitable.
The woman president of the board, Sarah Logan Wister Starr, revealed
the perilous circumstances to a meeting of the Alumnae Association
and challenged those present to match her own emergency loan.[67] One
by one, on the spot, a nucleus of loyal graduates pledged five hundred
or one thousand dollars. These were the Aesculapian daughters of the
1890s, now alumnae in mid-career and midlife, unwilling to envision
their youthful experiences and memories made unavailable to young
women of the future.

The Work of Golden Age Graduates

What did the turn-of-century graduates of WMC do with their degrees? A sampling of materials from their "deceased alumnae folders" at the archives of their alma mater reveals pathways similar to those in earlier decades, but with clearly greater opportunities.[68]

A report from 1914 shows that about 40 percent of the roughly 1,000 living graduates resided in Pennsylvania and 60 in New Jersey, 150 in the Far West, 270 in the middle and eastern states, only 50 in the South, and 75 in "Foreign Lands."[69] Most of the women entered private practice in general medicine, often with a special preference for obstetrics and gynecology. Many more than in the 1870s completed an internship or some other form of postgraduate work in the United States or Europe. The 1880s and 1890s were the first decades of specialism's efflorescence: a few WMC graduates chose work in psychiatry, dermatology, ophthalmology, otolaryngology, laboratory science, and of course obstetrics and gynecology.[70] A very few conducted research somewhere during their career, such as Lenore Gageby (WMC, 1901) on polio, Jessie Louise Herrick (1895) on epilepsy, Mary E. Lapham (1900) on tuberculosis, and Catharine Macfarlane (1898), who performed widely recognized investigations on cancer screening as a faculty member at WMC. As previously noted, WMC graduates, like other women physicians in the late nineteenth and early twentieth centuries, founded and worked in clinics or dispensaries for women, some held at night to accommodate work schedules. Sarah Tew Mayo (1898) founded the Woman's Dispensary of New Orleans, while Edith Hedges Matzke (1895) helped set up a health clinic for women in San Francisco with the support of that city's Western Women's Club.

Some of the turn-of-the-century graduates devoted all or most of their lives to institutional work, such as Mary McDowell Shick (1895) at the Elwyn Training School for retarded children and Elizabeth Quintard St. John (1900), who worked many years for the U.S. Bureau of Chemistry and the Mutual Life Insurance Company. Lillian South (or South-Tye; 1904) after a period of private practice served as director of the Bureau of Bacteriology and Epidemiology in Kentucky from 1910 to 1950. She carried out a survey of the hookworm problem in that state, which led to a Rockefeller Foundation grant to help eradicate it.[71] Also in Kentucky, Louise Healy (1897) spent some years in charge of women patients at the Eastern State Hospital. Many earlier WMC graduates had worked as staff physicians for female inmates of state hospitals: Alice Bennett (1851–1925), an 1876 graduate, in 1880 became the first woman physician to superintend the women's division of such an institution.[72]

All through the 1890s and well into the twentieth century the College continued to attract (and offered reduced charges) to missionary students, most of whom like their sisters of earlier decades went to China or India.

Many women's careers showed remarkable durability: they commonly worked for at least fifty years.[73] Sometimes a professional life was spent in one town or city; others sought diversity. Josephine Phelps Broadhead (1895) did some postgraduate courses in homeopathy, practiced for a time in the Germantown section of Philadelphia, then did missionary work among the Navajos of Arizona and New Mexico; she is said to have mastered the language. She also married a clergyman and had two children. Arley Munson Hare's (1902) serpentine trajectory found her briefly at a mission hospital in India, then physician for women at the Southern Indiana Hospital for the Insane, next in private practice in New Jersey. During World War I she became a serologist and bacteriologist at Red Cross hospitals in France, where she remained to work in tuberculosis control under a Rockefeller Foundation program. Back in the United States, she practiced until 1941 in New York City! The remarkable Ellen Culver Potter (1903), even before entering WMC, had worked in a mission in New York City's Chinatown and organized a settlement in the mill district of Norwich, Connecticut. She conducted private practice in the Germantown section of Philadelphia (a favorite choice for WMC graduates) until 1920, when she became head of Pennsylvania's Child Health Division. This post led to her appointment as the Commonwealth's secretary of welfare in 1923; hers is said to be the first state cabinet appointment of a woman anywhere in the United States. She also served on the WMC faculty and briefly as acting president in the 1940s.

Careers of African-American Graduates in the Nineteenth Century

With its early roots in that Quaker activism which so vigorously fired the antislavery campaigns, it is perhaps not surprising that the nineteenth-century WMC admitted some African-American students: by 1900, at least ten had received the M.D. The identified black graduates included (with years of birth, death, and graduation) Rebecca Cole (1846–1922; 1867), Caroline Still Wiley Anderson (1848–1919; 1878) Georgianna E. Patterson Young (1845–1887; 1878), Verina M. Harris Morton Jones (1857–1943; 1888), Juan Bennett-Drummond (?; 1888); Halle Tanner Dillon Johnson (1863–1901; 1891), Alice Woodby-McKane (1863–1946; 1892), Lucy Hughes-Brown (1863–?; 1894), Lulu Cecilia Fleming (1862–1899; 1895), Eliza Grier (1864–1902; 1897) and Matilda Evans (1872–1935; 1897).[74] Their presence gave further testimony to the "door of opportunity" that the school provided and that Clara Marshall cherished, though the fact that most were middle class and actively Christian no doubt favored their admission; the 1890s was not a decade of favorable feelings toward blacks.[75] The lives of the African-American graduates reveal an interesting variation on the work of the woman physician in the nineteenth century, a variation in which clinical practice frequently yielded to a desire to serve within the race. Often sustained by a deeply felt Christianity, that service centered on education and social progress, and linked medicine, religion, race, and gender. Both wedding a minister and founding a clinic, hospital, or nursing school recur in the lives of the early African-American graduates, several of whom were born into slavery.

Rebecca Cole, the first known African-American to receive her M.D. from WMC, practiced in Philadelphia; Columbia, South Carolina; and Washington, D.C. Early in her career, she worked for Elizabeth and Emily Blackwell's New York Infirmary for Women and Children as its "sanitary visitor," an assignment that entailed visiting poor women in their tenement homes. Later, Cole returned to Philadelphia, where with Dr. Charlotte Abbey, an English-born 1887 WMC graduate, she founded the "Woman's Directory," an entity offering social, medical, and legal services to pregnant women, aimed at avoiding "feticide and infanticide" and providing help to mothers who had been abandoned by their partners. Cole was also active in the black women's club movement.[76] Following marriage to a clergyman, Lucy Hughes Brown practiced in Charleston, South Carolina, where she helped establish the Cannon Hospital and Training School. Matilda Evans, one of the most accomplished of early southern women physicians, founded the Taylor Lane Hospital and Nurses' Training School in Columbia, South Carolina, where she also conducted a free clinic for black children.

Alice Woodby-McKane first practiced in Augusta, Georgia, then married Dr. Cornelius McKane of Savannah; she and her husband set up a small dispensary, a hospital, and a training program for nurses, which they kept going despite meager financial support. Most of their first patients were "women in service" with little means and sometimes no other place to be cared for when ill. The McKanes' lives suggest a thirst for change and adventure: they spent a year doing medical missionary work in Liberia before settling in Savannah. Later, they moved to Boston where practice brought them wealth and prominence. In 1922, Alice Woodby-McKane still practiced, and worked actively for the local Republican Party. Verina M. Harris Morton Jones also married a physician, and the two practiced for many years in Brooklyn, New York. Another of the nineteenth-century African-American women physicians who went to the missionary field, Lulu Cecilia Fleming, gained her WMC degree in 1895 then returned to the Congo as a medical missionary supported by the Baptist Missionary Union (she had worked there previously as a nonmedical emissary). Following a devastating illness (said to have been "sleeping sickness"), Fleming returned to Philadelphia in 1899 and died the same year. The celebrated Philadelphia Baptist pastor and orator, and founder of Temple University, Russell H. Conwell presided at her memorial service held at the great Baptist Temple on Broad Street.

Halle Tanner Dillon Johnson was born into Philadelphia's African-American elite: her father, Bishop Benjamin Tanner, was a leader of the African Methodist Episcopal Church, and her brother was the noted painter Henry Ossawa Tanner. Some months after her graduation in 1891, she wrote a letter to Clara Marshall from Tuskegee, Alabama, in which she thanked the dean for the good wishes earlier conveyed and described her successful sitting for the Alabama state board examination—the first African-American and the first woman to do so. The recent graduate expressed satisfaction with her new position as resident physician for the students of the Tuskegee Normal and Industrial School.[77] Dr. Johnson also founded a free clinic (the Lafayette Dispensary) after discovering that the beautiful and seemingly healthful vicinity of Tuskegee, in the "Black Belt" of the South, was black "not only with people of this despised hue, but black with disease and death." She saw adults and children in the countryside sick with disease and "abject poverty," unable to afford the two-dollar per mile fee that doctors charged.[78] She later married a minister and moved to Nashville, where she died.

Caroline Still Wiley Anderson, another native Philadelphian from an upper-caste family, was the daughter of William and Letitia Still; William was a leading black merchant, an activist, and the author of a history of the Underground Railroad, which he had served. Following her 1878 graduation from WMC and a year as intern at the New England Hospital for Women and Children, Dr. Anderson practiced briefly in Philadelphia. After her marriage to Matthew Anderson, a Presbyterian minister, she joined him in the work of his Berean Manual Training and Industrial School (later Berean Institute), which offered (as it still does) a variety of educational services to its community. Dr. Caroline Anderson served as one of its teachers and as vice principal for many years, and she ran its dispensary. She somehow found time to read a paper on "Popliteal Aneurysm" to the WMC Alumnae Association in 1888.[79]

Earlier in this chapter we recorded the letter of Eliza Grier, declaring herself an emancipated slave as she wrote to WMC in search of medical education and a way to pay for it. Hers was the saddest story of these pioneering black women. Grier did receive some financial aid from the College, and she graduated in 1897, already thirty-three years of age. She attempted practice first in Atlanta, then in Greenville, South Carolina. In March of 1901, she again wrote for help, this time to Susan B. Anthony, who forwarded the letter to Dean Marshall:

> I am a young Negro woman. I am engaged in the practice of medicine in this city [Greenville]. I have made a pretty good practice, but mostly among the very poor and in neglected districts. By and by I hope to get something from that source. I

have been quite ill for six weeks with La Grippe. I have not
been able to make a single dollar. My expenses are going on just
the same. I cannot retain my place of business unless someone
will help me.[80]

Grier died in 1901, before she could achieve a synthesis of self-
realization and service enjoyed by others of these early black women
professionals.

Little can be known about the reception the African-American
women found at the College, but some evidence suggests it was not unfavorable in this period, despite the prevailing discrimination of 1890s
Philadelphia, which through northward migration had gained, but not
entirely welcomed, the largest black population of any northern city.[81]
The minutes book for the class of 1897 shows that Matilda Evans for a
time served as the class recording secretary and also on the committee
for visiting the sick.[82] At least five of the group joined the Alumnae
Association; Caroline Wiley Still Anderson served as its treasurer in
1888, and Halle Tanner Dillon Johnson described her dispensary to one
of its meetings. We have already noted that Johnson wrote to Clara
Marshall soon after settling in Tuskegee. It is reasonable to conclude
that the early African-American graduates acquired an education at
WMC well able to support their later evolution as physicians and educators and that they did so in a sufficiently respectful environment that
they too could comfortably look upon the school as their alma mater.

The presence of black women in the College also allowed the other
students, most of whom were white and Protestant at this time, to encounter an African-American as peer, rather than as servant or laborer.
A freshman student of the 1920s, who "had been carrying the torch
for racial tolerance and goodwill," when attending a kind of orientation weekend agreed to share a room with the only African-American
woman in the class. Her liberal resolve softened when she discovered
the room contained one double bed; she went outside to walk and think
about the situation:

> I got so in earnest that I started talking to myself. "You got
> yourself into this, It's your own decision and its right. It's what
> you believe in, so go ahead." Right here I came to a little bridge
> over a brook, and saw someone sitting there scuffing her foot

on the path, and saying just as earnestly, "You've got to do it whether you like it or not." At the same moment we recognized each other, my roommate and I, and threw back our heads, and laughed and laughed at ourselves. From that time on we were fast friends.[83]

While this charming tale seems perhaps too theatrically perfect, at least a trifle improbable, it suggests the potential for yet another outcome of four years at WMC in the shaping of future women physicians. Opportunity existed to encounter students from diverse backgrounds, which necessarily meant *women* from diverse backgrounds, such as African-Americans, Jews, Catholics, the celebrated visitors from Asia or India, and the white, Protestant majority. This opportunity no doubt fostered among the open-minded matriculants a sense of women physicians as an enlarging, broadly based group, even a "network." At the same time, of course, students also enjoyed the benefit of seeing women practice, teach, and manage, and collegially share authority and expertise with liberal men. All this added up to a distinctiveness of experience at WMC that, as already suggested, created for at least some graduates meaningful memories and a sense of association that would long persist.

Chapter 7	The Age of
	Educational Reform

1900–1920

The small school founded in 1850 had set out on a course fundamentally new, though it modeled its organization on the typical American nineteenth-century medical school. Within twenty-five years, it had matured well, despite opposition and paltry means. The crises and demands of the early twentieth century forced the College to reinvent itself, and the new "Flexnerian" exemplar of the American medical school required, as we will see, a far more difficult job of emulation.[1] WMC tried to fulfill some of the new expectations, while ignoring or deferring others (in this it was not alone). It increased clinical and laboratory work and raised entrance requirements, but could afford few "full-time" faculty and undertook no research. With these limitations the College managed to stay afloat and even physically rebuild, largely under the direction of Clara Marshall.

By the end of 1910, all the other strong women's medical schools in the United States had closed their doors—*so the existence of WMC represented the continuation of separate medical education for women as a choice.*[2] From 1910 through the 1960s, the question of sustaining the College became inseparable from the debate over coeducation. The rhetoric of survival voiced in fund-raising campaigns and pleas for moral support employed arguments for the right of women to learn medicine with women if they so chose. Clara Marshall, like her nineteenth-century predecessors Preston and Bodley, had grown into a powerful champion and articulate voice of the College, and indeed of American medical women.

Mandated Reform

What new demands would the reform of medical education bring to WMC? The reform and upgrading of medical education expanded as centralized organizations and philanthropies assumed a role previously unknown.[3] The rise of new state licensing boards in the late nineteenth century has been discussed earlier. In 1905 the American Medical Association formed its Council on Medical Education, which undertook to inspect and assess medical schools. In 1906 the council created its rating system, used by many state boards to determine which schools' students could sit for examinations. In the AMA system, as it evolved, Class A+ rewarded a superior program, A meant acceptable, B denoted need for certain improvements, while C designated a demand for complete reorganization. The ratings depended mainly on the amount of a school's endowment, whether it controlled a teaching hospital, and the number of full-time faculty members. In addition to its application to licensing, any such rating system at a national level no doubt affected a college's prestige and ability to attract students.

The Council on Medical Education to further its goals quietly approached the Carnegie Foundation for the Advancement of Teaching to carry out a seemingly independent, and more detailed, inspection of all North American schools of medicine.[4] Professional educator Abraham Flexner was hired to carry out the project. The product of this inspection was the celebrated *Medical Education in the United States and Canada: A Report to the Carnegie Foundation for the Advancement of Teaching*, published in 1910 and widely known since as the "Flexner Report."[5] Flexner actually exerted his most powerful influence subsequent to the publication of the *Report*: in 1913, he joined the General Education Board of the Rockefeller Foundation, from which flowed the massive funds that would pay for the reshaping of many American medical schools into one image. That image gave enormous weight to the university environment, the presence of salaried full-time faculty members in both basic science and clinical departments ("full-time" became nearly an obsession with Flexner), and the conduct of research.

Flexner's assessment of WMC in his *Report* was largely favorable

("There is striking evidence of a genuine effort to do the best possible with limited resources"). But his concept of a system of medical education housed in universities predicted only two medical schools in Pennsylvania, one at the University of Pennsylvania and the other with the University of Pittsburgh.[6] No such winnowing of Pennsylvania medical education ensued, and no major Rockefeller money came to Philadelphia medical schools. WMC nonetheless had to face the external demands for reforming medical education, and in several ways stood particularly vulnerable.

Why vulnerable? First, WMC was not a university school of medicine. Second, research at WMC had never been developed. And, third, although numerous faculty received salaries, few were "full-time"; that is, paid to devote their entire professional work to the College. Paying for more full-time faculty would greatly accelerate expenses at the very time when student applications and enrollments were declining. This decline occurred as formerly all-male schools admitted women, while fewer women overall sought medical training.[7] Raising entrance requirements, another mandate to medical schools from state boards and the national bodies, had the potential to further reduce enrollment, and therefore income. Finally, insistence on control of a teaching hospital emerged precisely when the bonds between WMC and Woman's Hospital of Philadelphia finally separated, as will be seen.

As noted previously, the College had acquired about $280,000 of "permanent production funds" by the end of the nineteenth century. The fifteen thousand or so dollars produced annually from investments was more than many schools could claim, but not enough to support rising expenses and diminishing student income.[8] Lack of funds slowed the construction of the College's own hospital and limited the ability to hire nationally known women or men for the faculty. In May of 1903, the executive committee of the board discussed the "critical condition of the finances of the College" and recent deficits.[9] And this was before the sharp drop in enrollment that occurred from 1903 to 1910.[10] While the board managed to keep the institution solvent for much of the troubled 1900s and 1910s, financial collapse finally occurred in 1921. Although the specific events leading up to that unhappy moment will be reviewed later, perhaps this is the appropriate place to pause and explore the context of the chronic financial woes of WMC.

WMC was not alone in its financial struggles. In 1908 the president of the Association of American Medical Colleges declared that "the greatest single difficulty in the way of progress in medical education is undoubtedly poverty. Beside it all other difficulties appear trivial."[11] In the nineteenth century, neither individuals nor government saw medical schools as public enterprises warranting support. The women's schools may have actually fared better, since they clearly did embody a cause and therefore attracted some charitable assistance.

But certain factors having to do with its friends, its alumnae, and its city specifically limited WMC in acquiring endowment. In 1890, responding to a letter of friendly criticism from an alumna, Clara Marshall stated that what she needed more than criticism was *money*: "The college is not sufficiently 'fashionable' to awaken the interest of those who are working in the direction of Johns Hopkins. The substantial aid has heretofore come from Quakers who though careful business managers, number few very rich men."[12] Indeed, members of the Society of Friends provided the College's most steadfast backing during the nineteenth century. But, as the prominent Quaker educator Isaac Sharpless lamented in 1909, Friends' philanthropy in Philadelphia represented only the "generous gifts of a few" rather than "the spontaneous outpouring of the many."[13] And the "few" had to choose from many worthy causes: Friend Anna T. Jeanes and her family (mainly dry goods merchants) aided WMC faithfully, but her million-dollar estate eventually went to fund education for southern blacks.[14]

More than a few wealthy businessmen, Quakers and non-Quakers, lived in Philadelphia. But the region could claim no one like John D. Rockefeller, J. P. Morgan, or C. P. Huntington, ready to make massive gifts of money, such as those that fed the investment accounts of the medical schools of Harvard and Cornell.[15]

Finally, and most important, a woman's medical college would expect its strongest financial patronage from women, but unlike Anna T. Jeanes, few women in the United States have controlled great wealth. Furthermore, American women never identified women's medical education as a cause to support, as they had for temperance and foreign Christian missions. And, although most alumnae probably made an acceptable living or better, not many became rich.[16] Few women physicians had access to those pathways—prestigious residencies and hospital appointments—leading to extremely lucrative specialty practices. At least some alumnae always came through when the College needed their help most, but alumnae alone never could build a major endowment.

The Need for a New Hospital

Understanding some of the sources of the chronic lack of sufficient funds, let us now return to WMC in the new century, and one source of fiscal demand—the imperative to build a College hospital. In previous chapters, it was mentioned that a general failure of the teaching arrangements for WMC students at the neighboring Woman's Hospital of Philadelphia occurred early in 1896.[17] Over the ensuing years the College and the hospital attempted to resolve differences and agree upon a teaching program satisfactory to both.[18] Though periodic improvements occurred, a firm solution proved elusive. The final dissolution came in 1903 when the hospital refused privileges to Ella Everitt (1866–1922) and Edith Cadwallader, whom the College had appointed as successors to Hannah Croasdale and Anna Broomall, professors of gynecology and obstetrics respectively, who had resigned in 1902.[19] Everitt was a first-rate operator and teacher, while the younger Cadwallader had solid credentials but less experience. In addition, the hospital dropped the College's professor of surgery, William L. Rodman, from its staff, accusing him of some action that brought "disrepute to the Hospital."[20] Woman's Hospital had effectively excluded all major clinical faculty of the College, though it offered to teach students using its own staff, on its terms.

Such an arrangement would not meet the external requirements that a medical school control the teaching elements of a general hospital. The Woman's Hospital in any case did not function as a general hospital, admitting only women and children; this also presented a difficulty for the College.[21]

What issues produced the split between hospital and medical school? We have already seen that in the 1890s medical students on the floors of Woman's Hospital were seen as disruptive of routine and annoying to patients. In 1903, Mrs. E. F. Halloway, secretary of the hospital's board of managers, in responding to a plea by the College for more ward teaching, complained that the "devotion of so much time to bedside instruction is detrimental to the work of the hospital in other directions, interfering unwarrantably with arrangements for private pa-tients, with the work of Internes, with both the routine work and the training of nurses."[22] The managers assigned priority to their intern-ship and their historic training school for nurses. These were their own programs, and useful ones: interns and nursing students carried out the daily work; medical students got in the way.

Another problem in the view of the College faculty was the hospital's unwillingness to encourage general medical and surgical work or to admit men. Halloway stated that the managers did not wish to see a "shrinkage of the Gynecological work, which has always been . . . the characteristic and preponderating work of the Hospital."[23] "Gyne-cological work" meant a large amount of surgery. By 1900 surgery had become the crux of hospital existence, and many disputes centered on access to this arena.[24] Women surgeons did not seem immune to surgi-cal fervor: Catharine Macfarlane wrote that Marie Formad, master sur-geon at the Woman's Hospital and one of her mentors, "would rather operate than eat."[25]

The dispute between WMC and the Woman's Hospital revealed that women physicians and surgeons were flourishing in Philadelphia by 1910—enough to staff and support *two* major institutions. Like WMC, the Woman's Hospital saw itself as a venerable and complex institution. Pride and proprietary identity were at stake. Efforts by the College to meet its pedagogic needs led some hospital managers to feel "that the independence of their institution was assailed."[26] The women physicians of Philadelphia here displayed not the putative female virtue of cooperation, but rather typical professional and proprietary attitudes. Institutional bonding can be powerfully motivating: only the force and folly of human ardor could have divided these two sister institutions.[27]

Merger?

The board of corporators of the Woman's Medical College faced the absolute necessity of constructing its own hospital. Knowing that such a move would strain the already limited financial capacity, the board first requested that the faculty offer its opinion on the possibility of an "affiliation of the Woman's Medical College of Pennsylvania with some other medical school of Philadelphia." A committee of two was appointed in 1903 or early 1904 to report on the question: Frederick P. Henry, a senior, widely known male professor, and Ella Everitt, a newly appointed woman and WMC alumna.[28] These choices would seem hardly accidental, pairing a woman and alumna with a senior male faculty member.

The Henry-Everitt report concluded that the College should carry on independently. The writers believed that one of Philadelphia's male medical schools might accept women but only with the motivation of receiving the College's endowment.[29] More positively, Everitt and Henry proposed that women students can receive more "individual attention" in a smaller institution.[30] The facilities for learning obstetrics were superior. Women ought to have the choice between coeducation and separate-sex medical education in a strong college. Finally, the committee of two gathered data on female faculty positions at "six prominent coeducational schools of medicine" showing that none of them had appointed more than one or two women, and virtually all at the lowest ranks. The provision of choice, a small, helpful environment, and opportunities for women doctors to become teachers, would continue as the primary arguments to maintain the autonomous "Woman's Med" in the twentieth century.

New Hospital, Class A Rating, and Fund-Raising

With its idea of merger rejected for the time, the board of corporators authorized building a College hospital, which the faculty had been seeking since at least the early 1890s.[31] The alumnae permitted their dispensary (which was legally established as "Hospital and Dispensary") to merge with the College, thus avoiding the need to seek a new charter.[32] By early September of 1904, a small, one-story "hospital pavilion" attached to the north side of the College building neared completion.[33] Board members, alumnae, faculty, friends, and students all contributed money to help build the little structure; the students raised over two hundred dollars from a "Theatre Benefit."[34] The hospital included male and female wards with ten beds each and an operating room, certainly better than nothing but inadequate for the amount of clinical instruction desired. Outpatient work continued in south Philadelphia.

With the intent of constructing a larger, permanent hospital on a

lot between the College and the Woman's Hospital, the College sought
to raise further funds, and won in 1905 its first stipend ($25,000) from
the Commonwealth of Pennsylvania.[35] Later, Andrew Carnegie provided a like amount. Yearly, the Alumnae Association, board, faculty,
and students offered their support, while Clara Marshall pleaded for
funds to whoever would listen, as Ann Preston had done for Woman's
Hospital in the 1850s.[36] Construction began on the permanent hospital in 1907 and proceeded a floor at a time as money became available,
with sections placed in use along the way. It was not complete until
1913, but its visible progress satisfied the Council on Medical Education.

About the same time as the completion of the hospital in 1913,
the College learned with disappointment that the AMA rating system
failed to list it as "Class A+," a designation bestowed on only the few
most progressive schools. Dean Marshall requested a statement of explanation. The reply from N. P. Colwell, the AMA secretary for the
Council of Medical Education, based on an earlier inspection, brought
unwelcome attention to real deficiencies that even threatened the Class
A (acceptable) rating. First, WMC still required for entrance only a
high-school diploma plus a course in inorganic chemistry, while Class
A+ schools demanded a year of "college grade" physics, chemistry, and
biology. The faculty and board periodically discussed a higher standard,
but moved slowly, always fearful of a consequent loss of enrollment.[37]
Second, "your college did not have as many expert, full-time, salaried
professors as the majority of colleges included in Class A." Third, there
was inadequate "clinical material," though Colwell recognized that this
need would improve with completion of the hospital. Fourth, asserted
the secretary, the College lacked certain desirable equipment, such as
a "balopticon, embryologic models, a microphotographic outfit, a
projectoscope." Fifth, there is little or no research, and no "atmosphere
of investigation." Sixth, the curriculum provided no "modern course in
pharmacology," a relatively new science in 1913.[38]

Colwell acknowledged that there were "of course, many fine points
about your school which are worthy of the highest commendation," and
offered his help by way of letters to encourage endowment. Only increased funding could correct the deficiencies.

In 1911 under Dr. Blanca Hillman (a 1905 graduate), the Alumnae Association initiated a Committee on Endowment.[39] They could hardly do otherwise: at each annual meeting Dean Marshall sounded the word and cast it in upper case for the printed version: "ENDOW-MENT!"[40] In cooperation with the corporators, the association issued a handsomely printed pamphlet to make the College better known and gather support. It began with a brief historical outline stressing the lineage of heroines and one hero (Isaac Barton). Subsequent pages displayed photographs of each laboratory filled with conspicuously diligent students and instructors. Finally appeared a colored map showing "the Importance of this College to Christian Missions." The messages were clear: the Woman's Medical College claims a distinctive past; in the present it scientifically prepares women for medicine; and—a continuity with that past—readies some for medical service to women throughout the world, a Christian mission.[41] In 1914 a new Joint Committee on Endowment contracted with a "public-relations" firm, News Distributing Company: the quest for "good copy" had begun in earnest and never would cease.[42]

Adding an extraordinary component to the publicity program, the College paid to have made "a film of motion pictures, illustrating the activities of the College." It was shown at the Panama Exposition in San Francisco, and extensively at women's colleges, high schools, and private homes. The film followed the activities of a student as she first entered the College, working in laboratories and on the wards, competing in a basketball game, and at last attending commencement. Another sequence featured the maternity practice on Washington Avenue. The film concluded with a tableau exactly recreating the famous sentimental painting "The Doctor" by Luke Fildes, except, of course, that a woman practitioner holds vigil.[43]

Alumna mailboxes received direct appeals to "catch anew the spirit of the dear old College that graduated Ann Preston, Emmeline [sic] Cleveland, Clara Swain, Anna E. Broomall—and you!"—and send a donation.[44] Many alumnae did, even if large gifts were few. The school's distinctive history and its promise of current opportunity for women became forever linked in its self-presentation to the world: its leaders wanted students to come and friends to endow based on what WMC had been and what it still could be.

At the conclusion of this campaign in 1917, over $200,000 had been pledged, with over $114,000 in hand, a testimony to alumnae loyalty.[45] Another campaign launched in early 1920 also led to over $200,000 in pledges or contributions. Yet, somehow, the financial health of the school and its hospital continued to decline. Following the elevation of entrance requirements in 1915 to at least the equivalent of two years of college, enrollment slipped (to under fifty total students at its worst) and with it tuition dollars.[46]

Also, not all the money raised in the campaigns actually entered general endowment: much of it went to designated funds and categorical scholarships that could not always be used. Hospital expenses continued to increase. By the end of May 1918, the "accumulated deficiency in income" totaled $29,980.[47]

The pressure of financial peril led the College to again consider merger. Apparently some quiet communication went to the University of Pennsylvania in 1916, perhaps through a third party. But Clara Marshall was shown a letter in which the dean of Penn's medical school said this about possible merger with WMC: "I don't think it would be worth the while to talk about a 'union.' The University must dominate, so that the only thing we could consider would be a complete absorption. If there is any one who cares to speak to me along that line, I will be glad to meet them."[48] Whatever sentiments existed for merging into Penn no doubt vanished when this letter appeared. Despite the obstacles, faculty, board members, and active alumnae stubbornly insisted on the independent survival of the College, and of single-sex medical education for women.

At the Fiscal Brink

But the deficits continued, bringing on a crisis in the spring of 1921. The board approved borrowing from special funds (such as scholarship trusts) to pay operating costs. In addition, the College had yet to pay twenty-five thousand dollars in bills and the hospital faced a twenty-thousand-dollar deficit.[49] The president of the board since 1913, Emily Sargent Lewis, resigned, and a new administration took over in June, headed by Mrs. Sarah Logan Wister Starr (1874–1956).

Philadelphians will recognize in that appellation a string of familiar names long associated with the city. Mrs. Starr was a Philadelphia patrician and club woman, a member and often leader of correct and useful organizations of all sorts, with access to Philadelphia's upper crust. No doubt Starr, like the College's first woman president, Mary Mumford, had acquired administrative skill through club work.[50] Her father was a man of business, and her husband for a time worked for a coal-mining concern, so she knew something of methods and customs of the business world. Walter Lee Sheppard, a lawyer and member of the board, and friend of Dean Martha Tracy, became her faithful right-hand man. Mrs. Starr's first action was to lend the College six thousand dollars to pay salaries.[51]

It so happened that the annual meetings of the board of corporators and of the Alumnae Association took place concurrently in 1921 in different rooms of the College. Mrs. Starr on 17 June dramatically walked from one to the other to address the alumnae and seek their immediate aid; she herself had already announced her loan. She began: "[L]ast night I was your guest on a perfectly delightful occasion [presumably the annual alumnae dinner] in which you instructed me in the form in which you are so familiar and about which I know nothing, so it is a comfort to me at this time to come and tell you something about which you know nothing"—the desperate and disordered state of College finances. She challenged the alumnae to immediately pledge ten thousand dollars in loans. First Ellen C. Potter declared her one thousand dollars "without interest"; then Frances C. Van Gasken, Martha Schetky, Eleanor C. Jones, Bertha Connely, Catharine Macfarlane, and others pledged money or securities.[52] They had attended WMC during the last years of the nineteenth century and first of the twentieth, what we have referred to as its golden period. Their teachers, and in some cases friends, had been Clara Marshall, Anna Broomall, Henry Leffmann, Frances Emily White, Arthur Stevens. WMC had provided them their profession and uncommon memories of youth: now they acted to save their alma mater.

This "Emergency Loan Fund," added to larger bank loans and other actions, stabilized the College's precarious fiscal deterioration. The Woman's Medical College was saved—saved by women. And indeed by 1921 it had become in some ways more of a Woman's Medical College than ever before. The head of the new board (most old members had resigned) and actual chief executive—Starr—was female. The March 1921 issue of the *Bulletin* began with a photograph of "The Major Faculty," showing thirteen women and only three men.[53] When most of women's medical education moved toward coeducation, the remaining women's school became more fully than ever a place run by women for women. In a way, this made for a clearer choice and placed more at stake for those reviving the nearly insolvent survivor. At least one women's school had managed to tack around Flexner, the American Medical Association, hospital disputes, and near-bankruptcy.

Survival came, as it always would, at some costs. "Centralized, executive control" became the watchword of recovery. Mrs. Starr insisted that she as chief executive and the new executive committee oversee all fiscal dealings of the College and hospital.[54] In addition, according to Starr, "as might have been expected, a deeply rooted individualism permeated the institution, enabling the strongest and most aggressive personalities in the Faculty and Staff to dominate."[55] She wanted rational management and fiscal control from the top down.

Sarah Logan Wister Starr did not invent phrases or notions such as "centralized executive control," "chief executive," nor "individualism," though they were new to the minutes and publications of the Woman's Medical College. The so-called "Progressive Era" (roughly the 1890s to 1915) accentuated the value of expertise, methodology, and the application of science and rationality to the conduct of all aspects of society. The growth of giant business generated a set of principles of "scientific management," built of centralized oversight and coordination.[56] "Individualism," which when "rugged" had once denoted the American spirit, now could be seen as an impediment to rational planning and management. And Mrs. Starr probably wrote correctly, for only strong individuals could have guided a woman's medical school through so many years of struggle.

Some Faculty of the New Century

By 1905 the faculty had lost to retirement Frances Emily White, Anna Broomall, and Hannah Croasdale, all of whom invested the late nineteenth-century WMC with their distinction and varied personalities. Adelaide Ward Peckham in bacteriology and Ruth Webster Lathrop in physiology spanned the first two decades of the century as stalwarts of the teaching staff, though neither became notable as researchers.[57] Alice Weld Tallant (1875–1968), a medical graduate of Johns Hopkins University, assumed the chair of obstetrics in 1905 and proved as teacher and practitioner a worthy successor to Broomall.

The year 1917 saw the retirement of three pillars of the College. Clara Marshall stepped down as dean, no doubt worn out from battles and begging, but aware of her accomplishments. Marshall had begun classes at WMC when students still learned from Ann Preston, the first woman dean—abolitionist, poet, practitioner; Marshall turned over *her* deanship to Martha Tracy (1876–1942), also a WMC graduate, physiological chemist, and doctorate in public health. Marshall lived until the age of eighty-three and maintained a deep interest in her College.

Second only to Dr. Marshall's tenure on the faculty was the long association of the polymath Henry Leffmann, who counted among Philadelphia's most resolute male friends of the College and the cause of medical women. Leffmann's graceful letter of resignation in 1917 assured his "dear friends and former colleagues" of his "respect and esteem," and that the "interests of the Woman's Medical College of Pa. will be prominent in my mind." He concluded with verse:

> The play is done, the curtain drops,
> Slow falling to the prompter's bell.
> A moment yet the actor stops,
> And looks around to say—
> > farewell.[58]

In fact, Leffmann reprised his part briefly, returning from retirement to lecture when the faculty lost many of its members to war work in 1918–1919. Frederick P. Henry, professor of the principles and practice of medicine since 1891, also stepped down in 1917.[59] Henry recommended that Frances C. Van Gasken succeed him, she having worked "faithfully in the interests of the College for many years."[60] Ruth Webster Lathrop also favored Van Gasken. Van Gasken (WMC, 1890) was chief of the medical service at Woman's Hospital of Philadelphia, and held the College title of "professor of clinical medicine." The other faculty, however, favored an internist and educator named George Morris Piersol, who was elected. Van Gasken's position was elevated to a seat in the major faculty, with voting right in the absence of the chair of medicine. It seems that some unwritten rule called for a male in this post. In any case, Van Gasken remained actively involved in College and alumnae affairs, and a memorable teacher.[61]

Curriculum

WMC certainly aspired to Flexnerian ideals with its laboratory work, already substantial in the 1890s and abounding by the twentieth century. First year brought immediate elevation to the "sky parlor," the students' name for the old skylit dissection rooms on the top floor of the College. Osteology ("bones") seemed a particularly onerous challenge. According to the annual announcements, physiology prescribed a great deal of practical work ("frogs and turtles became our daily torture and delight"), as did histology, for which each student was expected to prepare one hundred to two hundred slides to be kept as a personal reference library. Microbiology work comprised ten hours weekly for twelve weeks during which students gained acquaintance with a wide variety of bacteria and parasites and learned the techniques for culturing "pus, sputum, blood, etc."[62] Almost all the materia medica-pharmacology course was taught in the laboratory. A committee to review "laboratory instruction" in 1915 concluded that the total hours of laboratory exercises equaled those of the University of Pennsylvania or Johns Hopkins, but practical, diagnostic instruction might be improved.[63]

Of course, the curriculum still contained large numbers of lectures and recitations (quizzes) throughout the four years, though the fourth offered most of the clinical activity. Students attended clinical lectures and did hospital work at the College hospital, the nearby German Hospital (later called Lankenau Hospital), and at the city hospitals. In fourth-year medicine "the students are assigned cases which they follow and study carefully, making the routine clinical and laboratory examinations."[64] Beginning with the Annual Announcement for 1916–17, students were promised "service as clinical clerks," though it is unclear

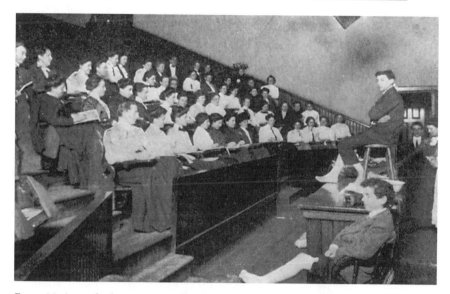

Figure 14. A standard component of medical education in the nineteenth and early twentieth century was the demonstration clinic, such as this one in which WMC students observed orthopedic cases. *Scalpel,* 1911.

what this actually entailed. A class historian wrote that "section work, whose intricacies taxed our ingenuity to keep in order, has, nevertheless, given broad and valuable lessons in practical work."[65] Outpatient work probably proved of even more value in the period we are exploring. "Need we recall Barton Dispensary, with its varied crowd?" rhetorically asked the class historian of 1911 about work in the College's outpost within the immigrant district of South Philadelphia. "There we obtained practical work; applied bandages; examined babies; took histories, in all languages except our own; saw a new phase of humanity, perhaps for the first time. Things we considered impossible to be accomplished, came to lose their formidable appearance."[66]

Pediatrics and Preventive Medicine

Two curricular initiatives that resonated with the times and with the need of WMC to further its arguments for existence were the expansion of pediatrics and of preventive and social medicine. But each of these undertakings showed that timeliness could not easily overcome inertia and institutional poverty.

"If humanitarian progressivism had a central theme," wrote historian Robert H. Wiebe, "it was the child. He united the campaigns for health, education, and a richer city environment, and he dominated much of the interest in labor legislation."[67] In the Progressive Era, the child was seen as a malleable potential for good and a resource for a better future. The nation witnessed the passage of long-sought child labor laws, innovations in education, and attention to the mother's "efficiency" in her maternal responsibilities.

The "child-saving" movements of the Progressive Era were largely the work of women reformers and social workers, including Philadelphia native Florence Kelley, a Quaker turned socialist who headed the National Consumers League, which led the campaign for child labor limitations. Another was Julia Lathrop, who directed a largely female staff in the Children's Bureau. This federal agency attempted to reduce infant mortality through programs of research and education in childhood nutrition and maternal health. Many women physicians of the Progressive Era participated in the various child welfare endeavors including working for the Children's Bureau. The specialty of pediatrics has always assumed an advocacy role as well as curative one. In this great period of child-saving, and with WMC aiming to demonstrate its special role in educating women physicians for *their* special roles, it is no surprise that the building of a pediatrics department turns up in the various minutes and announcements of the 1910s and 1920s.

Although there had been lectures on diseases of children going well back into the nineteenth century, by 1904 pediatrician Eleanor C. Jones (1861–1925) was conducting clinics at the college dispensary twice weekly for sections of students, and also presenting one amphitheater clinic for seniors.[68] Jones, one of the forgotten heroines of WMC, graduated from the College in 1887, as had her mother in 1856. At the Woman's Hospital of Philadelphia Jones developed the children's ward and later the children's building (Children's House).

Possibly because of Jones's primary affiliation with Woman's Hospital, a young physician named Theodore LeBoutillier was appointed professor of pediatrics beginning in 1908. By 1915 instruction included a variety of lectures, demonstration clinics, and quizzes throughout the third and fourth year. Twice weekly, students had some opportunity to examine children and infants. In 1918, LeBoutillier headed off to war service.[69] Eleanor Jones was appointed acting professor of pediatrics, and the Woman's Hospital (selectively cooperating again with WMC) agreed to the provision "of instruction by Dr. Eleanor C. Jones in dispensary and ward as she deems advisable."[70] On his return in March of 1919, LeBoutillier offered to relinquish his chair in favor of Jones, though he agreed to stay on as an adjunct in pediatrics; the latter arrangement allowed him to continue instruction at the Municipal Hospital (a hospital for infectious diseases run by the city).[71] Here occurred another example of bi-gender agreement and good will familiar to the College.

Dr. Jones wrote in accepting the faculty's nomination that she hoped the "Department of Pediatrics will continue to develop, and that in a few years we shall have full hospital and dispensary service."[72] Unfortunately, her hopes arose exactly at the nadir of the College's ability to pay for expansion. And even with Dr. Jones as chief of pediatrics at both the College and the Woman's Hospital, the latter's busy "Children's House" became only minimally available for instruction. Thus financial and political encumbrances prevented what might have been a powerful attraction for WMC—a premier department in service to the child and to pediatric instruction. Still, pediatrics had secured a foothold under a capable chief.

Even more agonizingly slow was progress toward a strong program in preventive medicine which would build on Frances Emily White's early efforts. During the first decades of the twentieth century, many women physicians embraced both older melioristic and newer laboratory-based approaches to public health and disease prevention. Though numerically men dominated the professional field of public health, according to Regina Morantz-Sanchez "women physicians' concerns were wide-ranging," encompassing both science-based prevention, health education, and social welfare.[73] In many of these efforts women doctors and women's clubs collaborated.

For some years during the 1910s, a faculty member named Randall Rosenberger served as professor of hygiene and preventive medicine at WMC. His course of one lecture weekly throughout the second year comprised "personal hygiene" (e.g., effects of food, exercise, and bathing);

"domestic hygiene" (e.g., water supply, ventilation, food poisoning); and "public hygiene" (e.g., prevention of infectious diseases, purification of water, school hygiene).[74] When Rosenberger left, Henry Leffmann looked after this course for several years, adding at least one site visit.

When Leffmann retired in 1917, Martha Tracy added the direction of the hygiene course to her responsibilities as professor of physiological chemistry and dean. Her intellectual interests had indeed moved toward public health, and it was also in 1917 that Tracy received a doctorate in public hygiene from the University of Pennsylvania. She began immediate efforts to expand the College's presence in both public health and related social medicine. Already in the 1916–17 session, the school provided for senior students a new elective course in social medicine which comprised mainly site visits to observe the city's Bureau of Child Hygiene, health inspection at schools, and a "correctional institution for girls."[75] The College also offered a series of public lectures on topics dealing with public health and prevention, in a modest way reviving a role—going back to its founding and Ann Preston's public lectures—as educator for health. Tracy envisioned an expanded undergraduate curriculum and a postgraduate program that would comprise modern instruction and research in "child hygiene," inspection of school children, nutrition, industrial hygiene with emphasis on women employees, control of infectious disease, and other topics "which especially claim the attention of women physicians."[76] With funds from the National American Woman Suffrage Association she began in 1932 the Anna Howard Shaw Health Service for Women, a "health Clinic where women of moderate means may receive for a moderate fee a careful, detailed physical examination and advice."[77] This initiative marked one of the first incidents of support for the College by women outside Philadelphia.

Martha Tracy maintained an enduring interest in preventive medicine, but she relinquished the professorship in 1931 to Sarah I. Morris (1879–1969), a 1910 graduate of WMC, who did advanced training in preventive medicine and public health at the Johns Hopkins School of Hygiene and Public Health. Morris left a faculty position at the University of Wisconsin, a progressive environment, when recruited by

Tracy. Morris established a four-year curriculum in prevention, conducted the student health service, and directed the diagnostic clinic for women. While the curriculum relied on the didactic lecture, Morris resumed or expanded field trips to sewage plants, factories, water treatment facilities, and other sites.[78] She added new topics to the third- and fourth-year lectures, including what she referred to, in a phrase suitable for the annual announcements, as "certain controversial problems confronting the medical profession." The country was deep in the Great Depression, so one may presume these topics included the organization of medical care and perhaps even health insurance. Martha Tracy had some years earlier revived the senior thesis, designating that it address a topic in prevention. Morris continued to supervise them. One year she upheld, against general faculty opposition, the choice of one student of the 1930s to write on medical care in the Soviet Union.[79]

Despite her earnest efforts, in the 1930s Morris encountered only mixed enthusiasm for her department's work. In fact, when Tracy and Morris eventually left the College (Tracy in 1940, Morris in 1945), the department of preventive medicine virtually collapsed.[80] Even at the Woman's Medical College, whose historic mission looked back to the ideal of women educating women for the maintenance of health, preventive medicine remained fragile. Especially in the period after World War II, medicine increasingly honored surgical and technologic cure, not prevention. Students read this message, and few could feel excitement contemplating a visit to the local filtration plant. But the tradition of incorporating preventive medicine had taken root, and the small but progressive department would revive under Katherine Boucot Sturgis in the 1950s.

From the Students' Perspective

Despite the ever-expanding quantity of work in laboratory, lecture hall, and clinic, students of the period 1900 to 1920 continued most of the traditions established by their predecessors.[81] The annual Halloween masque and dance given by the sophomores remained popular. The event always included some sort of "skits" at the expense of faculty. The gymnasium housed social events and basketball games: each class generated a team, and games attracted students and faculty. Some of the more ethereal collegiate customs we encountered in the 1890s, such as the class color and class cheer, apparently died out, replaced by parodies— the class cough, class giggle, and class blush.

From 1910 through 1914, students published a small monthly magazine full of stories, vignettes, and news, as well as countless puns and bad jokes. The thirty-two graduates of 1911 even managed to prepare and publish the College's first "annual," or yearbook, a remarkable treasure of almost two hundred pages.[82] Its photographs documented collegiate activities and that Fairmount Park's ageless beauty continued to beckon WMC students for walks, excursions, and canoeing on the Wissahickon Creek.

In contrast to the 1890s, but consistent with trends in the extra-collegiate world, suffrage appeared regularly in the College. Several editorials turned up in the school magazine, including one by faculty member Ellen Culver Potter.[83] Rita S. Finkler, a 1915 graduate, recalled "many parades in which some of us participated, carried banners, wore sashes across our chest with slogans of 'Votes for Women.'"[84] At one Halloween send-up, there appeared in "neurology clinic" a suffragette, who, in her "ardor and enthusiasm, raged and raved, struggled and fought."[85]

Minutes of the Student Association and faculty document that like their predecessors, the early twentieth-century students showed no hesitation in bringing complaints to the dean and the teaching corps, but no bitter discord arose. The yearbooks' contents suggest considerable affection for the teaching staff (and for Alfred Congo, the African-American custodian and practical advisor to students). Class votes recorded in the yearbooks from 1911 and 1914 ("Votes by Women: Winners in the Great Contest!") showed that the most popular professors included Arthur Stevens, Alice Tallant, Ellen Culver Potter, F. P. Henry, and Henry Leffmann.[86] From 1900 into the early 1920s, WMC still enjoyed a cohesive sense of unity and purpose shared by most students and faculty.

And WMC of the early twentieth century occasionally afforded its students a transcendent experience nowhere else available to the young woman preparing for a medical life. Let us extract one student's story that perfectly declares the meaning of WMC for much of its existence, and embodies the arguments it always pleaded when defending its being as the sole surviving women's medical school. In "Our Evening In," senior student Frances Petty Manship recounted for 1912 readers of the *Iatrian* an evening when she and several students were called by telephone to attend a Cesarean section at Blockley, where the WMC professor of gynecology, Ella Everitt, was on staff.

"The trolley crawled down town, then rushed through its Subway tube and landed us at Thirty-Fourth Street, and presently we were before the bleak white walls of old Blockley." The WMC students climbed the spiral staircase to the amphitheater, where "off in the wings were groups of internes, looking like nice white clad boy angels." The ether was being administered and other preliminaries attended to. From the front row, which the WMC students occupied, Manship, senior "med" and reporter, described the scene:

> Bestowed modestly in a corner was Dr. Everitt, swathed like a surgeon to be sure—but remote and detached, looking a good deal as if she had never done a day's work, and had no interest in the present occasion. In a nook on the other side loomed up Dr. Potter, also in official raiment. . . . We had the delicious knowledge that when the other people finished monkeying around, these two demure ones would move together in the center of the scene and *do* things.
>
> So it turned out. The anaesthetist began to give ether by the eye of faith, his physical ocular apparatus being glued to the field of operation; the young interne (male sex) gathered up his sponges in business-like fashion. And then Dr. Potter draped herself over the table, ready for her famous strangle hold on the uterine arteries. Dr. Everitt picked up the knife—and the rest writes itself in the minds of all of us who have seen her operate.
>
> When the operation was over, after the patient and attendants had left, we Seniors and Juniors swarmed down into the arena. We did not actually hug Dr. Everitt in the flesh, though we certainly did in spirit. Also we limbered up our tongues and said something of what we really felt. We didn't get called down for it, either. There are times when the real sentiments come to the surface. . . .

It's a little different proposition to see our leaders work in
alien climes and still keep the colors nailed to the masthead. We
just naturally get some edema of the glottis and cardiac tissue.[87]

There is a good deal that invites analysis in this tale: the quality of
adventure; the adulation of surgical skill; the virtual absence of the patient from the writer's sensibility. But the essential meaning is clear:
though she refers to "our leaders" rather than directly to gender,
Manship does not fail to twice point out that men were present—interns, *taking orders* from Everitt and Potter. She and her companions
witnessed women surgeons, their professors, display consummate skill
in what was still a male stronghold, where female faltering would still
have been for some a welcome exhibition. "Role model" fails to capture the heady exhilaration of the moment. For at least some students
like Manship, who in another article called WMC "a great old school,"
the early twentieth-century College retained the capacity to win an
emotionally vital allegiance.[88]

Manship documented an event that not every WMC student had
the opportunity to witness. But, in the period we are reviewing, when
students chose to write, one particular activity known to every graduate most attracted their literary effort—acquiring their ten cases (up
from the six required in the 1890s) at the "South Pole."

South Pole was the name the WMC students gave to the maternity practice in the poor district of south Philadelphia, begun by Anna
Broomall in 1887. During the first two decades of the twentieth century, the flow of immigrants into the district accelerated, especially Ital-
ians and Russian Jews. Seniors had to dwell for one or two slots of time
at the old building at 333 Washington Avenue. There they lived and
slept, on call to be fetched for deliveries at home, which, unless difficulty arose, they managed on their own. Accompanied by the husband,
the student accoucheurs visited the "vermin-infested matchboxes, boil-
ing in summer, freezing in winter," that the countless immigrant families endured.[89]

The South Pole expedition unquestionably formed the most un-
forgettable phase of clinical work at WMC from the late 1880s through
the late 1920s. "My baby work was pulled off successfully—two Jews
(one on Christmas Eve!) one Italian, one Greek and a Swiss. I man-

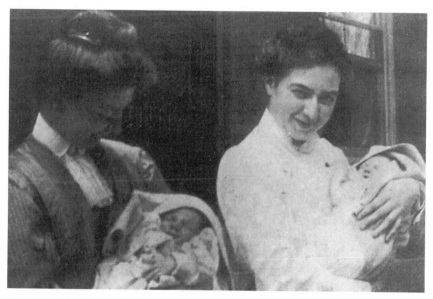

Figure 15. WMC senior students c. 1910 show off infants they helped deliver during their stay at the maternity outpost. *Scalpel*, 1911.

aged to save the father in each case," student Elizabeth Clark told a friend in 1909.[90] "Nothing I have ever done since has quite equaled that time in colour and unexpectedness," wrote another graduate of her summer days at the maternity in 1926.[91] Frances Petty Manship, evidently open to the variety of life's offerings, addressed her Washington Avenue days in another essay for the *Iatrian*. Framed as an open letter to a friend and recent graduate, Manship wrote, "I can't get the words to express just what the experience meant to me. To put it palely, I had a very large time."[92] She confided her fascination with the old "senior bags," the ancient containers of needed utensils and medications handed down from student to student to be carried to each delivery.[93] Manship enjoyed the camaraderie of the "Barton bunch—a little group of educated, cultivated women with no frills or pretensions, just trying to run two hospital adjuncts creditably and helpfully. And, after all, they are just girls alone here in the unlovely slums."[94] She described some of the actual maternity work as follows:

> As to the work itself, you know how it is to be on call and lie
> awake nights scared stiff, and to feel that the hurrying footsteps
> of the night nurse are treading on your vitals.

All my cases were normal except a placenta previa case, on which I had to have help. I doubt if I ever saw anything that looked quite so good as the sight of Dr. Kraker [an assistant in the obstetrics faculty] speeding around the street corner in the gray morning light with a bundle-laden Junior in tow.

A 1911 class historian summarized some of the meaning found in the south Philadelphia maternity service:

We were shut off from the world—from *our world*—but not from another, which was quite as real, although as much novelty to us as the South Pole might be. . . . We were entrusted with responsibility, "just like a real doctor" for the first time; we were entrusted with human lives; we had the opportunity to put in practice the knowledge we had gained during our course. Oh, how we sat down on our dusty, rickety chair in the Senior room, which should have been called the *Senior cell*, to wait for that first call![95]

The maternity rotation in the southeast district had the allure of adventure and exploration as students made an expedition from the familiar regions of North College Avenue to the bustling, noisy slums of south Philadelphia. Though there to deliver babies, they could not help but receive an introductory education in poverty and its consequences; how "the other half lived" became apparent in unavoidable detail. No doubt some students gained a new social awareness, while others felt merely disgust. Even graduates of the 1930s and late 1940s remembered the shock of immersion into unimagined domestic squalor as they tended to their home deliveries.[96]

More important, the experience was for the WMC students their first as "real doctors": the initial occasion when they were charged with using what they had learned to take care of patients on their own—with help available, but not always in sight. Gathering the ten delivery cases formed a rite of outward passage for seniors that far exceeded in emotional content the entry rite of freshmen bone study. In the small crowded houses of German, Italian, or Russian families on South Fourth, Fitzwater, and even Catherine Street (near William Mullen's old House of Industry), students shared in a usually blissful event. Birth was a happy display of normal physiology despite the deprivation of the surroundings (one adds "usually" since no doubt many immigrant parents did not covet a seventh or eighth child). But always looming was the unexpected, the uncommon obstetrical calamity that threatened two young lives. Such an event sent the husband off to fetch the resident physician or even the staff obstetrician back at Washington Avenue, while the fearful senior student tried to maintain composure and initiate treatment based on firm guidelines acquired through study and no lack of drilling back at North College Avenue.

Attending births placed the young WMC student into a traditionally female event. Until the emergence of obstetrics as a medical specialty dominated by men, in Western society (and others), when a baby was due, women gathered—and men were dispatched to secondary chores. The young student from the Woman's Med owned the privilege to join some of these timeless women's gatherings, somewhat in the role of midwife, but certainly lacking in that practitioner's experience and authority. Indeed, we have no record of what the mothers thought of their tyro physicians, though some used the College service for many pregnancies.[97] Since many women physicians did not marry, the student could not help but reflect that the birth of a child was something she may—or may not—herself experience one day.

So the outdoor maternity work meant all of this, and also an opportunity to relate as junior colleague to an older sister of the medical profession—one of the "Barton bunch," or even the Chief herself. "You remember her," wrote Frances Petty Manship, "her smile, her voice, her superhuman patience."[98] The 1911 class historian wrote of this admired teacher: "Finally, we had the ten cases and then decided that, after all, the sojourn in the slums was not so bad, and that as long as Dr. Tallant was the chief, we should always be able to find a silver lining in every cloud."[99]

Johns Hopkins medical graduate Alice Weld Tallant in 1906 had inherited the chair of obstetrics and the outpatient maternity service which Anna Broomall had created. Tallant proved herself eminently suitable to oversee this most important clinical chair and the outpatient baby work, for many years the most transformative and memorable experience of WMC students. To the grievous injury of the College and its traditions, it was Tallant, the Chief of the South Pole, who found herself dismissed from the faculty in 1923, perhaps the worst possible victim of a laity-versus-faculty struggle.

WMC from 1900 to 1920 had survived the loss of its longtime hospital partner, death or retirement of cherished faculty, the Flexner Report, organized external scrutiny, and financial collapse. It remained for a ruinous internal schism to next test the school's will to carry on, a determination implemented by individuals, yet increasingly seeming to assume a supervening life of its own.

Chapter 8

The Troubled 1920s and the Tallant Affair

The 1920s and 1930s proved perilous years for WMC. Now the only remaining women's medical college in the United States, it nonetheless did not enjoy wide national support, especially financially. These were decades (especially the 1920s) in which American women favored attempts to work with men as equals and establish "companionate marriages," not to express feminist separatism.[1] WMC was not part of a university, the setting Flexnerian ideology prescribed for the American medical school. Local enthusiasm kept the small school on its lonely course as it encountered outside obstacles and the one near-suicidal internal conflict forming the main subject of this chapter. Increasingly, it attracted a segment of young women seeking medical training who did not choose to or could not fit into the major coeducational university medical schools that opened a few places to women.

The Tallant Affair

Alumnae and others interested in the Woman's Medical College in 1923 suffered the opportunity to read extraordinary passages such as the following:

> The introduction of business methods of administration of the
> Hospital was extremely difficult. The rules and orders of the

Executive Committee . . . were often ignored. The most frequent offences occurred in the Department of Obstetrics, and repeated interviews between Dr. Tallant, the Chief of that Department, and Mrs. Starr, the President of the Corporation, produced no appreciable results. She conducted her department as if it were a separate unit, altogether independent of the control of the Corporation Executive. [A statement of the board of corporators.][2]

We submit that these results of arbitrary "adoption of central administrative policy" are appropriate to Soviet Russia and not to the ethical conduct of an American College. . . . To fail to re-elect a prominent member of the faculty, an honored and distinguished physician, and then in face of a storm of protest, to fail to give any reason for this action, shows insolent abuse of power. [Expression of protest by a group of alumnae][3]

To the corporation of the Woman's Medical College of Pennsylvania:
We, the students of the Woman's Medical College, feel that injustice has been done Dr. Tallant. . . . We feel that the honor of the School as it has been upheld by our faithful Faculty members in the past is at stake. We therefore withdraw as a Student Body until a plain statement of justifiable cause be given Dr. Tallant and us or reinstatement to her former position be made.
(signed) "THE STUDENT BODY" 13 March 1923[4]

Not since the feisty years of the early 1850s had WMC community known such words of angry resolve. What triggered this monumental battle within the school was the board of corporator's immutable decision to not reappoint Alice Weld Tallant to a nineteenth year as professor of obstetrics and chief of the inpatient and outdoor maternity work. It pitted the new president and chair of the executive committee, Sarah Logan Wister Starr, against most of the faculty, an outspoken segment of the alumnae, and the students.

Starr was one of three sisters born into a branch of the prominent and affluent Pennsylvania Wister family and received her education at the elite Agnes Irwin School. Within their family, they became known as the "iron sisters": all were tough and commanding. It is safe to say that Mrs. Starr, tall and assured, was not the sort of person to whom one readily said "no": this enhanced her fund-raising effectiveness. Her grandfather's will enjoined that no women in the family work for a living, but that they place their efforts in philanthropy.[5] Mrs. Starr owned a great amount of innate ability and a deep desire to manage—to run a business—that was not adequately met by her work in various women's clubs and civic campaigns. Virtually excluded in 1921 as a woman aristocrat from actually starting and directing a business, Starr found one in WMC, at least in her mind.

Although the complicated controversy stormed from February to June of 1923, thoroughly covered by the press, an attempt will be made here to present a concise account of the incident. During the summer of 1922, the board advised Dr. Tallant that she was not complying with management's rulings in her conduct of the hospital's obstetrics service. Mrs. Starr had agreed to step in and save the College from total financial collapse on the "platform and declared policy of centralized executive control and sound business management."[6] "Centralized executive control" became almost a mantra for Mrs. Starr and her committee, business management the watchword. But Alice Weld Tallant had "proved herself altogether impossible as a subordinate."[7]

In midwinter of 1922–23, the executive committee of the board advised Tallant that she would not receive reappointment by the board for the following academic year. As word of this decision spread, so did a sense of outrage and a variety of protests. Frances C. Van Gasken, professor of clinical medicine and stalwart alumna, one unafraid of battle, led the challenge from the faculty.[8] On 13 March the students, who rated Dr. Tallant as one of their favorite professors, sent their letter of protest to the corporation. Virtually the entire enrollment signed it and followed with what now would be called a strike: they refused to appear for classes for one week.

The alumnae issued a petition, signed by about two hundred of those present at a meeting on 21 March, to the board of corporators. The document insisted only on a written statement of the "reasons for its failure to re-elect Doctor Tallant," so that if the board's decision were "just," the "widespread criticism of the College may be successfully combated and harmony restored among Corporators, Faculty, Students, and

Alumnae."[9] The board's unwillingness to reveal Tallant's transgressions in the management of her hospital department infuriated her supporters. In the absence of firm details, all manner of suspicion had arisen.

On 4 April 1923, the board supported the executive committee's decision to not reappoint Dr. Tallant by a narrow margin of nine to seven. By 9 April, a number of the senior faculty had resigned in protest, including such faithful teachers as Ruth Webster Lathrop, Frances Van Gasken, Arthur Stevens, Harry Deaver, George Peirsol, and Berta Meine; these included the professors of physiology, bacteriology, medicine, and surgery! (They would all carry out their remaining work for the academic year, however.) No doubt for some—or all—of the departing faculty, the decision to resign was poignant and painful. Van Gasken wrote to alumna Mary Riggs Noble: "However, Mrs. Starr says we are all 'old' 'they will replace us with young ones'—This is a study. But I can not tell you how this all has made me feel. My glory in and zeal for the W.M.C. to have such an inglorious ending."[10]

On 12 April, a sad and simply worded communication from the no doubt dazed and fearful students restated support for Tallant and reported that "many of us desire to make application to other colleges and feel that we cannot delay much longer. . . . While we have always felt a loyalty to the College in the past we do not feel that at present her ideals are being upheld."[11] Faculty resignations continued; Adelaide Ward Peckham, Henry Leffmann, and even Clara Marshall repudiated their emeritus titles.[12] The College seemed headed for autolysis.

A few of the senior faculty did support Mrs. Starr and "the Corporation" (Mrs. Starr favored that phrase). These included Martha Tracy, who was a close friend of Walter Sheppard, the board's vice president and counsel, and Mrs. Starr's most faithful retainer. Alumna and recently appointed professor of gynecology Catharine Macfarlane, later one of the preeminent figures of the faculty, did not much care for Tallant and stood firmly with Starr and the board, as did senior clinicians Margaret Butler in otolaryngology and Eleanor Jones in pediatrics.[13] Bolstered by this support, the executive committee would neither yield nor ever publicly provide details of its displeasure with the professor of obstetrics.

Who was the individual over whom this storm broke? Born in 1875, Alice Weld Tallant graduated from Smith College, did graduate work at Massachusetts Institute of Technology, then obtained her M.D. from

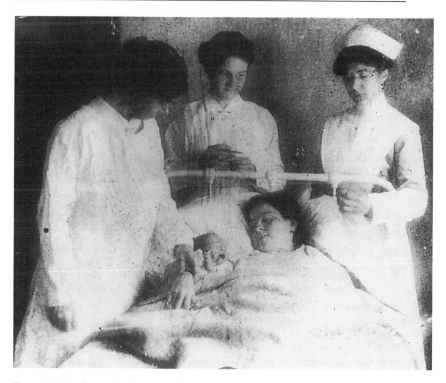

Figure 16. Professor of obstetrics Alice Weld Tallant in 1915 examines a mother, accompanied by intern Helen Taylor and an unidentified nurse. Tallant practiced, taught at WMC, and was active in national "child-saving" efforts.

Johns Hopkins in 1902.[14] She did an internship at the New England Hospital for Women and Children, then eventually came to WMC in 1905 as professor of obstetrics. In 1909 Tallant spent a summer at the Charité Hospital in Berlin, and during World War I served in France with the Smith College Relief Unit and the American Committee for Devastated France, then with two French evacuation hospitals. France awarded her the Croix de Guerre.

By 1923, Tallant had served nearly twenty years on the faculty. She became known beyond the College for her prominence in the "child-saving" crusades of the Progressive Era.[15] Tallant also authored a *Text-book of Obstetrical Nursing* in 1922, and dedicated it to the "nurses who have worked with me for the welfare of our patients in the Maternity of the Woman's Medical College of Pennsylvania."[16] Aware of her elite educational background and attainments, Tallant indeed probably

evinced indifference to hospital regulations and the niceties of accounting. Three medical directors of the College's hospital attested that she
could be uncooperative in following directives aimed at enhancing revenue to the hospital of the WMC.[17]

Although the board never publicly revealed examples of its complaints, archival files shed light on some of Tallant's perceived offenses.[18]
A "Mrs. Steel" required a uterine curettage following miscarriage. Dr.
Tallant wanted to do the procedure in a treatment room rather than in
the operating room, and sought to have an intern give the anesthetic.
"This was an attempt to save the patient all possible hospital expense
and secure for her private patients' privileges," wrote the hospital's medical director. In other cited examples the chief of obstetrics apparently
circumvented rules to reduce hospital charges for women seen by administration as capable of paying full rates.

Tallant for many years had been attending physician at the girls'
division of the Philadelphia House of Refuge, later called Sleighton
Farm, a progressive "reform" school.[19] When state reimbursement to the
hospital for care of Sleighton Farm girls was threatened, Dr. Tallant several times still admitted them, against management's directive, "because
they were interesting cases for interns, needed observation, etc." One
young woman on probation was admitted when "those whom she lived
with were unwilling to care for her." So it would seem that Alice Tallant
ignored some fiscal rules because she did not care to be bothered, and
others to reduce costs for women of modest means. At other times, she
was looking after the needs of young offenders, presumably pregnant
while unwed.

Starr and her circle by no means opposed *any* form of help to the
poor, but had acutely in mind the fiscal collapse of 1921 and the rising
expenses of the hospital. The executive committee's position was far
from arbitrary, even if objection to admitting Sleighton Farm girls also
reflected typical class attitudes.

On the other hand, Tallant's supporters—most of the faculty, students, and many alumnae—also argued from strength: the dismissal of
a senior professor based on ill-defined charges unrelated (by admission)
to academic performance defied professional custom and could prove
highly injurious to the school, as well as to the individual. And by the
worse chance, the nationally known professor under attack was the chair

of *obstetrics*—the much admired "chief" of the traditionally and symbolically most important clinical department of the College, who oversaw the students' most transforming clinical experience.

Mrs. Starr and the board held out, and prevailed. Unfortunately, the entire battle received prolific coverage in the regional press, calling attention to the school's parochial leadership.

The Tallant dispute points out some of the underlying issues that would confront WMC for decades. WMC was not a university school and had to rely on its own form of internal governance. While a university also has a board of trustees ultimately responsible for financial integrity and overall policy, the layers of academic process and custom might have prevented the direct lay involvement that led to the Tallant disaster and would later attract the displeasure of the AMA Council on Medical Education. WMC was not affluent: if it were, Tallant's offenses might have been overlooked. Tallant's behavior also revealed the potential for conflict in the medical school hospital's conflated roles as charity, business, and academic enterprise.

Antagonists Tallant and Starr may be seen as two examples of the public woman of the 1920s. Both sought and earned standing and power rarely ceded to women before this time. Tallant's authority derived from professional training and recognition; Starr's from ability, but mainly from money and family stature—enduring and ponderous determinants in the city of Biddles and Logans.

The nearly suicidal Tallant incident proved once again the strength of feeling that WMC had the capacity to induce in students, faculty, alumnae, and even board members. Of course, the awful business interrupted the saga and dissolved internal harmony. It took time for the College to reconstitute itself as a distinctive and worthy entity. Eventually, it did so, but in some ways would never be the same.

Reorganization

The work of the College continued and students enrolled, though in diminished numbers. The executive committee was somehow able to recruit new major faculty, some of considerable reputation. Philadelphia housed a large pool of experienced and aspiring medical teachers, men and women. Among the newcomers were internist Henry Jump

(1867–1949), next in the succession of male clinical faculty who developed strong allegiance to WMC. He became a favorite teacher, participated fully in College affairs, and even served as dean during Martha Tracy's sabbatical. Lida Stewart-Cogill (1869?–1943), chief of obstetrics at the Woman's Hospital of Philadelphia, replaced Tallant in the critical professorship of obstetrics, while Tallant herself remained in practice in Philadelphia. Stewart-Cogill, a WMC graduate of 1890, continued the interest in prenatal care pioneered by her friend and teacher Anna Broomall.[20]

Perhaps the most celebrated addition, whose recruitment negotiations actually began in 1919, was the Canadian pathologist Maude Abbott (1869–1940), an authority on congenital heart defects and one of the most recognized women medical scientists of the 1920s and 1930s. Dr. Abbott came literally "on loan" to the College from McGill University to build a modern department of pathology.[21] The ebullient "Maudie" became known as "the Big Chief of Hearts" at WMC, where, according to her successor, Helen Ingleby, she "did a wonderful job. It was just after the great schism, and she set herself to reconcile warring factions and heal the breach. No one could resist that amazing personality for long, and members of rival camps would forget their differences sitting side by side at her jolly parties. Her interest in the institution never waned."[22] Indeed, through two years of energetic work the famous pathologist and Oslerian secured a small place in the College saga.[23]

In part aided by the Canadian visitor, some degree of harmony reemerged within the WMC faculty. Despite the creation of a new board-faculty joint committee to oversee faculty affairs,[24] however, WMC entered a long period of near autocratic rule by a small clique headed by Sarah Logan Wister Starr that included Dean Martha Tracy, Walter Lee Sheppard, board secretary Vida Hunt Francis, Catharine Macfarlane, and a few others.[25] When Marion Fay, later dean and president of the College, came as head of physiological chemistry in 1935, she found that Mrs. Starr ("an amazing character") "took the place as her private charity . . . which had some advantages—because every year, when the College came out in the red, she would go and press all her wealthy friends."[26] Of the commitment to the College of Starr and her

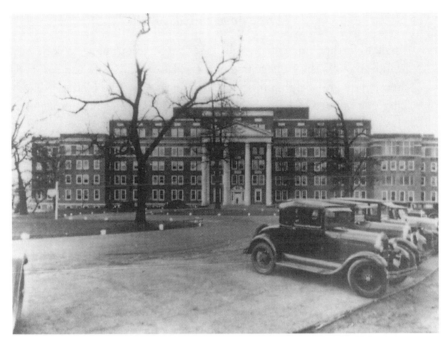

Figure 17. In 1930 Woman's Medical College left North College Avenue after seventy years to occupy this building in the East Falls section of Philadelphia. It remains part of MCP Hahnemann School of Medicine and Medical College of Pennsylvania Hospital.

coterie, no doubt exists: if near tyranny won out, it was of the sort weakly condoned as benign.

Yet a kind of hardness became part of WMC. Mrs. Starr certainly owned this attribute even before the Tallant battle; and Martha Tracy, though a sterling woman endowed with humor and wisdom, is recalled as stern in class and often rigid as dean. A 1929 graduate remembered how Tracy sat down the new freshmen and told them "you've got to measure up or you'll be out."[27] The dominant figure of "Kitty Mac" (Catharine Macfarlane) could also display an imperious manner on occasions, though most alumnae recall her with affection and sometimes reverence.[28] To some extent, such toughness proved necessary for the struggles that immediately followed the reconstitution of the school, which had—against daunting odds—survived a hectic first quarter of the twentieth century to celebrate its seventy-fifth anniversary in 1925.

The Move to East Falls

As if to further vindicate herself and her group, Starr undertook to raise funds to move the College to a new and larger campus in the East Falls section of Philadelphia in its northwest reaches. The College's building that opened in 1875 increasingly showed its age; and although the hospital was relatively new, its small size limited clinical work. Part of the justification for moving was, however, related to perceived deterioration of the College's old district. The alumnae representative to the board of corporators, in describing the proposed new location to the Alumnae Association in 1926, casually noted that the clinical "material is excellent and of a quality far superior to that of the negro neighborhood in which we are now situated."[29] A fund-raising brochure of 1925 merely referred to the neighborhood having "completely changed since the present buildings were erected."[30] The economic decline meant few paying patients to help support the hospital.

Philadelphia, like other large northern cities, showed a massive influx of southern African-Americans during the early twentieth century and especially during World War I—that hungry movement in search of jobs referred to as the Great Migration. The intense competition for jobs and housing heightened what were already ungenerous racial attitudes nationally prevalent in the 1910s and 1920s, though Philadelphia managed to avoid the race riots known to East St. Louis and Chicago.[31] The women and men of WMC and its board simply thought as others in their society thought, showing prejudicial attitudes typical of the times.

An official published statement gives an accurate sense of the East Falls neighborhood in 1926 and of the perceived needs of the College:

> It is the site of an old-time mansion, and the trees which were planted many years ago have grown to magnificent proportions. To the south and southwest lies the river and Fairmount Park. To the northwest is a city reservoir. The light and air and sunshine, so necessary to the College, as well as to the Hospital, can never be shut off.
>
> The site is especially well adapted for its accessibility to clinical material for the Hospital and the dispensaries. It will be the only hospital within a wide radius. The nearness of large

industrial plants such as the Midvale Steel, the Pencoyd Iron
Works, the Atwater Kent Manufacturing Company, the Budd
Wheel Company, to name but a few, as well as such industrial
centers as the mills of the Falls of the Schuylkill [an earlier
name for East Falls] and the Manayunk Mill district, will insure
plenty of patients to the accident wards of the Hospital. Within
easy access by street car is a large Italian district, which will be
served by the dispensary and clinics. A rapidly developing
neighborhood of modest homes is immediately adjacent to the
site, and if the Hospital can place private and semi-private
rooms within the financial reach of families of modest incomes,
it will render a great service. Finally, the site is sufficiently near
Germantown, with its population of well-to-do families, to
insure the use of its private rooms.[32]

To raise funds for the new building, Mrs. Starr and the corporators
launched yet another campaign under the name "The Greater Woman's
Medical College."[33] A small pamphlet from 1925 listed "twenty-one reasons for giving the Woman's Medical College of Pennsylvania your support." These included a putative need for more places to educate women
in medicine; meeting the need for women doctors in special fields, such
as child health work and the missionary field; the opportunity for
women to study in small classes with women "holding major positions
on both teaching and hospital staffs"; "the privilege of choice" as men
have who choose one of the medical schools yet to admit women; the
College's strength in obstetrics, gynecology, and pediatrics; and its intent to increase opportunities in a "health maintenance division."

In 1926 the College produced another promotional booklet called
Natural Guardians of the Race—meaning women and women physicians,
but in retrospect a somewhat alarming title. Eugenics, at least as a general concept if not implemented practice, attracted the attention of a
wide spectrum of Americans in the 1920s. In addition to recalling forebears such as the Longshores and Ann Preston (reunited in memory),
the publication presented perhaps for the first time a charming illus-
tration purporting to be the original Arch Street building. The quaint
image has claimed its place in institutional publications ever since. The
first home of the College appears to be a house, the structure which
nurtures a family. Yet from the little house would symbolically grow

larger buildings and lofty works. That drawing has pleaded this message to generations: however much WMC might grow or change, the heroic founding family would not be forgotten, and students would be as daughters, not just of Aesculapius, but of their alma mater.

Although the money-raising campaign did not reach its one and one-half million-dollar goal, enough was raised to build the "Greater Woman's Medical College." The board engaged the versatile Philadelphia architectural firm Ritter and Shay, best known for some of Philadelphia's better excursions into the Art Deco style, though such would assuredly *not* be the choice for the new College campus.[34] Costs defeated ambitious proposals from the designer. The final plans combined the College and hospital into a single building of five stories and basement, with a business-like flat roof. The colossal portico was retained as the only ornamental feature, and still proclaims "temple of learning and healing" symbolically, and—unalterably carved into stone—"WOMAN'S MEDICAL COLLEGE."

In anticipation of the move to East Falls, in 1927 the College had moved the Barton Dispensary, including the outpatient maternity work, to the new neighborhood from south Philadelphia. Dean Tracy recorded this event for the alumnae with "mingled feelings of regret and expectancy."[35] Like her predecessors in the deanship, Tracy knew and honored the College's history, saw it as inextricable from the school's contemporary purpose, and recognized it as a necessary commodity in gaining support for that purpose. In 1931 she told alumnae about moving the College: "The hard work was lightened by the discovery of unexpected treasures, official records, letters, photographs and relics which were and are still a continuing source of interest and inspiration."[36] Shards of the past, from a building that sheltered many pioneer medical women, had surfaced to encourage those moving to the future.

Since the opening of the new campus in 1930, the East Falls section of Philadelphia has known the tragic de-industrialization of American cities—factory doors closed at the textile mills, at the massive Atwater Kent factory which produced fine radios, at historic Midvale Steel, even at Hohenadel, the neighborhood brewery. With rising unemployment and further demographic shifts in Philadelphia, indigent regions arose in nearby north Philadelphia and Germantown; before fifty years were spent in East Falls, the transplanted hospital of WMC again had to deal with the provision of an immense amount of free care. But the nearby streets remain green and pleasant, with an unusual admixture of modest row houses, "twins," and many English-style single homes of great beauty. The College would share East Falls with judges, senators, mayors, and even one princess—as well as the numerous hardy families of working "Fallsers."[37]

The selection of the new site had merit. Yet it was also an idiosyncratic choice of the small governing group, most of whom lived in nearby affluent sections known as Germantown and Chestnut Hill. The move to East Falls meant withdrawal into partial isolation—away from the actual and implicit competition of the large downtown medical schools and hospitals, away from the medical societies, away from the center of gravity of Philadelphia and Philadelphia medicine.[38]

The Students of the 1920s and Early 1930s

Despite the work expended in organizationally and spiritually rebuilding the school after the Tallant disruption, and raising funds to physically reconstruct it in 1928–1930, the number of students knocking on the door during the 1920s and 1930s disappointed the leaders of the College and even seemed to belie the repeated assertions that there remained a critical need for such a school. The total enrollment fell below one hundred in 1925. Only eleven students graduated in 1928, eighteen in 1929, the year of breaking ground at the new site, and fourteen in 1930, when the new complex opened.[39] Historians of American women see the 1920s as a period in which the public women's movement cooled after finally capturing the vote. Ideals of separatism, of women working together, yielded to a cultivation of individual opportunity and freedom. Much of popular culture, especially films, endorsed the widest range of heterosexual experiences, including coeducation, casual sex, and the companionate marriage. The vast majority of women attending college (and large numbers did in the 1920s and 1930s) studied and played in coeducational institutions.[40]

The Woman's Medical College did provide what its rhetoric claimed: excellent instruction in the areas of supposedly greatest interest to women physicians, the opportunity to learn in an environment free of gender-based annoyance or dominance, the daily experience of seeing capable women manage the institution, teach, and carry out medical and surgical care. But the times simply did not favor large numbers of women choosing to come to the surviving women's medical school, or to medical school at all; and the horrid publicity of 1923 almost surely hindered recruitment.

Of those who did come, many had no easy time of it. The attrition rate was high in the 1920s and 1930s: the faculty minutes devote page after page to detailed discussion of problem students. One easily perceives a tension between the resolve to maintain firm standards for graduation and the willingness to give each student a reasonable opportunity to succeed.

The desire to increase class size with potentially successful students no doubt encouraged what would now be called "diversity" within the classes. WMC maintained its international character through admission of students from the orient and Europe. The class that entered in 1928 recalled the 1890s with its cosmopolitan quartet of young women from India, Russia via Turkey (but looking in a photograph every inch the American flapper), Syria, and "Porto Rico."[41] That remarkable class also included several Jewish students, and the Italian-American Alma Dea Morani, who would become a pioneer plastic surgeon, artist, and staunch friend of her alma mater and the interests of medical women.[42] A steady stream of graduates still went into missionary work.

Jewish Students at the Woman's Medical College

The class rolls of the 1930s reveal a number of Jewish names: just as qualified young Jewish women pressed for admission to universities and the "seven sisters," so did they set their sites on medical education.[43] By 1927, even the lower ranks of the auxiliary faculty included some Jews, such as Marie Finkelstein in pediatrics and Yetta Deitch, Eleanor Goldberg, and Goldie Fink in gynecology.[44] There had been earlier Jewish students. Sarah Cohen-May (1857–1934), an 1879 graduate, practiced with her brothers among Philadelphia's growing Jewish immigrant population. After finishing her work at WMC in 1886, Rebecca Fleisher

(1854–1906) spent a year as intern at the Nursery and Child's Hospital on Staten Island, then returned to Philadelphia to practice among her co-religionists; she also founded a Jewish Maternity Association. Fleisher regularly attended and participated in the annual meetings of the Alumnae Association. Cornelia Kahn (1850–1928) came from an affluent and religiously observant German-Jewish family. Following her graduation in 1887, she practiced only for a few years. Kahn later turned her attention to Jewish philanthropy.[45] But it was the 1920s and 1930s that saw a steady influx of Jewish women to the College.

On the other hand, a list of "Negro Graduates" of WMC, prepared for unknown reasons in 1962, identifies only four African-American graduates during the 1920s and none during the 1930s. The compiler of the list points out, however, that no official records recorded race, and there may well have been others.[46] Among the most distinguished graduates of WMC in the 1920s was one of the African-American women, Virginia M. Alexander (1899–1949), a member of Philadelphia's black elite. After graduation, Dr. Alexander practiced in Philadelphia, opened a small maternity hospital for African-Americans, and carried out a survey of the health status of that segment of the city's population. Later she acquired a master's in public health from Yale and continued to mix practice and public health work in Washington, D.C., and in Alabama. Though WMC provided her the opportunity to gain the M.D. (and even allowed her to repeat the first year when outside distractions caused her to initially founder), she did encounter racism, but also friendship and help from several white alumnae.[47]

The faculty debated more than once the practice of accepting into the College students who had flunked out of prominent coeducational schools. Several professors decried this elasticity, but Catharine Macfarlane urged that these occasional exceptions be allowed. Always challenging gender discrimination, she believed that "persisting prejudice in some medical schools . . . may, in some instances at least, result in an injustice which denies to a woman student the right of promotion in those schools." She therefore felt it to be of great importance "for us to deal critically with each individual case of this sort in order that this only surviving medical school for women may still be fulfilling its purpose of freedom of opportunity for women."[48] In effect, with its eagerness to fill places in order to survive and further its original mission, the College of the 1920s and 1930s did provide opportunities to many non-elite students whose pathway might otherwise have been blocked: many Jews, immigrants, a few African-Americans, even occasional students of only modest academic capacity who nonetheless might in the right setting succeed with medical training. Perhaps there were some who, as Macfarlane suspected, had failed elsewhere in part owing to actual discrimination or at least a male-shaped environment too intimidating for their needs. This niche, training women medical students on the social or even academic margin, had in no way been coveted by the upper-crust leaders or the faculty of the 1920s and 1930s WMC. But it was a role the College did not repudiate.

On the other hand, numerous women of superior ability attended the College in the 1920s and 1930s: the senior class of 1935–1936, for example, included graduates of Vassar, Wellesley, Barnard, Radcliffe, Hunter, Geneva, Penn, and other prominent colleges and universities.[49] Needless to say, graduates from this period, regardless of their premedical college, succeeded in all areas of practice and some in academics and research. Class notes and obituaries in issues of the College's *Alumnae News* fifty years later record careers in private practice, general and state hospitals, the armed forces, industry, public health, and research. WMC graduates of the 1920s and 1930s worked as general practitioners, pediatricians, obstetricians, internists, and surgeons. Anesthesiology, psychiatry, and school health proved especially popular choices. Several alumnae of the 1920s and 1930s devoted their careers to the care of retarded or troubled children and adolescents, persons with alcoholism, and the disabled. Others taught at medical schools in New York, Alabama, Illinois, Maryland, Texas, and of course at their alma mater. They took care of patients in China, India, Nepal, Syria, Tunisia, and all over the United States, exactly as had been the case fifty years earlier.

Although the students' Halloween party, dances, and benefit concerts continued into the 1920s, available sources suggest—more by their lack—that student life was less rich than in the 1890s and pre–World War I years. Still, some customs and experiences spanned the decades and schisms. Mabel Emery of the class of 1929 later wrote with pride that her class's basketball team suffered no defeats. She loved the "cheering and yelling, everyone there and such rivalry. . . . We were fighting for the crown and I sprained my ankle. Dr. Macfarlane insisted on bandaging my ankle—I begging, pleading, insisting I must play."[50] A 1932 graduate, Mary Bruins Allison, recalled sharing an apartment with students from South America and Jamaica. With a friend, she "took long walks in the beautiful Wissahickon Valley and Fairmount Park."[51] Allison crammed for exams, did twenty home deliveries, ate lunch with her apartment-mates on the floor of the autopsy room while awaiting the professor, and discovered a twinkle in the eye of Mollie Geiss, a demanding but compelling professor who at various times taught both pharmacology and pathology.[52] Allison enjoyed the graduation reception given by the faculty "at a garden inn where we entertained them with skits and stunts."[53] Other students of the 1920s and early 1930s utilized their full energy to keep up with course work. No doubt some of those who did excise occasional free time from their schedules chose to spend it in ways newly condoned by the spirit of the 1920s—as individuals, sometimes with boyfriends (Mary Bruins Allison and her two friends all had them at one time or another), and less regularly at school events or church.

The College continued to nurture and display its own saga, renewing through history the sense of continuity and distinctiveness which so much motivated its leaders and alumnae. The Founders' Day pageant for 1931 utilized a "picture frame illuminated from above. Dr. Tracy represented Dr. Ann Preston the first woman dean. Dr. Tracy[,] dressed in an authentic costume of 1860[,] sat at a small table scattered with papers from which she read bits of the early College history and as she read—Deans, College Professors and Students stepped into the frame as their names were read."

First-year students carried out the costumed impersonations. There followed a "tableau of the College 'in the gay nineties'" and a showing of the publicity film from twenty years earlier.[54]

Many students of the rebuilt WMC in East Falls from 1930 on would devote spare hours not to tableaux or athletics, but to whatever part-time work they could find. For Woman's Med, in debt and too-little in demand, had by sorry chance entered its new and hopeful home just in time for the Great Depression. And through that grim interval it continued to struggle along, a small, private school, its doors kept open as they always had been to teach medicine to women and to house women medical teachers. Now perched on a hill from which the center of its natal city could be seen only in the distance, through an unexpected vista of trees and river, the College followed an increasingly isolated pathway, cognizant of but separate from the main currents of American academic medicine.

Chapter 9

As One Hundred Years Approached

Woman's Medical College and the Great Depression

Philadelphia felt the impact of the Great Depression slightly less than many other cities owing to its great diversity of manufactures. Nonetheless, and despite philanthropic aid, poor and middle-class Philadelphians, and even a few of the upper crust, suffered long and onerously.[1] Institutions and constituencies looked more than ever for local philanthropic and governmental support. WMC remained as always dependent on such beneficence. Its class size remained small, and its endowment limited. Little national support came from American women or even American medical women.[2] A "plan of soliciting the aid of the women of the United States through the Federated Women's Clubs" did not materialize.[3] Undeterred, and well acquainted with adversity, WMC entered the Great Depression.

In her 1932 report to the Alumnae Association, Dean Martha Tracy found some good news. The College had recruited Sarah I. Morris (a 1910 WMC graduate) from the University of Wisconsin to head preventive medicine and a talented scientist named Helene Wastl for physiology. Surprisingly, the first-year class had reached its capacity of fifty-one. The new tennis courts were proving "a wonderful source of happiness and health," and the "adventure of our Health Clinic for women has been an interesting one."[4] But she also told of these ominous events: "The effects of the financial depression became apparent early in the year, as word came to one student after another of failure of home banks and disappearance of funds depended upon for college fees and maintenance expenses."[5]

Indeed some students withdrew, unable to pay. Recollections of WMC students of the 1930s confirm the deprivations but also the determination to stay in school and the daily selflessness that sometimes made doing so possible. Lillian Seitsiv, a 1931 graduate, found work selling millinery and another job as a sort of nurse's aid. She recalls vividly the difficulty of making ends meet, and that some students literally did not have enough to eat.[6] Alma Morani of the same class managed to "eke out a living" with another student, Elizabeth Veach, by sharing resources depending upon whose family had come through with help. Morani earned an occasional few dollars or a meal tutoring some of the foreign students.[7] Angie Connor, who received her WMC degree in 1937, cooked for a faculty member and remembers that students seemed always pressed by work and sometimes hungry.[8] To Morani WMC of 1928 to 1932 was "a small, sort of private institution where everybody was supportive and friendly; the faculty was interested in you as an individual and would invite you to their homes for an occasional meal."[9]

In 1933, both Dean Tracy and Florence H. Richards, alumnae member of the board of corporators, told the gathered graduates of further financial peril.[10] College investment income fell as did governmental allocations and private donations. Faculty salaries, already low, were reduced. Strenuous efforts of Mrs. Starr and the Finance Committee managed to cover an annual deficit of twelve thousand dollars. Martha Tracy concluded her remarks on as positive note as she could manage: "The Woman's Medical College has faced many a crisis and, like the Phoenix, has always arisen triumphant from the fire of adversity. Confident in the support of its Alumnae and its friends we look forward cheerfully to the future."[11]

The indefatigable president begged of her friends and collected; deficits remained worrisome but not calamitous. Classes and clinics carried on. Tracy again found some favorable facts to tell the alumnae in 1933. The internationally known Philadelphia specialist in bronchoscopy, Chevalier Jackson (1865–1968), had joined the College faculty. Some social events lightened the weight of those burdensome years: Tracy noted the president's fund-raising garden party in May and the theatrical performance of Helen Ingleby, the professor of pathology, a flamboyant personality and ardent amateur actress.[12]

The Weiskotten Inspection of 1935

Indirectly, the Great Depression brought on the next academic crisis for WMC: the withholding of approval in 1935 by the Council on Medical Education and Hospitals of the American Medical Association and loss of membership in the Association of American Medical Colleges (AAMC). This devastating result followed the council's inspection of all medical schools, the first such careful look in many years. As Martha Tracy wrote to the board in late 1934, to acquaint them with the import of the new survey, "this year, 1934, in view of the economic situation which is pressing heavily upon the earnings of the practicing physicians, the question of graduating too many doctors has come to fore, and some have challenged the advisability of maintaining as many medical schools as now exist."[13] According to historian Rosemary Stevens, the financial concerns of depression-era doctors about overcrowding induced the AMA to discover ways to reduce the number of "students and immigrant physicians" and eliminate the "poorest and least desirable" men from entering the profession.[14]

In the 1930s, the American Medical Association promoted the cultural paradigm of one, orthodox medical profession whose authority derived from science. Almost all AMA officers and council members had been white and male.[15] On 14, 15, and 16 January 1935, the WMC found itself under the intense gaze of H. G. Weiskotten, M.D., director of the new AMA survey, and M. W. Ireland, M.D.[16] By 20 February 1935 came the official communication from the council reporting its resolution that approval of the Woman's Medical College of Pennsylvania "be withdrawn with the provision that this decision will not prejudice the students now enrolled."[17] Loss of membership in the AAMC followed.

The inspectors gave praise to most of the clinical departments and clinical instruction, but objected to much else they saw. The pre-clinical departments needed full-time heads (most were part-time) and reorganization of their programs. Salaries for faculty were ridiculously low. The

caliber of students (asserted the council) was weak because no applicant meeting the minimal requirements seemed to be turned away. As
a presumed indicator in their eyes of the marginality of many in the
classes, the AMA inspectors noted "that about 40 per cent of the students are hebrews [sic]," a figure erroneously high.[18] The library was inadequate and lacked a full-time librarian. Finally, Weiskotten and
Ireland correctly perceived the unbalanced governance of the College:
"Apparently the attitude of the board is such that it participates too
much in the administration of the educational aspects of the medical
college. Their entire institution, both medical college and hospital, is
dominated by the president of the board."[19]

Responding to the 1935 Inspection

Martha Tracy requested from Ray Lyman Wilbur, chairman of the Council on Medical Education and Hospitals, a more detailed "bill of facts"
to back up her "insistence on corrective measures."[20] Professor of surgery John Stewart Rodman (?–1958), a nationally known figure and
president of the National Board of Medical Examiners, rallied to the
cause of the College using his ties to the male medical establishment.[21]
Rodman wrote to (among others) Walter L. Bierring, then president of
the AMA. In his response, Bierring admitted to being "considerably dis-
turbed" by the council's decision regarding WMC. He summarized the
concerns about lack of full-time science chairs and "that certain departments were controlled by lay (lady) members of the Board of Trustees."
"Much good may result" from the inspection, advised Bierring, and "the
end is not yet."[22]

The main "lady" in question was at the moment aboard the SS
Southern Prince on a round-the-world, or nearly round-the-world, cruise.
The vice president and counsel Walter Lee Sheppard gamely took
charge. He wired William D. Cutter, secretary of the council, vehemently protesting the "unfair action of Council" and requesting "deferment until opportunity is afforded for conference and removal of
causes of criticism."[23] Then he convened an emergency meeting of the
executive committee to which were invited Tracy, Rodman, Catharine
Macfarlane, and Henry Jump. It was another pivotal juncture in the epic
life of Woman's Med. "We sat until nearly twelve o'clock in canvass-

ing the whole situation and agreed to make the effort to find a way to meet the large increases in the budget next year that would be involved in the reorganization of the Pre-Clinical Departments [*sic*] to conform to what Dr. Tracy and Dr. Rodman stated would be the minimum requirements of the Council."[24] They heard a chilling calculation: the additional funding needed would approach $50,000. "While this would appear to be an impossible task under present conditions, we all determined last night to make the effort," wrote Sheppard to Mrs. Starr, hoping his letter would reach her in Buenos Aires.[25]

At its meeting of 20 March 1935 the board of corporators authorized the executive committee to "take whatever action it may deem necessary" to correct the deficiencies.[26] Meanwhile, the efficient board secretary Vida Hunt Francis discussed with her contacts in Harrisburg the urgent need for hospital appropriations from the state.[27]

Mrs. Starr's Interpretation

Sheppard's first letter to Sarah Logan Wister Starr, dispatched in February, finally caught up with the seafaring president on 18 March in Capetown, South Africa. Hastily she penned a response ("we sail in one hour"), offering her unequivocal interpretation of the events: "I felt we were doomed as a Class A institution since our interview [with Weiskotten; Starr was present at the time of the visit]. A contempt for women as an intelligent group was evidenced by his every word. I was sick at heart so kept in the background as much as possible."

Starr concluded the letter by declaring that she would "devote the rest of my trip to gathering strength for the battle ahead, for I am fully conscious of the fact that it is war to the finish, and death to the College is a tragic end to the efforts we have all made."[28] She proposed to Sheppard that *he* head the College, and she work under him. She pursued this theme—that the Weiskotten report represented outright sexism—in another letter of 30 March (from Montevideo Harbor): "This is a man equation, anti-feminists are in the saddle, we must cater to that situation and I believe that we can win with you as President. . . . Dr. Weiskotten will be immensely flattered, and may be won over to our cause by the complete withdrawal of women from Executive control."[29]

While she did not deny that defects existed at the College, Mrs. Starr saw the issue not as one primarily of education and economics, but of what now would be called gender politics. To what extent might she have been correct?

In fact, WMC hardly stood alone in receiving low marks after Weiskotten's scrutiny: twenty out of seventy-seven American medical schools ended up flagged, especially for lack of full-time staff, and several were attacked even more sharply than was WMC.[30] This understanding does not, however, exclude gender as a variable. Though its curriculum matched those of other schools, Woman's Med did not fit the chosen model of medical education. It had no university parent, stressed clinical teaching over research, relied on part-time faculty—and was run and largely staffed by women. To the male, conservative AMA hegemony, or to the medical academy, anything so different had to be suspect.[31]

The historian Sarah Evans and others have suggested that during the depression, some of the frustration and humiliation men felt when facing loss of income and status turned into anger against women, especially visible, nonsubmissive women.[32] Might women physicians in the 1930s have been seen by the male establishment of organized medicine as a poorly qualified source of unwanted competition in difficult times, almost like the "foreign doctors" noted above by Rosemary Stevens? The historian Margaret Rossiter in discussing discrimination against women scientists in the United States argued that "ejecting women in the name of 'higher standards' was one way to reassert strongly the male dominance over the burgeoning feminine presence."[33]

Among the extant correspondence centered on the 1935 disapproval, the most sarcastic and putatively sexist tone is found in a letter of William D. Cutter, secretary of the Council on Medical Education, responding to Martha Tracy's request for a detailed statement of the deficits. After impatiently noting that "it would be impossible, as well as unnecessary, for me to enumerate all of the items in which your school is lacking," Cutter suggested that WMC was not needed, and ought to give up: "In order that your Trustees may be informed as to the opportunities now existing for women to obtain a medical education in institutions other than your own, may I suggest that you bring to their notice the fact that during the academic year 1933–1934, 1,017 women were enrolled in 75 of the 87 approved medical schools of the United States and Canada."[34]

Clearly Cutter disdained the idea of women conducting their own medical school.[35]

A possible gender bias is revealed when Weiskotten and Ireland discussed the need for full-time faculty in the basic science departments. They recorded that in pharmacology "a Mrs. Helen Wilson, Ph.D., who is married and has a family comes to the college one day a week and assumes charge of the laboratory period."[36] Given the societal arrangements prevailing in 1935, clearly married mothers could less easily than husbands sustain a full-time science career. Mary Bickings-Thornton, the much admired but part-time professor and head of anatomy, also had a family, and in fact would relinquish her position so that the College could appoint the requisite full-time chair.[37] Bickings-Thornton had remained part-time because she not only looked after a family, but also maintained a private practice of medicine!

Bickings-Thornton's truncated career raises questions about the dominant model for medical education that extend beyond those of gender. No one had proved that "full-time" necessarily implied better education. For most medical students, who will become practitioners and not scientists, a "part-time" professor of anatomy who was also a doctor might prove the superior teacher, being better able to relate anatomical knowledge to the needs of clinical work. And for women students, such a professor *who also managed to combine family life with a career* showed that option possible. Two senior medical educators who came in April of 1935 for a second look at WMC on behalf of the Council on Medical Education indeed had to conclude that the school's product surpassed the limitations of its resources: "Full credit must also be given to the loyalty and fine spirit of the small group of instructors and teachers. . . . The results which have been obtained by this small faculty . . . with the many handicaps of inadequate equipment and lack of sufficient personnel is [sic] striking."[38]

Furthermore, Martha Tracy gathered data to show that despite its small size, by 1935 the WMC was surpassed by only eleven schools in number of graduates (not percentage, but actual total numbers) winning the then prestigious diploma of the National Board of Medical Examiners.[39]

Starr remained insistent in her belief that sexist attitudes had cata-
lyzed the AMA's disapproval. She promulgated her plan to step down
as president at a board meeting of 8 May 1935 and to the faculty on 10
May. Mrs. Starr would remain chair of the executive committee and
devote much of her time to finding revenues. "I simply have a gift of
going out and collecting money and making people give it," she told
the faculty as part of a long and rambling statement.[40] Since this "gift"
had proved itself in the past, her pledge found eager acceptance.

Mrs. Starr favored as the new, male president Chevalier Jackson,
the recently appointed professor of bronchoscopy. He ranked unequivo-
cally as a Philadelphia medical gentleman "of the old school" but
showed sympathetic interest in the city's medical women and their college. The seventy-year old Jackson offered this unprepossessing acceptance speech after election to presidency of WMC on 19 June 1935:

> A weak small voice tells me that I do not deserve the honor
> and am incapable of doing the work that should be done by the
> President. Among the many things I cannot do is raise
> money. . . .
>
> The Second Vice-President is able to do the work better
> than I can myself, so I choose Miss Francis to do the work.
>
> In conclusion I hope we are all agreed that you are all to do
> the work and I get the glory.[41]

Mrs. Starr, in fact, continued to run the College as chair of the executive committee, and Chevalier Jackson appears to have helped where
he could, though his election probably impaired, rather than enhanced,
credibility among knowledgeable medical educators.[42] Vida Hunt
Francis remained a faithful and capable administrator for many years.

New Faculty to Fulfill the Mandate

At the June 1935 meeting of the board of corporators Martha Tracy
announced the first addition to the full-time corps. Esther Greisheimer
(1892?–1982) came from the University of Minnesota to become the
new chair of physiology. Greisheimer held both the M.D. (from the
University of Minnesota) and Ph.D. (from the University of Chicago)
and had studied in Berlin, London, and the Marine Biological Labora-

tory at Wood's Hole. Research productivity allowed her to become an early woman member of the American Physiological Society (elected in 1925).[43] Already in the small Department of Physiology was associate professor Roberta Hafkesbring, who succeeded Greisheimer in 1943.

Other full-time appointments followed. From the University of Texas Medical Branch at Galveston came Marion Fay (1896–1990) to head physiological chemistry; she would eventually serve WMC as dean and president. Fay held the Ph.D. in biochemistry from Yale and could list numerous publications from her years at Galveston. Another recruit of 1935 who became a central figure at the College over decades was the extraordinary German émigré Hartwig Kuhlenbeck (1897–1984), who might be described (incompletely) as physician, anatomist, philosopher, prodigious author, teacher, polyglot, world traveler, soldier, pilot, Japanophile, and mountain climber. Opposed to Nazism, Kuhlenbeck became a voluntary exile, and, after considerable travel, spent 1934–1935 as a fellow in anatomy at the University of Pennsylvania. Providentially, the young anatomist needed a post just when WMC needed a full-time head of its department. While carrying out his teaching and administrative responsibilities, Kuhlenbeck pursued to completion (in the 1970s) the colossal intellectual program he had outlined for himself as a youth—a comprehensive account of the structure of the nervous system and its relation to human consciousness.

Probably no more monumental intellect than Kuhlenbeck's ever dwelled at the Woman's Medical College; yet, despite his sometimes austere "Germanic" style, the professor of anatomy is recalled by many alumnae as an effective and dedicated teacher, and one who displayed early respect for the callow freshmen.[44]

Completing the four appointments of 1935–1936 to fulfill the demand for full-time chairs in science was Ben King Harned in pharmacology, a Ph.D. recipient from Washington University, recently on the faculty of the University of Tennessee.[45] In 1937 Linda Bartels Lange, a medical graduate of Johns Hopkins, came as full-time head of bacteriology; she had done considerable research on the tubercle bacillus while on the faculty of Johns Hopkins but unfortunately retired after a few years at WMC because of illness.

By 1937 the WMC had assembled a promising cadre of full-time science faculty comprising twelve women and two men (here including pathologists Helen Ingleby and Mollie Geiss). Several began to win small research grants, such as Greisheimer's award of twenty-five hundred dollars in 1936 from the American Philosophical Society.[46] For the first time, WMC acknowledged the expectation that the modern medical school carry out fundamental research. At the same time, the appointments markedly altered the social environment of the College. The new professors came from outside and mostly from beyond Philadelphia. They brought to the parochially conducted school potential for new viewpoints and expectations and familiarity with the broadly accepted customs of academic institutions. They also brought color and literally diverse voices, as students adjusted to Marion Fay's gentle New Orleans modulations and Kuhlenbeck's German accent.

Building Science at WMC

Before 1935, the small science faculty could not find time to add serious research to their extensive teaching and service work. The long-time professor of bacteriology Adelaide Ward Peckham wrote in 1911 that she did "regret very much that I have had no time for research work since I came to the Woman's Medical College in 1898. When not engaged in the duties of this position I am at the Woman's Hospital where I am the pathologist."[47] But a critical mass existed after the 1935 expansion. Despite the heavy load of teaching in the anatomy department, Kuhlenbeck was able to initiate research and aid his two assistant professors in doing so. Fay, Greisheimer, and Hafkesbring collaborated on some studies of anesthetics.[48] In 1941, Phyllis Bott (1899–1991), a biochemist and physiologist, came from the University of Pennsylvania to the College as associate professor of physiologic chemistry under Marion Fay. During the 1940s she alone kept alive micropuncture, an elegant but daunting technique for investigating renal function, and published several papers of lasting importance.[49] Bacteriologist Ruth E. Miller, who came as assistant instructor in 1934, would later also publish regularly.

Although research lagged within the clinical departments, a notable exception began in 1938 when Catharine Macfarlane received a grant from the Committee on Scientific Research of the AMA to initiate her landmark study "of the value of periodic examinations of 1,000 women during a period of five years for the purpose of determining the possibility of detecting the early appearance of carcinoma [of the uterus]."[50] This successful long-term study would bring wide recognition to Macfarlane, her colleagues, and the College. Its objective suitably recalled one of the founding missions of the Woman's Medical College, the preventive care of women, and implicitly helped justify the continuation of a women's medical college.

The expansion of basic science at WMC beginning in 1935 held another gendered meaning, indicated succinctly by looking more closely at the careers of Phyllis Bott and Linda Bartels Lange. After obtaining her Ph.D. at the University of Pennsylvania in 1930, Bott spent two years as a research fellow at Princeton, then returned to Penn to work from 1933 until 1941 in the laboratory of A. Newton Richards, a major figure in renal physiology. There she devised ingenious chemical measurements on tiny samples of fluids and mastered the extraordinarily difficult micropuncture technique to study the function of single nephrons of the kidney. Her name appeared on some of the most important papers in renal physiology. Yet her title at the University of Pennsylvania never rose above "research associate." On coming to WMC, she achieved faculty rank, and eventually full professorship. Linda Bartels Lange, who came to WMC in 1937 as professor of bacteriology, had spent twenty years at Johns Hopkins University reaching only associate professorship.[51]

The careers of Bott and Lange tell much about the status of women in American medical education and the significance of WMC beyond undergraduate education. In the inter-war years, discrimination in hiring, salary, and rank pervasively frustrated the career aspirations of women scientists in the United States. Medical schools hired few female scientists as faculty members, though many qualified women worked, like Bott, as research associates or technicians. Remarkably, after the new appointments beginning in 1935, the tiny Woman's Medical College became one of the leading employers of female medical science faculty, and certainly the leader among United States medical schools.[52] Thus, in consonance with its founding mission, when research came to WMC, it brought a new demonstration of opportunity's door. The efforts provoked by the possibly misogynist AMA inspection of 1935 ended up strengthening WMC and making it more of a women's institution.

Further Struggles with the AMA and Paying for the Reforms

Despite the increase in science faculty begun in 1935, the AMA still refused to fully endorse WMC, leading to well over a year of frustrating and burdensome negotiations by the College officers. The board of corporators then eliminated its offending joint board-faculty Committee for Appointment, Promotion, and Tenure to address the correct perception of excess lay control. Finally, the bureaucratic harassment ceased as the council notified Chevalier Jackson that it had, on 6 June 1937, restored WMC to its approved list.[53]

The College emerged from this ordeal in fact considerably improved, if not transformed. Excellent new full-time faculty had come on board, and with them a foundation for research. Lay interference with academic governance lessened. The library enjoyed needed improvement. And, the College had once again shown a determination to endure that matched the latest set of external demands and provocations. Of course, the improvements required more funds. Mrs. Starr turned to the familiar device of a "sale of bricks" to associate the fundraising campaign with the new building and the need to reduce mortgage debt. Adopting a perhaps more than necessary literalism, she took the trouble in March of 1937 to ascertain from the architect the total number of bricks used in the East Falls building.[54] The board hoped that the brick sale would win "a large number of new friends" but planned to seek larger donors once local support could be shown.[55]

Such was a plausible strategy; but the dollar-a-brick sale, when considered in contrast to the Rockefeller millions that endowed certain medical schools outside Philadelphia, underscores the localism of the WMC, and to a great extent of Philadelphia medical education in this period. By December of 1938 the Brick Fund reached fifty-five thousand dollars.[56] Mrs. Starr and her allies found enough other contributions to pay the bills.

Nonetheless, troubles still brewed and reached a head in 1941. In 1940 Martha Tracy stepped down as dean to become an assistant director of the Philadelphia Board of Health.[57] She died unexpectedly the next year. Saddened friends and students recalled her decades of selfless and diligent service to the school, her polish and humor, the summers she looked forward to at her beloved Rocky Pond Camp in Maine, her automobile aptly named "Trotula." Some fortunate classmates and friends could remember her through their copy of *Ye Medical Student's Primer,* an engaging little book of doggerel and drawings she created while herself a pupil at WMC.

For its next dean the College turned to a promising woman physician from outside the institution, Margaret Craighill (1899–1977). Craighill, a Johns Hopkins medical graduate of 1924, had done considerable postgraduate work before practicing gynecology and general surgery in New York City and Greenwich, Connecticut.[58] Craighill drafted a progressive plan encompassing curriculum, student-faculty relationships, and the conduct of the teaching hospital. Old and new faculty unanimously and "heartily" endorsed it in March of 1941.[59] The many new faculty who had come to WMC from outside the school probably favored the acceptance of a non-alumna dean with an agenda for reform.

By this time, a faction had developed within the board not favorable to Sarah Logan Wister Starr, whose rule, after twenty years, perhaps had begun to falter. With so much energy devoted to basic sciences and the College during the late 1930s, administration of the hospital received inadequate attention. In particular, the quality of the hospital's internship had deteriorated.[60] While women in the 1930s could, with difficulty, find a place in a medical school, internships and residencies remained less open. Thus the positions provided by the Hospital of WMC remained extremely vital to the training of women physicians. In July of 1940, Craighill requested that the positions of dean and hospital director be combined; Mrs. Starr felt her authority threatened.[61] Discord between Starr and the new dean arose and grew.[62]

The hospital represented only one element in a renewed struggle for academic control within the school. Margaret Craighill, a more forceful personality than Tracy, claimed the power to manage the school and work toward the changes she had outlined, without lay interference. In a strategic move that succeeded, though at some risk, she in effect invited the AMA Council on Medical Education and Hospitals to again visit the campus in East Falls.[63] Its officers did so on 31 January 1941. Their criticisms indeed centered on the conduct of the hospital and internship.[64] The executive committee of the board on 12 March 1941—the day after Founders' Day!—concluded that it could not assure the raising of needed funds for another round of improvements requested by the AMA council, and resolved that "the advice and counsel be sought of the representatives of the Alumnae Society and of the Faculty for the purpose of ascertaining whether it is necessary to close the College."[65] (Probably this maneuver was aimed at saving face, not really at shutting the doors.) On 19 March 1941, a "Communication to the Board of Corporators" carried a resolution "that the undersigned Alumnae and Faculty being convinced of its importance hereby go on record as wishing this College to Continue."[66] The communication was signed by 115 alumnae and faculty. Mrs. Starr and much of the board resigned, to be replaced by a new group representing a broad range of Philadelphia constituencies.[67] The transition was necessary but painful: with her faults, Sarah Logan Wister Starr loved the College unselfishly.

Margaret Kelly (Mrs. John B. Kelly, 1899–1990), one of the board members who did not resign, became chair of the executive committee. Kelly was a prominent resident of the College's East Falls neighborhood, as were numerous other members of Philadelphia's colorful Kelly family. Her wealthy husband owned a major construction company and brickworks and had helped build an effective Democratic Party in Philadelphia. It was microcosmically perfect that at WMC—internationally known but deeply rooted in Philadelphia hardpan—a representative of the ascending Philadelphia Irish-Americans, with "new" money, would replace a Logan Wister Starr.[68]

Mrs. Kelly adopted WMC as had Mrs. Starr, but with less of a sense of presumptive ownership or inclination to meddle in its academic affairs. Along with Margaret Kelly's philanthropy and leadership came the affection and service of some of her family, exactly as occurred with Starr's. One Kelly daughter, Lizanne LeVine, became active at the school at several levels. And, from time to time, the Henry Avenue campus would welcome the neighborhood's lustrous film star and princess, Grace, another of Margaret and John B. Kelly's offspring.

"They Came on Crutches and Canes"

Mrs. Kelly decisively voiced her loyalty to WMC at the school's next contretemps, the 1946 aborted merger into Jefferson Medical College. Presuming that there are only so many serial crises that a college or chapter can absorb, this episode will be related briefly.

In 1943 Margaret Craighill went on leave from her deanship to become the first woman commissioned in the United States Army Medical Corps. Head of biochemistry Marion Fay stepped in as acting dean, with the expectation she said later, of "officiating at a funeral."[69] She supposed that as men went to war, vacancies at coeducational medical schools would draw away applicants from the WMC. Instead (and for unclear reasons), the number of well-qualified applicants actually increased, to Fay's delight. The College lost some faculty to the armed services, but far fewer than the dominantly male schools. Indeed the faculty worked gallantly, even conducting an evening refresher course for physicians—mostly women—wishing to reenter practice during the national emergency.[70] The institution came through the war years academically and fiscally intact, with more and stronger students.

When Margaret Craighill returned from her war work in 1946, however, she and the board's president, Judge Herbert Goodridge, without consulting faculty, alumnae, or the board of corporators, initiated discussions with Jefferson Medical College to effect a merger that would require Jefferson to accept 20 percent women students.[71] The plan amounted to more of an absorption than merger, with no provision secured for WMC faculty. Craighill argued that the financial circumstances of the school precluded further development and that without major improvement it would soon be unable to provide an excellent medical education to women. In early April, Craighill announced the plan as a *fait accompli* to the astounded faculty. Marion Fay met with a group of much perturbed students (who learned of the proposal) when the dean refused to speak with them directly.

Under pressure to do so, the board of corporators called a meeting for 10 April 1946, held at the College of Physicians of Philadelphia, and sent invitations to all faculty and regional alumnae of the College. As Katharine Boucot Sturgis later recalled, "they came on crutches and on canes. There was this tremendous loyalty to Woman's Medical, especially on the part of the Old Guard."[72] It was Catharine Macfarlane who had rallied the alumnae. One hundred and eighty nine persons squeezed into the meeting room, including the board, nearly the entire faculty, and a strong showing of alumnae. A letter was read from Mary Griscom, an 1891 graduate, "against the merger." Marion Fay spoke on behalf of faculty; they had already expressed their nearly unanimous opposition to the plan in letters. Longtime professor of surgery John Stewart Rodman, whose father had also served WMC, became "almost moved to tears in decrying the plan to merge at this time and before our centennial anniversary."[73]

Board treasurer William Price stood in response to questions about College finances. He declared them sound: other than mortgage, the College had no outside debt. Though he promised to "adhere to the economic end of this," he concluded with the sound of fury: "Now, if the Board wants to destroy the efforts of heroic women for 96 years by the abject surrender of the Woman's Medical College, that is their privilege."[74] A telegram of protest, though not read at the meeting, came in from prominent surgeon Bertha Van Hoosen, founder of the American Medical Women's Association, and not a WMC graduate. "The Woman's Medical College is not only the most historic institution for women in medicine," she declared, "it is a stockade for protecting their rights. Among the score of reasons why it is still needed is that it gives opportunities for medical women as professors and heads of departments." She signed it "with astonishment."[75]

Margaret Kelly finally moved that the proposal of merger be dropped, and that a committee be formed to work on funding needed expansion. Catharine Macfarlane seconded it. After further discussion, the board voted twelve to six to drop the merger plan. Another signal event, another part of the College saga, concluded. No one present would forget the meeting. Margaret Kelly and Marion Fay emerged as the school's leaders, with Catharine Macfarlane still a persuasive voice. The hundred-year mark, and beyond, would be easily reached.

Some time later, William Harvey Perkins, dean of Jefferson, smoothed an awkward moment when attending a dinner party hosted by Marion Fay, with this epigram: "Ancient Jefferson had dared to look with the eyes of longing on the beautiful young Woman's Medical, and, unfortunately, the marriage was never consummated; but he hoped they would continue to be very good friends."[76] No animosity arose between WMC and Jefferson Medical College; the latter school would not admit women to its classes for fifteen more years.

"The Patient's Will-to-Live"

Over the first half of the twentieth century, the WMC endured loss of its teaching hospital, multiple visits to the fiscal brink, an internal schism, the ascent of medical coeducation, the Great Depression, external academic mandates, and multiple explorations of merger. The first medical school for women, it also became the last, outliving as a single-sex program its sisters by fifty years. In referring to its refusal to collapse or merge, Catharine Macfarlane wrote: "In world affairs as in medicine, there is an important asset called 'the Patient's Will-to-Live.' The Woman's Medical College had no intention of dying or of losing its identity."[77] "The College that wins and never fails, is the Woman's Medical," boasted a class song from 1910. What explains the improbable survival of the College—or, at least one can ask, what are the characteristics of its astonishing durability?

Of course, for most of its history few women faculty of WMC could have won entry at other Philadelphia medical schools: a perfectly justified self-interest was at work. But this does not fully explain the tenacious resiliency and allegiance of many alumnae. As a way of suggesting some broader answers, we return to the work of sociologist of education Burton Clark, cited briefly in earlier chapters. Clark formulated the concept of the "distinctive college," usually a small school set off from the average by singularity of purpose and by a cumulation of history, ideology, and personalities constituting what he calls its "saga."[78] A saga requires an "intrinsically historical" sense of unique accomplishment over time, often won in the face of opposition. "The more special the empirical history and the more forceful a claim to a place in history, the more intensely cultivated are the ways of sharing memory and symbolizing the institution."[79] Usually, some central cause or curricular ideology forms the basis of the saga as it plays out; for WMC, this would be, of course, its mission to train women in medicine. But specific curricular innovations sustained over time also claim a part in the organizational saga; for example, the maternity program founded by Anna Broomall, or the development of preventive medicine. And one hardly need list the events, legends, memories, aspirations, and persons forming the empowering saga—from the quiet determination of Ann Preston to the explosive temper of the revered "Kitty Mac," from the jeering episode of 1869 to the shouting down of merger in 1946, from delivering babies in the slums of south Philadelphia to the Germantown garden parties of Sarah Logan Wister Starr, from hotly contested basketball games to the steamy clinics of missionary graduates in India.

Clark finds several factors necessary in propagating a college's legend. Faculty must, of course, become believers in the mission and the special historical place. A student subculture needs to form in order to hand down the sense of the school from class to class. External supporters must emerge. Some alumni feel suffused with "loyalty beyond reason." "For them, the idea of the college, the warm legend, can buy everything."[80] So alumnae of WMC, some also faculty, built a dispensary, laid down thousand-dollar loans in 1921, defended an admired professor in 1923, and "came on crutches" to defeat merger in 1946.

Other attributes favoring the emergence of a shared and enduring sense of distinctiveness include a "singularity of purpose" (equivalent at WMC with its history) and "smallness of size."[81] In a small institution, leaders, faculty, and students regularly see one another and commingle; if other advantages are in place, a sense of unity and mutual regard can arise. To the extent Clark is correct about smallness, that characteristic of WMC (and later of MCP) which made it more vulnerable to fiscal and social pressures than almost all other modern American medical schools made it also more worthy of protection from those forces.

To sum up Clark's notion in his own words: "Distinctiveness captures loyalty."[82] Clearly, the WMC over long stretches of time won that loyalty, if not from every student, faculty member, and alumna, then from more than enough to assure its distinctiveness and secure its durability.

Loyalty energized the "will to live" of the WMC during the first half of the twentieth century. But the mechanism of its survival represented a particularly local and Philadelphia solution. For much of its three-hundred-year history, Philadelphia eschewed change: a segment of its population has always taken comfort in its familiar institutions, buildings, ways of doing things. Philadelphians like accustomed parts of the landscape to stay around. One need only consider some of the institutions and buildings associated with the women and men of the Woman's Medical College since its founding. Musical Fund Hall, where the first class graduated, still stands. A descendant of William Mullen's House of Industry yet functions, as does the prison society that first employed him in 1852. Opening their doors daily are the Ethical Society that attracted C. Newlin Peirce and Frances Emily White, and the perfectly intact Wagner Free Institute of Science, founded in 1855, where White and Henry Leffmann taught. Also active is the Berean Institute where Caroline Still Wiley Anderson, an African-American graduate of 1878, worked with her husband who had founded the school.

Like these and other perennial Philadelphia institutions, the Woman's Medical College of the 1920s through 1940s really did seem to show a living determination to survive. They endured out of affection for them and Philadelphia's unwillingness to discard; and the essential mechanism is simply this: when a few thousand dollars were needed to keep going, the few thousand dollars turned up. It has not been unusual for a member of Philadelphia's aristocracy or one of its families to adopt an institution as Mrs. Starr adopted WMC. Such an arrangement expressed a local display of dogged loyalty and affection, though often tinged with eagerness to control beyond the patron's expertise. In short, the focused energy of faculty and alumnae melded with the loyal and local philanthropy of a few Philadelphians to keep WMC alive. The College's distinctive saga fueled both. Consider that in the bleakest years of the 1920s and 1930s strenuous efforts kept open a small but complete medical school and hospital that each spring awarded the M.D. to as few as fifteen young women! The valiant effort to maintain Woman's Med during these decades refused answer to timid reason, as it stubbornly honored a founding mission many outside the school thought anachronistic. It was, in one true and correct sense of the word, a thoroughly romantic campaign.

Yet it was also a strategic one for women, for by the 1920s the College had become more of a women's enterprise than ever before, with female executive management and a higher proportion of women faculty than previously known. Martha Tracy, Vida Hunt Francis, Sarah

Logan Wister Starr, Marion Fay, Catharine Macfarlane and other alumnae, and Margaret Kelly—capable women of diverse backgrounds—
managed to maintain an independent WMC. The mandated expansion
of faculty begun in 1935 created a corps of women scientists. The College served not only as a locus of professional work but also as a place
of longtime female friendships and alliances, such as between Martha
Tracy and Ellen Culver Potter, internist Frieda Baumann and pediatrician Jean Crump. Still, as always, men found their way to WMC and
attached themselves to its cause and its history, but played less essential roles than their predecessors of the nineteenth century. The grand
open meeting in 1946 that aborted merger into Jefferson Medical College,
only a few years before the College's centennial, dramatically symbolized the alliance that so long sustained the institution and its particular saga: determined, competent women, progressive and persuaded male
allies, and a dependable pocket of maternal Philadelphia patronage.

Chapter 10	The Marion Fay Years

Reshaping the "Good Medical School"

The Postwar Years

Saved from dissolution by the alliance of alumnae, faculty, and local patrons, WMC in the postwar period faced a sharply changing medical and social environment. During and after World War II, Americans felt a deepening confidence in science, medicine, and technology, stimulated by such seeming wonders as penicillin, atomic energy, television, artificial lungs and kidneys, and the Salk polio vaccine. A belief arose that many more doctors and hospitals would be needed to administer the new scientific medicine to Americans, while medical educators called attention to the costliness of producing a physician.[1] Fearing government aid and "socialized medicine" in the new Cold War sensibility, medical and business leaders created an independent granting agency known as the National Fund for Medical Education (NFME). The Ford Foundation briefly adopted medical education as a major beneficiary of its philanthropy.[2] The small and underendowed WMC welcomed these new sources of funds.

But eventually, much more support came from government. Despite initial skepticism, the presence of the federal government in medicine grew enormously during the 1950s, mainly through the development of a system of Veterans Administration hospitals, legislation to build or expand private hospitals (the so-called Hill-Burton Act), and research and training programs within the rapidly growing National Institutes of Health (NIH).[3] The overall NIH budget for research and training grants grew from about 13 million dollars in 1949 to over 300 million by 1960.[4] Research productivity became a critical criterion for the selection and promotion of medical school faculty. Research was deemed a good in itself, something a medical school *should* do, and came to be seen as a way of helping to pay bills.

All American medical schools experienced these changes. But WMC remained unique as the sole surviving women's medical college. What were the status and attitudes of American women during the 1950s—the context of gender?[5] A partial reality became embellished into a cultural norm that saw women again centered contently in the domestic sphere, now located in the lawned suburbs: the wartime riveter would return to motherhood and homemaking. Yet during the 1950s more and more women, including married women, did in fact work outside the home, though mainly in service positions. Certainly many individual women achieved public recognition in arts, politics, science, and other realms; while organized activism strengthened unions, challenged racism, and focused on other issues. But public feminism as such seemed largely dormant. Women of the 1950s were generally not expanding claims on traditionally male professions. While a sharp increase in women's applications to medical schools occurred during the war years, these numbers declined by 1951 and remained static throughout the 1950s.[6] WMC remained a rare example of an institution for women largely managed by women, but it displayed little medical-feminist fervor and, as we will see, became in some ways less of a women's college between 1947 and 1966 than it had been from 1926 to 1946.

Philadelphia with other American cities enjoyed a favorable postwar economy. Margaret Kelly, the first lady of East Falls, remained a steady friend to the school as lay leader and fund-raiser and helped cement its neighborhood attachments. The hospital, however, serving a larger region that included many poor persons, provided large amounts of costly free care during the 1950s and beyond.

Though WMC remained very much a Philadelphia survivor, for the first time the College gained broader support by American women in the form of a "National Board" and a "Commonwealth Committee," successful associations of prominent women nationally and in Pennsylvania willing to raise funds for Woman's Med and help make it better known.

The College Centennial and Its Messages

Four years after the reaffirmation of independence, Woman's Medical College celebrated its hundredth birthday. What public statements were advanced at the centennial? How did the College look backward and forward?

Following several years of planning, the events began with a dinner for four hundred persons on 10 March 1950, the evening before Founders' Day. Joining the College family were "leaders in medicine, education and community affairs" and four descendants of College founders. The speaker was Judge Dorothy Kenyon, a prominent activist and advocate for women's legal and economic rights. Founders' Day itself saw the gathering of a "family reunion, evoking memories of student days and bringing friends long separated together again . . . on the College campus."[7]

"Alumnae Days" occupied 13 and 14 June 1950. Scientific sessions offered new information on common gynecologic problems, asthma, RH factor, toxemia of pregnancy, cancer detection, cardiology, and diabetes. Alumna Katharine Horsburgh Hain (1945) lectured on her work using circulating eosinophils as an index of adrenal response in children. At the annual banquet the first Alumnae Achievement Award went to Jane Sands Robb (1918), widely known for her research in physiology. Also at the banquet, alumnae could watch an ice sculpture "in the form '100' melting slowly," symbolizing "the passing of the first century." A "huge Birthday Cake" made its ritual appearance.[8]

At the Centennial Commencement, thirty-four women received their M.D. in the presence of representatives from forty-five past classes and a variety of special guests and recipients of honorary degrees. Following lunch, ground was broken for a new nurses' home, the first postwar building project, with Margaret Kelly lifting the first spadeful of earth. Making this small ceremony a centennial element further connected the past with the future, while Mrs. Kelly's prominent role symbolized the tradition of lay support for the College and its foundation in Philadelphia.

The school's international reputation, its record of training mission-aries and women from all over the world, found suitable commemora-tion in September of 1950 as the College hosted the sixth congress of the Medical Women's International Association (MWIA), an organi-zation founded in 1919.[9] Were all this not enough, a two-day academic convocation in October concluded the centennial activities. Those at-tending the convocation dinner heard Captain Charles F. Behrens of the Naval Research Institute of the National Medical Center in Bethesda speak on "Medical Aspects of the Atomic Age." At the final ceremony WMC family and guests from seventy-five colleges and soci-eties heard famed African-American contralto Marian Anderson sing two Schubert songs and a spiritual.[10]

Clearly the centennial program looked both to the College's past and to medicine's future. That this was the centennial of a women's institution did not go unmarked: honorary degrees brought notable women to the school, while hosting the MWIA recalled the College's long-standing presence as an international contributor to the dissemi-nation of women physicians. Alumna Gulielma Fell Alsop's affection-ate and hagiographic *History of the Woman's Medical College* paid homage to the hundred-year College saga and the dynasty of women deans. But the bulk of energy and time honored the future—the auspicious prom-ise of science and modern medicine. Convened audiences learned about eosinophils and atomic energy. The Alumnae Association presented its first Achievement Award to a graduate known for her laboratory work. Women recipients of honorary degrees prominently included scientific workers such as Florence Seibert and Florence Sabin.

This emphasis on science in the centennial commemorations re-flected the College's leadership; scientists occupied both the presidency (Louise Pearce) and dean's office (Marion Fay).[11] But others might have made the same choices. Those guiding the College felt need to declare that a women's medical school can be a scientific medical school. The faculty minutes for the 1950s reveal Fay announcing each new or re-newed research grant.[12] She reported to alumnae in 1957 "a great feel-ing of pride in our faculty" who have carried on "such interesting and important experimental programs" despite heavy teaching loads and little laboratory space.[13] Though the dean certainly attended equally to developments in education and curriculum, her endorsement of re-

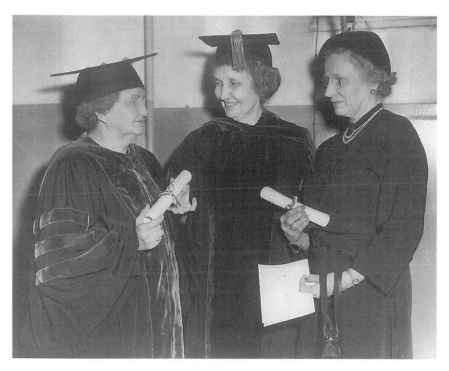

Figure 18. It's Founders' Day in the centennial year (1950); Dean Marion Fay (center) presents awards to longtime professor of pediatrics Jean Crump (left [WMC, 1923]) and professor of obstetrics Ann Gray Taylor (WMC, 1918).

search influenced both selection of new faculty and expansion of the campus.

New Buildings and New Revenues

In June of 1950, ground was broken for a new $450,000 nurses' home and nursing school building, which opened in January of 1952 as Ann Preston Hall.[14] Why a nurses' home? A severe nursing shortage existed in the postwar years as the expansion of hospital services and technology generated demand for more and varied nursing care. The College hospital had to rely on the services of student nurses and try to recruit new staff nurses from graduates of the school. The board and management hoped that a new facility, the "last word in comfort" with "fireplaces, game room, snack rooms, sun deck, television . . . picture window, built-in desk" would help attract students to the nursing school.[15] At the time, student nurses were housed in rented quarters off campus.

Though nursing in the 1950s was still a service occupation largely subservient to men, the College could claim that a modern *woman* architect—even more scarce than the woman physician—had designed its newest building. Elizabeth Fleisher, an accomplished architect of homes, institutional buildings, and theaters, also served on the College's board of corporators.[16] Fleisher and her colleagues looked visually to the future in their choice of the International Style with its horizontal emphasis, minimal ornament, and typical continuous bands of windows.

Paying for the construction of Ann Preston Hall also pointed to the future. The College had successfully applied for a grant from the federal Hill-Burton program, and received $166,666 toward the project.[17] Dollars from government also paid in good part for subsequent physical enlargements of the 1950s and 1960s.[18]

A small wing for the Department of Preventive Medicine would be the next new structure: it opened in 1954 as the Martha Tracy Memorial. But a more ambitious enlargement of the College seemed necessary to house expanding educational and research activities.[19] WMC applied for and received $500,000 from the Public Health Service, which offered money to help erect research facilities. The board of corporators accepted the mandate to raise three times this much privately. A new wing, dedicated in October of 1960, comprised mainly research space but also an enlarged teaching laboratory.[20] Even before the research addition opened, preliminary discussions commenced for a major addition to the hospital. Eventually begun in 1964 and opened in 1968, this project was also accomplished through a combination of public and private funds.[21] The nine-story addition transformed the institution's clinical scale and face; it is difficult to imagine how the College could have continued to attract patients and recruit students and house officers without it. Indeed, WMC could not have survived in the new medical milieu without the new buildings of the 1950s and 1960s.

Construction grants represented only one category of the new federal support of medical schools and of WMC. With attention in medicine shifting from acute infectious diseases to chronic disorders, the Public Health Service beginning in 1948 provided stipends to support education in cancer, cardiovascular disease, and "mental health"; WMC regularly obtained these grants during the 1950s.[22] Several faculty members won individual or project grants of modest amounts from the National Institutes of Health. The new chair of the Department of Pathology, I. Nathan Dubin (?–1980), received funding from the National Cancer Institute for a major project investigating the use of cytology in the detection and understanding of cervical cancer.[23] Upon returning from a national meeting of medical school deans, in January of 1960 Marion Fay told her faculty that in the future research funding would play an indispensable role in subsidizing medical schools. With the research wing now available, she urged her colleagues to "think very seriously about research grants and to take advantage of them in every way we can in order to strengthen our budgetary structure."[24]

WMC also enjoyed generous support from the Commonwealth of Pennsylvania, as did all the state's medical schools.[25] WMC in the 1950s and 1960s drank at the governmental troughs no more than other medical schools—in fact, less than many. But in doing so at all, it alone unwittingly threatened its founding mission, as will be seen in the next chapter.

The College joined all American medical schools in receiving private funding from the National Fund for Medical Education and the Ford Foundation.[26] The National Board, comprising over one hundred prominent women throughout the country, and the statewide Commonwealth Committee, both initiated in 1953, added substantially to the traditionally Philadelphia-based fund-raising on which the College had so long depended and aided WMC in many other ways.[27]

Curriculum

At least one entirely new short course appeared in the 1950s as a reflection of new scientific trends, the addition of genetics in 1959.[28] New faculty members in the basic sciences modified lectures and laboratory exercises to reflect changes in knowledge.[29] Nineteen-fifty-eight brought a major new second-year course, "Introduction to Clinical Medicine," a complicated transitional affair intended to pull together clinical lectures and enhance them with preliminary experiences with patients.[30]

Much discussion at faculty meetings in the late 1940s centered on a plan emanating from the Association of American Medical Colleges that would place junior students entirely into hospital work as clinical clerks, where they would "to all intents and purposes become a doctor."[31] Fourth-year students would spend most of their time in the out-patient clinics, where they would look after selected patients as if in a practice.[32] The WMC faculty partly adopted this ambitious plan.[33] But in the early 1950s the College hospital was failing to attract sufficient interns to meet its need. Since the 1930s, internships had proliferated at community hospitals and many more hospitals than previously accepted women as interns. The internship of the hospital of WMC, once so critical a resource for women medical graduates, now could not fill its roster. So WMC seniors were returned to the hospital floors confusingly ranked as "junior interns."[34]

Possibly the opportunity to function as interns enhanced the practical training of WMC students in the 1950s. Marion Fay, who kept track of WMC graduates, in 1954 told the faculty of the "splendid reports which she has received on the intern performance of last year's graduates. Almost without exception we have exceedingly glowing reports on these graduates." Some of the 1955 graduates were reported "as being the absolutely best interns in the entire group."[35] Graduates of the 1940s and 1950s have confirmed to the author that they were often surprised (and pleased) to find that their small school's training fitted them for internship work sometimes "better than the Harvard boys."

They particularly noted that their adeptness in obstetrics far exceeded that of their co-interns.[36] The long-standing excellence in teaching obstetrics and gynecology continued under Ann Gray Taylor, Mary Dewitt Pettit, and their staffs; and the home delivery program persisted well into the 1940s. But the faculty minutes for the two decades following 1946 record no curricular innovation proposed as particularly suited to the current or future needs of the medical woman. In her dean's report for 1948–1949, Marion Fay did offer the suggestion that WMC might become a "research center in medical problems concerned with women," but she did not press for this, given limited space and money, nor seek other new ways for WMC to gain meaning as a women's medical school in a largely coeducational world.[37] Possibly this lack of initiative represented a lost opportunity to build on the founding mission, and thereby attract students, house staff, and women faculty favorable to a partly gendered environment.

Katharine Boucot Sturgis and the Rebirth of Preventive Medicine

The Department of Preventive Medicine effectively collapsed when Sarah I. Morris left WMC in 1945. In 1952 Marion Fay recruited Katharine R. Boucot (later Boucot Sturgis, 1903–1987), a 1942 WMC graduate, to revive the department. Boucot, who had acquired special expertise in chest diseases, had already been teaching in the Department of Medicine.[38] But her first love was preventive medicine which she often spoke of as an attitude more than a separate discipline, and a necessary facet of every physician's thinking and work.

Gradually, through curricular trial and error, she reshaped the teaching programs in preventive medicine and public health.[39] Boucot attempted to make the department's offerings more clinically relevant and appealing to students, whose attention as always favored the diagnostic and curative dimensions. Her attempts to infuse exercises in preventive medicine into students' clinical work did not always meet with success, but Boucot never lacked for creative ideas and energy. To achieve more active learning, she transformed a set of senior lectures on prevention into discussion sessions on a variety of topics in public health and social medicine. As the faculty grew,[40] the department attempted implementing its ideals of prevention and community medicine within the neighborhoods adjoining WMC, though such well-intended "outreach" efforts ran into more socioeconomic obstacles than even their knowledgeable designers had imagined.

Despite mixed feelings about her student years at WMC, Katharine Boucot (Sturgis) worked fervidly to build its Department of Preventive Medicine which, though small, became one of the most vigorous in the College. She in turn became one of the most progressive, forceful, and colorful faculty members of the twentieth-century Woman's Medical College. Some of her friends and supporters regretted that she was never offered the deanship. Her official portrait fittingly challenges the viewer with a bold, nontraditional style nowhere else seen in the gallery.

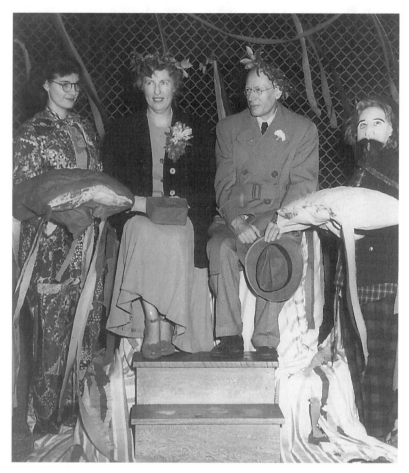

Figure 19. Katharine Boucot Sturgis (WMC, 1942), later professor of preventive medicine, and professor of anatomy Hartwig Kuhlenbeck tolerate ornamentation as Mardi Gras Queen and King in 1948.

Masculinization of the Faculty

At the June 1966 meeting of the Alumnae Association, members authorized a communication to the board of corporators which angrily reviewed some recent history:

> For one-hundred and ten years the Dean of the Woman's
> Medical College has been a woman. Today the Dean is a man.
> For approximately ninety years, the head of the Department of
> Physiology was a woman. Today the head is a man.

> For approximately ninety years, the head of the Department of Ophthalmology was a woman. Today the head is a man.

And so on for otolaryngology, biochemistry, and pathology. The letter went on to remind the board of the financial support recently provided by alumnae, and to "respectfully remind you that this is a Woman's Medical College—the only medical college for women in the western hemisphere. We ask you . . . to convey to the Dean and heads of Departments the Alumnae dissatisfaction with the small number of women on the Faculty."[41] By 1966, women directed only four of the twelve major departments, and a man had succeeded Marion Fay as dean. Also by this time, some of the most senior alumnae-faculty had retired, including internist Frieda Baumann, pediatrician Jean Crump, obstetrician Ann Gray Taylor, and otolaryngologist Emily Van Loon, though not all of these were directly replaced by men. Alumnae perceived the College to have declined as a demonstration of what women could accomplish in medical academics and as a secure "homeland" for the woman doctor.[42] What had happened to the status of women at Woman's Med?

The story emerges as more complex than understandably angry alumnae realized. By 1954, efforts had been underway for several years to find a replacement for Mollie Geiss, chairman of pathology, then sixty-eight years old and a faculty member since 1922. Records indicate serious interest in a woman candidate named Lalla Iverson, but she declined consideration on two occasions six months apart.[43] In March 1955 the selection committee finally proposed I. Nathan Dubin, M.D., a medical graduate of McGill University and recently on staff at the Armed Forces Institute of Pathology. Dubin, an acknowledged authority on liver disease, half-owned the eponymous Dubin-Johnson Syndrome, a disorder of bilirubin metabolism. He brought to his new post erudition and the potential for research and publication. Considered an engaging teacher by some (but not all) students, the feisty Dubin unfortunately indulged in occasional ribald and erratic behavior which would create much trouble later in his long career at WMC.[44] The job might well have gone to Lalla Iverson had she been amenable to persuasion.

When Marion Fay nominated Armand Guarino, an associate professor at the University of Michigan, to succeed the retiring Phyllis Bott as head of biochemistry, the seconds came from two women faculty, Katharine Boucot and Miriam Clarke.[45] For unclear reasons, Guarino was recommended by a search committee over Patricia J. Keller, a "research assistant professor" at the University of Washington. In March of 1964 a strong candidate for the chair of physiology, Jean M. Marshall of Harvard Medical School, became the second woman to decline an offer for that post. She stated that she did not wish to assume the administrative responsibilities, but expressed her "respect for Woman's Medical College and all the enthusiastic and capable staff members you have assembled there."[46] So, in August of 1964, this professorship too went to a qualified man, Edward Masoro.

Marion Fay felt frustration in not being able to appoint more women and some pique that alumnae seemed not to grasp the difficulties. "One of the hardest jobs I had when I was in the Deanship," Fay later recalled, "was to convince the alumnae that we had honestly tried to find a qualified woman and hadn't been able to. One of the pluses in this whole situation has been the very interesting number of very good men who have been willing to come here."[47] Indeed, some "very good men" had always found welcome on the WMC faculty. But when Marion Fay retired from the deanship in 1963, the gender makeup of the senior faculty had shifted alarmingly. What about the 1950s and early 1960s, or about Marion Fay, might have accounted for this marked change?

Marion Fay believed that during her years "the standards that we required of our professorial appointments were raised considerably." As she saw it, with only partial accuracy, in the past the essential criteria had been an eagerness to teach and the M.D. from WMC.[48] But in recruiting heads of science departments in the 1950s research credibility became a paramount determinant. Prestige and funding depended upon research. Gradually, this criterion applied in part to clinical chiefs.

Relatively few women pursued careers in science in the 1920s through the 1930s; and, as pointed out in the previous chapter, fewer still found an easy pathway to academic advance in medical schools and universities. Thus, by the 1950s, the pool of women scientists with desirable track records would have been tiny in relation to available men. Potential recruits who were married had to consider husbands' careers before relocating. Furthermore, in the 1960s coeducational medical schools began to hire and promote a few women, offering perhaps more money or prestige than did WMC.[49] So even search committees at WMC eager to see women appointed had no easy time of it, as some of the events related above suggest.

The letter from alumnae to the board, quoted at the beginning of this section, concluded, however, with this concise and apposite phrase: "We believe in the old adage 'Where there is a will, there is a way.'" Had the search committees, dean, and board shown enough will—tried hard enough to find women faculty for the last Woman's Medical College? Could not women have been found for *some* of the major professorships beyond pediatrics and obstetrics-gynecology? The questions remain unanswered—unless one believes they answer themselves—and the issue would continue to arise at the College even into the years of undergraduate coeducation.

An undoubted factor in the selection of new faculty and, more broadly, in setting the course for WMC in the post–World War II years was Marion Fay's outlook as a professional and as a woman. Although she never married, Fay liked men and enjoyed their company and attention. Her wit and social ease, surely incubated by her upbringing and college years in the gracious city of New Orleans, could delight colleagues of both genders. And she confidently felt the equal of accomplished men. In short, men were welcome in her personal and professional world.[50]

In Fay's mind, as a professional medical educator, the fundamental priority had to be running a "good medical school." This even exceeded in importance leading a *women's* medical school, as she indicated in her 1949 report to the board of corporators:

> the constant demand for the services of our graduates in various
> fields proves that we are needed. A good medical school will
> always be needed—and if the other schools ever do begin to
> take such large numbers of women that a woman's school is no
> longer needed as such, there will be just that many more
> qualified men who need places and we can become a coeducational school. But for men or for women we must give as good
> an educational experience as we can.[51]

It is unknown if any board members or others hearing or reading this passage started at Fay's casual reference to coeducation. But her imperative for developing the teaching corps meant finding individuals with the needed credentials for the 1950s and 1960s, including the potential for research work. Preference should go to women, but within limits.[52]

The junior faculty continued to grow through the addition of younger women and men, and still far more women than in the typical American medical school. Many new women clinical faculty held their M.D. from WMC, such as Doris Bartuska, Mary Dratman, and June Klinghoffer in internal medicine, Phyllis Marciano in pediatrics, Ann Pike and Martha Biemuller in obstetrics-gynecology, and Eva Fernandez Fox in medicine and radiology. They continued the tradition of alumnae-teachers-mentors going literally back to Ann Preston and Emeline Horton Cleveland, but also reflected their own times. Frieda Baumann, Jean Crump, Ann Gray Taylor, and Catharine Macfarlane had remained single; Bartuska, Dratman, Fox, Klinghoffer, and Marciano all married and had children. Drs. Bartuska and Dratman combined sophisticated laboratory research—unknown to earlier clinical faculty—with teaching and patient care.

Some of the new junior male faculty of the 1950s who in time became essential figures of the College were Andrew Beasley (anatomy and dean's office), Maurice Clifford (obstetrics-gynecology), Donald Cooper and James Bassett (surgery), Frederick DeMartinis (physiology), Ralph Myerson, Maurice Sones, and John Urbach (medicine). All won respect from students and colleagues. But it was beloved internist and diabetologist Harry Gottlieb (1925–1997) who so often received the supreme compliment: everyone at the College wanted this disheveled diagnostician to be their doctor.

A few instructors trained outside the United States appeared on the faculty in the 1950s, including some talented persons who might not have found positions at elite medical schools because of prejudice against foreign medical graduates. Gerardo Voci, from Italy, won considerable attention for carrying out the first, albeit makeshift, cardiac catheterization at WMC in 1958, performed in conjunction with Eva Fernandez Fox (WMC, 1943), hospital director and member of the Department of Radiology.[53] Cardiac catheterization typified the rise of high-technology medicine beginning in the 1950s, and it is of interest that its first tentative appearance at WMC grew out of the collaboration of a well-known WMC product and a male outsider with exotic background.

Also in the 1950s, a new class of de facto teachers grew in numbers and importance—hospital residents. A photograph of "House Staff, 1956–57" in the spring 1957 Alumnae Association *Newsletter* shows fifteen white-suited young physicians, of which six were men. Thus this valuable new segment of the College community began coeducationally.

The consequences of the masculinization of the WMC senior faculty during the 1950s and 1960s, from residents and fellows to department chiefs, can be readily surmised. When most other medical schools began to accept at least some women students, the College's provision of opportunity to women *faculty* helped justify its continuation. Although it still offered such opportunity, students and junior faculty alike saw fewer female role models enter the positions of greatest authority. Regardless of the adequacy of their medical training, would women students—at least those to whom it might matter—still be afforded the emotional apotheosis of the sort Frances Petty Manship knew in 1912 watching Ella Everitt and Ellen Potter operating at Philadelphia General Hospital?[54]

Was it enough for WMC to limit its M.D. enrollment to women if it began to look in other ways less and less like a women's institution? Would it appear, symbolically and invidiously, that women could no longer direct the affairs of a medical school or its departments in the complex new era of hospital expansion, programmatic research, juggling grants, and cardiac catheterization?

In the 1850s, the Longshores, Fussells, William J. Mullen, Ann Preston, and Emeline Horton Cleveland charted a "new and untried course," zealously motivated by a single idea: women might study medicine. WMC, the valiant survivor and idiosyncratic Philadelphia artifact, in the 1950s tacked directly toward the medical education mainstream. This movement began, almost unintentionally, with the mandated hiring of new science faculty, including Marion Fay, in the 1930s. Typical of 1950s mentality, a cautious focus on sound instruction, better science, and affordable growth guided the leaders of WMC, not any new sense of medical feminism. Marion Fay's "good medical school" became in important ways stronger, but at the expense of becoming more male. The intentions of the founders had been both expanded and muted.

From the Students' Perspective

A surprising continuity can be traced in the experience of WMC students from the late 1930s through the 1950s, and in fact some of what the 1950s students encountered and felt cannot be understood without looking back in time. Several of the most singular faculty members spanned this entire period, so graduates of 1938 and 1958 could compare recollections of Catharine Macfarlane, Mollie Geiss, Marion Fay, Hartwig Kuhlenbeck, Roberta Hafkesbring, Emily Van Loon, Ruth E. Miller, and others. Despite the curricular adjustments, the classroom and clinical work was not radically modified. A few old traditions, like the Halloween party, with some reconfiguration spanned these years. And, most important, from the point of view of students the College ambiance, both its appealing and irksome aspects, changed little from the 1930s into the early 1960s.[55]

Still a Door of Opportunity

Though most American women studying medicine in the mid-twentieth century did so in coeducational schools, WMC in many ways still provided the "door of opportunity" that Clara Marshall lauded early in the century. Even if the overall national rates of acceptance for men and women seeking a place in medical school did not differ in this period,[56] many women found rejection at universities they favored, in their native city, or even—most bitterly—at their own undergraduate university's medical college. One student of the late 1930s had been refused by Cornell, the University of Pennsylvania, and the University of Rochester, the latter her undergraduate school, which told her that "its quota for girls was limited." She won acceptance at WMC and felt "grateful for being here now."[57] Alumnae of the 1950s and early 1960s Doris Bartuska (1954), Lila Stein Kroser (1957), and Phyllis Marciano (1960) tell similar stories of enduring inquisitorial interviews by male officials at coeducational medical schools before deciding to come to Woman's Med. Bartuska kept a rejection letter from one medical school telling her that it had "accepted our two women for the year." Boots [Beaufort] Cooper (1965), who chose a medical career later in life, came to WMC from Dallas, Texas, after being refused admission by the university where she had both studied and worked professionally.[58] These last four women became WMC faculty and presidents of the Alumnae Association.

Even when medical coeducation had been long established, some women perceived the distinctive value of the small, single-sex school. In 1938, one student (responding to a survey issued by Catharine Macfarlane) said she valued WMC because "we are not treated as intruders as are women in the other schools." Katharine Boucot Sturgis (then Katharine R. Guest) acknowledged the "opportunity to study under the outstanding women in the profession."[59] Many WMC alumnae of the 1940s and 1950s speak of the importance of seeing women faculty doing everything medical and surgical. Another student noted the value of small size: "we have small clinic groups and therefore receive practically individual instruction, and we have the opportunity of seeing all the interesting cases that are admitted."[60]

Faculty and students readily came to know each other in such a setting. Not infrequently a faculty member or even the dean would respond to a student's urgent need. Two Japanese-American graduates of 1948, who had been in internment camps before coming to WMC, found themselves the only students in their class unable to obtain an internship, though one had graduated *cum laude*. Marion Fay used her connections to secure internships for both women in Pittsburgh. Lila Stein Kroser found a friend and mentor in Katharine Boucot Sturgis, who herself when a student had been aided by Catharine Macfarlane. These connections and experiences represented the finest potential of the small medical college, such as WMC. It was not at all unexpected that women would form personal friendships and alliances within the still largely male world of medicine. (Of course, student-faculty attachments certainly can and did occur in coeducational schools and across genders.)

An Array of Experiences and Feelings

Alumnae of the 1940s and 1950s, in union with their predecessors, almost invariably tell of a collegial, noncompetitive spirit among students. The intensity of the medical school experience induced the need for mutual support. The young women shared meals, apartments, study, notes, and cars. The increasing number of married students found one another and formed friendships as couples.

At the same time, WMC of the 1940s and 1950s did not leave its daughters with only warm and pleasing memories. Much depended, of course, on the outlooks and attitudes that the students brought to the institution, and the chance of experiences while there.[61] Memories proved kind to those easily given to institutional "bonding," or those crucially helped by classmate or instructor. But not so for others. Some students of the 1920s and beyond matriculated at Woman's Med following rejection by more prestigious medical schools. Many of these students recognized worthwhile qualities at the College or at least would never forget the school's provision of opportunity; but others in bitterness could never forgive the school for being their second choice.

From the 1930s into the early 1960s the educational programs at WMC, particularly in the basic science years, remained demanding, exhausting, and at times intimidating. It may not have been terribly difficult for a qualified student to enter the door of opportunity, but never did the faculty make it easy to get out with a degree four years later. Attrition was significant. The volume of material to learn grew ever more massive, spreading over five full days and half of Saturdays. Students passed countless weary and uninteresting hours in the laboratory and many more in endless memorization.

Such drudgery existed at other medical schools, but WMC had somehow come to rely on a particularly archaic and oppressive style of pedagogy in some of the basic science courses. In the words of inspectors from the Liaison Committee on Medical Education even as late as 1960, there was "little evidence of responsibility . . . given to the student for her own educational process. . . . There is still a high dependence upon examinations and quiz sessions of various sorts for motivating purposes."[62]

Furthermore, several longtime faculty members regularly resorted to abrasive classroom behaviors approaching ridicule. The motivation was to see students learn, but the method often looked like malice. Pathologist Mollie Geiss was notorious for this approach (though revered nonetheless by many graduates), and even Marion Fay herself, though gracious and caring in other settings, could frighten her chemistry pupils.

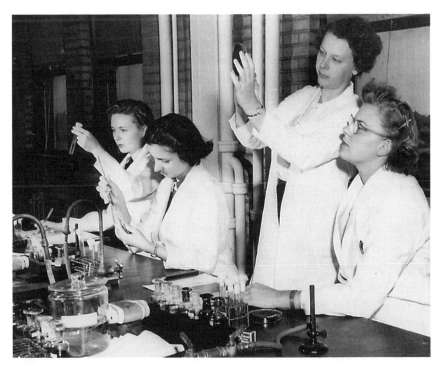

Figure 20. Among the best-liked and most respected of the basic science faculty from the 1930s to the 1960s was Ruth E. Miller, posed here in 1950. Emulating the best medical schools, WMC always insisted on a heavy dose of laboratory work.

Several other instructors are recalled as tough and daunting. Few students brought to tears by harsh classroom technique found a way to love the school during their first two years or became interested alumnae.

Exceptions, of course, certainly existed in the pre-clinical faculty. Alumnae particularly recall the microbiologist Ruth E. Miller as a gentle woman and thoroughly capable teacher. Anatomy head Hartwig Kuhlenbeck, initially terrifying to freshmen, could prove tolerant, helpful, and even humorous once one knew him.

The official conduct of the College in the 1940s and 1950s seems in retrospect also unnecessarily strict. The *Student Handbook* of the 1950s warned that "slacks and culottes are not worn on the college premises" and prescribed stockings when working in the wards or clinics.[63] Students eager to encounter patients were "discouraged from visiting the hospital unofficially."[64] The strictures on dress and deportment may have reflected the authoritarian 1950s as much as WMC, but still tell of an environment where the woman was too often treated like a girl.

What accounted for this stringency and the harsh instructional approach of some faculty? The basis goes back probably to the 1920s and partly to issues of gender. In 1921 when Sarah Logan Wister Starr agreed to rescue the College financially and manage it, she insisted on complete executive control by herself and the executive committee, resulting for a time in a tense and repressive atmosphere. The Tallant firing in part grew out of such a mind-set. That crisis was followed by further financial struggles during the Depression, then came the years of probation beginning in 1935. Mrs. Starr believed that the school came under attack because it was a women's place, led by women. WMC survived all this adversity, but not surprisingly it and Mrs. Starr acquired a defensiveness and "siege mentality" that propagated a custom of toughness and rigidity. "Woman's" would not equal weakness, and standards must remain high. Students had come to *work*, and no nonsense would be tolerated.

But why were certain women faculty particularly hard on the women students?[65] Many alumnae have suggested to the author that WMC over much of the twentieth century could not exorcize a tenacious "inferiority complex" as a "women's school." Some of the women faculty during this period probably without knowing it "internalized" slanted cultural beliefs about the value of women and women's institutions, and even, perhaps, about the ability of most women to learn science![66] This sensibility drove them to force learning on their students by whatever technique seemed to succeed. They either believed that their students needed this pressure or felt impelled to make absolutely sure that WMC graduates would know as much or more chemistry or pathology if compared to graduates of any other school. Finally, some of the acerbic behavior might have had its source simply in perplexing idiosyncrasies of personality.

Formative Faculty of the Clinical Years

The clinical years seemed an entirely different sphere, the hospital, a long-awaited promised land. Students of the 1950s assumed clinical responsibilities and autonomy as never before permitted at WMC, especially in those years when seniors filled the role of interns. But that responsibility meant long hours, often nocturnal, spent in completing "work-ups" and orders, drawing blood, doing laboratory tests, talking with families, investigating fevers and fits. Students on obstetrics rotation no longer delivered babies at home after about 1948, but certainly did so in the hospitals. Alumnae also remember work on the old obstetrics mannikin, reciting to the instructor "I stand to the right of the mother . . . I place my hands on the abdomen . . . I feel what I take to be the head." Others remembered the masterful surgery and teaching of "Polly" Pettit. Clinical rotations for juniors and seniors took them off the WMC campus to Philadelphia General Hospital, that great old museum of disease, familiar to Woman's Med students since the late 1860s. Students of the 1950s also went to the new Veterans Administration Hospital, where internist Ralph Myerson, a WMC faculty member literally by luck of a draw, became a favorite bedside instructor.[67] Outpatient work took place mainly in the clinics of WMC's hospital.

Clinical faculty appeared more as collegial teachers and comrades than stern taskmasters. Alumnae of the 1940s and 1950s reliably identify the same list of memorable clinical teachers and their characteristic stories or attributes. Internist Frieda Baumann represented solid competence and the essence of physicianship. Pediatrician Jean Crump extended her devotion to patients to raising chickens during World War II in order to provide eggs to her small charges. The Department of Pediatrics during the 1950s remained almost entirely female, its members all recalled with affection. Harriet Arey and Jean Gowing impressed with their diagnostic skill.[68] One alumna remembered the admired chief of surgery L. Kraeer Ferguson not for a particularly brilliant operation, but for his qualities as a person and even for apologizing to a class on discovering an error in his written examination.

Students and graduates revered the refined and ladylike chief of obstetrics Ann Gray Taylor (1893–1982), a master clinician and teacher. She could on occasion play the martinet—in many ways she replicated the progenitor of her lineage, Anna Broomall. Alumnae gleefully remember the contrast of Taylor's size and deportment with her penchant for fast and heedless driving, a challenge to Philadelphia police officers from East Falls to west Philadelphia.

Still very much in evidence was Catharine Macfarlane, the beloved

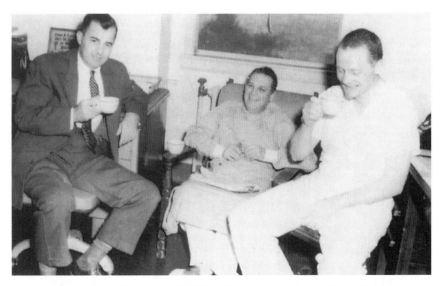

Figure 21. General surgery at WMC had been mainly the province of men, many of whom served the College steadfastly. Here professor and chair L. Kraeer Ferguson (center) and junior associates Donald Cooper (left) and James Bassett (both future chairs) sip coffee for a yearbook photographer in 1956. *Iatrian,* 1956.

Kitty Mac, retired as chair of gynecology but still active as "research professor" of that department, and grande dame of the medical school. Students and interns of the 1950s remember assisting Macfarlane at operations, aware of her temper and sometimes terrified by the opportunity. Her humor and kindnesses offset the occasional outbursts. Almost surely Kitty Mac operated well beyond her surgical prime: on hearing a suggestion to turn over such work to one of the gynecologists "as good at operating as you are," she replied that "I would if I knew anyone as good as I am!"[69] One alumna recalled that Kitty Mac in the 1950s displayed occasional lapses of sterile technique, but her patients somehow did well: residents joked that no bug would dare grow in any of Dr. Macfarlane's incisions.[70] Macfarlane had graduated from WMC in its "golden age" (1898), stood in 1921 to pledge a loan to save the school, rallied the opposition to merger in 1946, and in 1966 when eighty-nine years of age signed the protest concerning loss of women faculty. No one at WMC more vividly embodied the College saga and adherence to the cause of medical women.

Although the Liaison Council on Medical Education pressed for

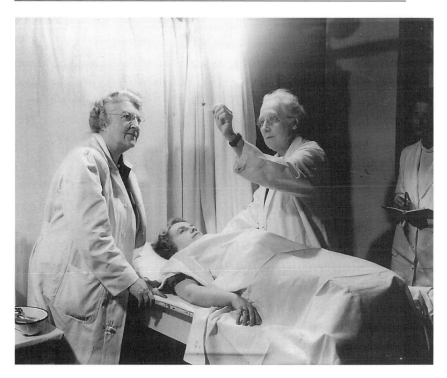

Figure 22. Professor of gynecology Catharine Macfarlane (WMC, 1898), the legendary "Kitty Mac" (holding slide), poses with collaborator Margaret Castex Sturgis for the *Saturday Evening Post* in the 1950s.

more full-time salaried clinical faculty, many alumnae of the 1940s and 1950s believed it an advantage that virtually all their clinical mentors actively practiced. They believed that what the faculty taught was what they daily did—real, not "ivory tower," medicine and surgery. The absence of true full-time clinical faculty did inhibit clinical research. Nonetheless, the reliance on volunteer faculty and "geographic full-times" generally served well.[71] At the College's hospital or at Philadelphia General, students generally found capable clinicians eager to teach, both women and men, seasoned faculty and newcomers. As mentioned earlier, residents increasingly contributed to practical instruction.

Like their predecessors, most WMC graduates of the 1940s and 1950s became private practitioners of medicine, either as generalists or in a specialty. Some attained unusual distinction. Joyce C. Lashof (1950) headed the University of California School of Public Health at Berkeley.

Lucy Frank Squire (1940) wrote what for years was the most popular introductory textbook of radiology. Edithe Levit (1951) rose to presidency of the National Board of Medical Examiners. Radiation oncologist Eleanor Montague (1950) published on the early diagnosis of breast cancer and treatment options. Ruth Bleier (1949) did research in neuroanatomy and published on gender bias in biological investigation. Enid Denbow (1955) became the chief medical officer in her native Guyana. This list, or one like it for any period, could be easily lengthened.

Student Life in the 1940s and 1950s

Organized student activities declined during the 1940s and 1950s, though a few traditions survived and interesting transformations occurred.[72] WMC students in the years immediately following World War II showed a continuation of wartime civic mindedness through activities analogous to those carried out by other women's groups. They sent clothing to students in postwar England and Italy and in the 1950s medical texts to Korea.[73] The WMC chapter of the Association of Internes and Medical Students (AIMS) gathered medical journals, textbooks, and used instruments to send through its national organization to Europe and China via Prague, headquarters of the International Union of Students (IUS).[74] AIMS had formed to improve the educational and general well-being of medical students and interns, but expanded its interests to the social and economic aspects of medical care. It attracted suspicion in those early cold war years for its generally leftward sympathies and its alliance with the IUS, considered by many an organization dominated by Communists.

The thirty or so WMC students in AIMS formed one of the larger chapters among Philadelphia's medical institutions. In late 1949 some AIMS literature from WMC found its way to Ivan H. Peterman, a writer for the *Philadelphia Inquirer*, who devoted a column to AIMS ("Young Medics Entangled in Pinkish Group"), singling out WMC for having one of the two "strongest chapters."[75] Soon after, fifty-five WMC students signed a petition objecting to the name of WMC appearing in AIMS literature. In the late 1940s, this protest exemplified spreading fear of Communism, or perhaps fear of the Communist-hunters. The student council proposed an open meeting to discuss AIMS. Marion Fay agreed to facilitate such a meeting, and urged faculty to attend; she also prepared a balanced report on AIMS for the board, even pointing out that some "outstanding graduates and some of the present good students" were members.[76] By the time the meeting was held on 5 January 1950, AIMS at the national level had voted to separate from the IUS. The brouhaha at WMC quietly died down. It was something of an anomaly that a vigorous AIMS chapter flourished for some time in the generally conservative atmosphere of WMC, and *not* surprising that with the conformist 1950s came its decline.

That hoary WMC tradition, the Halloween party, continued under sponsorship of alumnae, who warmly recalled it from their school days. But by 1953 it had evolved into a mixed dance with University of Pennsylvania medical students and later became a square dance.[77] The "skits" which had formed a highlight of the Halloween party since the nineteenth century moved to their own "April Fool" party in the spring; yearbook photographs from the late 1950s document elaborate and high-spirited productions for "skit night." Perhaps as a hint of the more rebellious 1960s, however, Dr. Fay in 1962 had to discuss with students and faculty one skit night whose angry satire had grown perhaps both too sharp and too coarse.[78]

In 1956 a yearbook, the *Iatrian*, appeared for the first time since 1914 and continued annually. Photographs from the yearbooks help construct a portrait of students at WMC in the 1950s. Group poses reveal that the two fraternities, Alpha Epsilon Iota and Zeta Phi, flourished, providing housing and aiding in the bonding of students with each other and with graduates. The active Christian Medical Society and the Marian Guild (a society of Roman Catholic students) recalled something of the religious cast of the nineteenth-century College. Various yearbook photographs demonstrate the continued presence of Asian and Asian-American students (another long tradition), while several African-Americans also appear. All classes included Jewish women as well, though they seemed not to have set up any formal organization.

Gazing at the 1950s yearbooks one finds other familiar photographs that, despite the 1950s clothing, transcend time: a small cluster of women around the anatomy lab's skeleton, others on an "inter-fraternity" outing in the park, a pair of students examining a child in clinic. True, some students had husbands, the Halloween dance was mixed, and men abounded on the faculty and house staff. Nonetheless, the "activities" pages of the *Iatrian* still evoke photographically a time and place of women together, sharing in some adventures of medicine and life, as long had occurred at WMC. None of the subjects of the *Iatrian*'s cameras in the late 1950s and 1960s could have known, as they sat for the Marian Guild portrait or cavorted in a chorus line at skit night, that theirs was a world soon to be lost or at least altered. Momentum for more change already existed, and Woman's Medical College was about to give way to Medical College of Pennsylvania.

Chapter 11   Coeducation

Background to the Debate

The search committee for a new dean and president to succeed Marion Fay in 1964 sought a woman candidate, but none was found. The committee solicited suggestions from alumnae, most of which Marion Fay later dismissed as not realistic.[1] Alumnae felt understandably disappointed and alarmed when Glen Leymaster, M.D., became the first male permanent dean of WMC since Ann Preston's predecessor in the 1860s. Trained in internal medicine and in public health, he had studied at and served on the faculties of the medical schools of Harvard and Johns Hopkins. He became chairman of the Department of Preventive Medicine and director of the health service at the University of Utah, Salt Lake City, and later (in 1960) Leymaster worked for the American Medical Association's Council on Medical Education and Hospitals.[2] He had gained familiarity with WMC as one of the council's site visitors in 1960.

Leymaster in his brief and largely unhappy tenure at WMC (he resigned in November of 1969) confronted rising dissatisfaction of faculty, student activism, as well as the usual financial worries. Not the source of all the problems, he lacked the charisma and forcefulness to overcome them. Though knowledgeable and at times poignantly introspective and frank in his self-assessment, Dr. Leymaster maintained few

supporters among faculty and alumnae at WMC and, despite some notable accomplishments, is remembered mainly as the leader who pressed
for the admission of men to the medical school's classes.[3]

What was the context, within and beyond the College, of Leymaster's proposal to consider coeducation? The 1960s saw the country
address discrimination and civil rights as had never been done before:
segregation (this was the word sometimes applied to single-sex education) of any sort became legally and socially suspect. By the early 1960s
all other medical schools admitted both men and women, though hardly
on an equal footing in many places. At the collegiate level coeducation advanced as Vassar and Bennington Colleges became among the
first of many women's schools to question their original policies and
purpose. The civil rights acts of 1964 prohibited discrimination in programs receiving federal funding, but only on the basis of race, color, or
ethnic background; might gender, however, not soon follow?[4]

Federal funding had become crucial to medical schools: by 1969,
this source supplied one-third of the College's income.[5] Another third
came from state appropriations, and here the single-sex admission policy
offered a different sort of threat. The Pennsylvania legislature repeatedly rebuked WMC for the relatively low number of Commonwealth
residents in its classes, and in 1967 a legislative "Task Force on Admission Policies of Schools of Medicine, Dentistry and Nursing" actually
recommended that the school consider admitting men to increase the
pool of Pennsylvanians who might win enrollment.[6] The College ran
deficits most years during the 1960s and could not chance loss of governmental funds.[7] Rising costs of indigent care in the College Hospital
accounted for much of the losses.

Deficits in morale and confidence also troubled Woman's Med in
the later 1960s. Discussion at a faculty meeting referred to the "anxiety and tension which our present system of grading, including a large
number of probations, seems to be producing," all remnants of the oppressive pedagogic approach detailed in earlier chapters.[8] The number
of superior students who sought transfer to other medical schools irked
the faculty and bred controversy, though some of these moves related
to marital circumstances.[9]

Faculty expressed other concerns. Increase in space and other facilities lagged behind the growth of faculty.[10] The delays in filling four

vacant departmental chairs, including the important chiefship of medicine, seemed a worrisome sign.[11] As WMC grew more complex, faculty perceived a failure of communications and an inability to achieve a voice in governance. Faculty morale had declined to a point of "mass pessimism," thought dean and president Leymaster in 1969, probably exaggerating. He partly blamed himself and the sometimes conflicting demands of his two offices: in serving the board and the budget, he neglected advocacy for the teaching corps.[12]

Leymaster and the Committee on Admissions Policies

Glen Leymaster and others of like mind never asserted that admitting men to the medical classes would solve all these problems, but they did come to see such a change as necessary to right some of them and prevent loss of funding. Leymaster may have moved to this conclusion over several years, though some alumnae opposed to coeducation believe he came to WMC, or indeed was hired, to end the single-sex tradition. His comments suggest at least ambivalence. In 1963 Leymaster stated his commitment to WMC "as a woman's school," but cautioned that "accepting men at Woman's Medical College is a subject of discussion."[13] A 1964 article in the *Medical World News* quoted Leymaster as stating that the College leadership was "not at all opposed" to coeducation, though he noted that "there's no point in our becoming coeducational while we're turning away so many qualified women."[14] Several articles and speeches during his first years in office advocated the role of women in medicine and conceived of the future WMC as "a National Center for Medical Education for Women."[15] Numerous obstacles—especially in recruitment of faculty and the financial picture—eroded what confidence he may have felt for the single-sex tradition.[16] By June of 1968 the president and dean presented to the executive committee of the board of corporators his assessment of how coeducation would positively and negatively influence the Woman's Medical College of Pennsylvania.[17] He concluded that the benefits would outweigh the costs.

In Leymaster's opinion, the central advantage would be improved morale among faculty and easier recruitment of both faculty (including chairs) and house staff (interns and residents). Since forty new medical colleges around the country had been organized in recent years he had good reason to worry that competition for qualified faculty could only increase.[18] Ironically, during the previous fifteen years a steady inflow of men had assumed most chairs, to the justifiable anger of many alumnae. But Leymaster did not invent his argument. One medical academician being wooed for the chair of medicine declined, citing the "sexual segregation" as a major impediment. The eventual successful candidate, Donald Kaye, wanted—and received—"assurance that the school will almost certainly become coeducational."[19]

In the late 1960s chairs of growing clinical departments at WMC believed that they were not recruiting the best possible candidates for their postgraduate training programs. Leymaster asserted, without citing evidence, that "the fact that this is a woman's institution, with the name of a woman's institution, does affect the number of applicants for residencies and internships."[20] American male physicians, he and others believed, were reluctant to become interns or residents at a medical college so "different" from all others.[21]

A medical student, when later offering her opinion to the Committee on Admissions Policies, turned the pivotal argument for coeducation on its ear: if faculty and potential house staff were indeed reluctant to come to WMC because it was a women's school, then prejudices against women in medicine must remain prevalent and the College should retain its exclusive admissions policy.[22] Those uncomfortable with the single-sex status of WMC would have argued that the issue was not sexism or opposition to women in medicine, but that a professional school accepting only women was "eccentric," an "oddity" in the world of science where supposedly "the mind has no sex."[23] Jay Roberts, who became chair of pharmacology at WMC in 1970, after the coeducation decision had been made, considered coeducation necessary and saw the single-sex status as linked with the past during a period of rapid change in science and medicine.[24] And to some extent, as suggested earlier in this book, WMC *did* constitute a gallant holdover from another era.

Yet this attitude—that the objection was to being different, "eccentric," or lost in the past, not to women per se—in some cases probably masked ingrained sexism of which some men were not even aware. One wonders how many male faculty at Jefferson Medical College thought the school "eccentric" until 1961 when it finally admitted women; or how many male chairs of the countless medical school departments throughout the country with no women as faculty or trainees thought *that* in any way odd or antiquated in 1970.

Even if linked to the past, the value of a women's medical school could not be dismissed even in 1968; women had not achieved full equality in medicine. Though the percentage of all male and female applicants to medical schools who found acceptance did not differ,[25] most coeducational schools maintained a quota for women admissions and employed few women on their faculties.[26] In 1970, it was still possible for a woman applicant at her medical school admissions interview to suffer questions about plans for a family and choice of contraception (one such student, whose husband had a job offer in Philadelphia, found instead at WMC a helpful assistant dean who expedited her application).[27] Furthermore, the College's status as a medical school traditionally for women still embodied its identity. Leymaster acknowledged that "it is extremely important that a private school today have a unique characteristic which sets it apart from the others," one of the ideas we have referred to earlier. The president and dean also recognized that an orientation to women did not necessarily preclude continued excellence and even national prominence, but believed "the College does not have the money to become the outstanding women's institution, and will not without substantial additional funds."[28]

Let us return to Glen Leymaster's other arguments for considering the admission of men. In his formal letter requesting the formation of a Committee on Admissions Policy, and in his written analysis of the issue, he called attention to the issue of state funding and number of Pennsylvania matriculants, but only briefly listed risk of losing federal funding. As earlier noted, in 1968 no law yet forbade federal funding to educational institutions segregated by gender, so the risk remained hypothetical. Nonetheless, members of the Committee certainly considered it, and (erroneously) stated that accepting men would allow the College to "conform to the Civil Rights Acts of 1964 and 1968."[29]

Board chair Louise Kaiser (Mrs. Paul Kaiser) on 4 October 1968 formed the Committee on Admissions Policies, already referred to.[30] Its membership comprised Kaiser and Leymaster (*ex officio*), two faculty representatives (Mary DeWitt Pettit of obstetrics and gynecology and William Riker of pharmacology), alumnae E. Cooper Bell (WMC, 1947, an internist and president of the Alumnae Association, and on the volunteer faculty), and Jean Gowing (WMC, 1926, a pediatrician and member of the volunteer faculty), administrators Charles Glanville and George Hay, and, as student members, class presidents Lourdes Corman and Lisa Luwisch.[31] The committee began to meet monthly.

In December of 1968 Louise Kaiser issued a letter to inform faculty, staff, alumnae, and members of the National Board and the Commonwealth Committee that leaders of the Woman's Medical College had appointed a committee "to recommend to the Board and President whether our goal of providing the highest quality medical education obtainable is best realized by remaining open only to women candidates or whether, like other institutions of higher education, we should be investigating procedures whereby we broaden this policy."[32]

She invited readers of her communication to offer their comments through any member of the committee. Seventy-five letters representing every group were received, three quarters of which expressed support for the admission of male medical students to the Woman's Medical College provided, in the opinion of most, that women's places *not* be reduced.[33] The committee would reflect this sentiment in its report.

Viewpoints of the Constituencies: Faculty and Alumnae

It is of interest to examine the opinions of the three major constituencies, faculty, alumnae, and students, as expressed both to the board's committee and through other vehicles. The faculty discussed the admission of men at its meeting of 15 January 1969. Senior faculty member Elizabeth Waugh (WMC, 1931) spoke of the "early founding of the College and its purpose," but advised her colleagues that "if the institution is to progress we must be open-minded," and again raised the concerns about state and federal funding.[34] According to the minutes of this meeting (signed by Dr. Leymaster), "a straw vote was taken by a showing of hands which indicated no opposition to the suggestion that the institution admit both men and women."[35] Of course, not all faculty members were present. Individual faculty members would, however, come to oppose the admission of men; these included Maria W. Kirber, professor of microbiology, committee member E. Cooper Bell—who eventually filed an articulate and astute dissenting opinion—and others. Analysis of twenty-one faculty letters to the committee showed that three opposed the proposed change, six favored it, and twelve favored it conditionally.[36]

Dr. Cooper Bell's objections probably represented her sentiments more as an alumna and medical feminist than as faculty member. Indeed, the response of alumnae to coeducation forms a more complex and passionate story. Of the forty alumnae responses to the committee, thirteen opposed coeducation, fourteen favored it, and thirteen favored it with the conditions noted earlier, that no places for women be lost. But the numbers hardly reflected the extremities of opinion. Frances Norris (WMC, 1958), a surgical pathologist then in Washington, D.C., unleashed her outrage in a letter to Glen Leymaster. She contended that College leadership was "attempting, by subterfuge and misrepresentation, to pervert the aims and purposes of our college through the influence of a misogynistic and turncoat male faculty."[37] Norris also published a vehement letter in the *New England Journal of Medicine*, accusing the College leadership of choosing to restrict the admission of women "so that male applicants rejected elsewhere can be admitted."[38] Alumna Marian Hall (WMC, 1926) beseeched Louise Kaiser to retain the exclusive admission policy because sexism still prevailed: "the very fact that I must address you as 'Mrs. Paul Kaiser'—with no resemblance to your name as a single woman . . . points up the basic fact that woman is still considered as subservient to the male."[39] Many other alumnae, already antagonized by the masculinization of the faculty and executive leadership, felt at the very least apprehension and distrust.

The Alumnae Association's executive committee offered its opinion in a letter to the Committee on Admissions Policies dated 7 February 1969, signed by Dr. Cooper Bell, association president. The alumnae leaders did not oppose "the admission of male students per se," but predicted that the number of women students would necessarily drop over the years unless vigilant efforts arose to prevent this happening. They pleaded the continued "need for an institution such as The Woman's Medical College to represent and protect the place of Women in Medicine and to provide special opportunities for them." Thus, "the admission of male students should be carefully controlled."[40]

On 29 August 1969, one week before the board was to vote on the committee's recommendation to admit men, the Delaware Valley Chapter of the Alumnae Association petitioned the board not to authorize doing so until facilities were constructed to accommodate additional students. The chapter vehemently insisted that sixty-six places in the freshman class—then the maximal number—be reserved for women and expressed displeasure that two male students had been recommended for admission before the new policy had been officially adopted.[41] On 4 September 1969, the night before the board voted to accept the report of the Committee on Admissions Policies, two hundred students and alumnae organized a panel discussion on coeducation. The alumnae magazine reported that though many individuals echoed the concerns of the Delaware Valley Chapter, administrators and faculty seemed to feel that coeducation could not wait.[42]

Student Views and Student Activism in the Late 1960s

How did the students currently enrolled at WMC look upon the possibility of admitting men to the school? Clearly during the late 1960s one would expect students to have opinions and press that their voices be heard. Indeed such was the case with many American medical students, including some at WMC, though the admission of men did not win the attention and activism seen with other issues.

In December 1967, nearly one hundred angry medical students from around the country interrupted a conference of medical school deans at the American Medical Association convention in Chicago, asserting that the organization was trying to "silence the anguished cries of the poor."[43] In September of 1968 a group of Philadelphia medical students within the activist Student Health Organization formed a Committee for Black Admissions. This committee wrote to the Deans of all six Philadelphia medical schools to demand that one-third of the entering freshman class consist of black students. In a "Public Statement of the Six Philadelphia Deans on the Matter of Disadvantaged Students in Medicine," the leadership agreed to work at finding qualified black applicants and encouraging high schools and colleges to offer black students better preparation for medical school. In early 1969 at WMC the Student American Medical Association chapter and the student council sponsored a Forum on Black Admissions.[44]

Though Glen Leymaster acknowledged that the activists represented "intelligent, socially concerned and articulate students," he also lamented, with the Chicago incident on his mind, that their techniques induced gray heads to "get a little grayer."[45] Focusing on intramural issues, fifty-eight WMC students in their "Open Letter to the Board of Corporators" called for replacement of vacant departmental chairs, better teaching, and—perhaps above all—"opening channels of communications on all levels."[46]

The students' petition to the board made no mention, however, of coeducation or the Committee on Admissions Policies. Lourdes Corman and Liza Luwisch, student members of the committee, used a careful written survey to assess student opinion. A total of 128 students responded (55 percent of enrollment). Corman and Luwisch summarized the opinions on coeducation at WMC as follows: "Assuming equal standards of admission, 73 students (or 57%) would like to see WMC accept men. However, of these students only 34 (or 47%) would favor admitting men without increasing the size of the entering class."[47] Sixty-four percent of those favoring the admission of men believed that a quota should limit their number. This stance was not surprising: a majority of WMC students had failed to gain entry to coeducational schools, while others chose WMC because it was a women's school.[48]

On 24 March 1969, twenty-eight senior students signed a letter to the Committee on Admissions Policies agreeing that WMC "should indeed become coeducational," but asking for a "ratio of around 50:50 male/female." This petition expressed alarm, however, that some faculty at WMC questioned "the validity of women in medicine." They sensed this attitude more among some "pre-clinical professors" than among the clinicians, and called for the latter group to gain a larger "say on the admissions committee."[49]

No overwhelming opposition to admitting men prevailed among WMC students of the late 1960s, though undoubtedly the majority wished to see the school's commitment to women maintained. The debate, however, held other meanings for a few students. *Vital Signs*, the student newspaper printed first in September 1968, described itself as a "Publication Sponsored by Students Who Provide a Voice for Those Who Feel Deeply and Think Seriously about the Practice of Medicine." Interested faculty also wrote for it. The initially leftist *Vital Signs* included art, literature, and commentary on current events within and without the Woman's Medical College. Curriculum critiques appeared alongside articles on abortion, equity of medical care, the effects of marijuana, and the horrors of the war in Vietnam. The inadequacies of the emergency room for patients, staff, and students in particular stimulated writers.

In one compelling editorial, founding editor and activist Nancy Coyne proposed reforms in the conduct of medical education and in the relations between the institution and its community. To correct wrongs and better serve patients and students, Coyne challenged the faculty and administration to "get the necessary staff and money before the hospital is burned, bombed, or 'sat-in.'"[50] She saw the proposal to admit men as a false issue, and suggested that "instead of just competing for State money by going co-ed, WMC could make a real contribution to medicine by creating a model of education whose goal is truly that of training students to see, define, and provide for the health of human beings and where 'academic excellence' has a chance to grow in a community of interested scientists and students."[51]

A less combative but equally pointed article by Lourdes Corman titled "Another Committee" appeared in the May 1969 issue of *Vital Signs*. Corman had intended to write an article on the progress of the admissions policies committee, but had been told by the committee that she could not yet do so. The experience led Corman, never one easily muffled, to evaluate the worth of student representation on committees at Woman's Medical College if the student cannot serve as a conduit of information to her peers.[52] Corman came to staunchly oppose the controversial change after weighing the arguments and reflecting on her own experience. Like Coyne she concluded that admitting men amounted to a false but "defendable" solution to problems at WMC. She feared that WMC would lose its identity and pointed out that regardless of national statistics, numerous future women physicians currently enrolled at the College had found acceptance at no other medical school.[53]

Few students, however, voiced unconditional opposition to the admission of men. Indeed, that segment of the student population given to forming and expressing distinct opinions—the activists—lent much of their energy to causes beyond WMC, such as civil rights, equal access to health care, the war in Vietnam. Within the College, concerned students cared about the well-being of the school, but found themselves focusing not on the question of admitting men, but rather on their access to authority and the decision-making process. Such access mattered as they condemned entrenched flaws—none unique to WMC—in the very process of medical education.[54] Maintaining all-women medical classes did not seem directly relevant to the causes at the College or in the world that won their attention.

The Decision Is Made

Clearly a large proportion of alumnae would agree to seeing men accepted *only* if no places were lost to women, but few seemed resolute in defending an absolute, complete status quo.[55] Thus no major constituency—students, faculty, alumnae—put forward firm, unqualified, and unified opposition to coeducation at Woman's Med. In this setting members of the Committee on Admissions Policies and the board of corporators—many of whom were probably convinced before the process began—had little difficulty in favoring the proposed change.

Meanwhile, the board of corporators made some preliminary efforts to improve the sense of distrust and deficient communications fouling the College air. The board's executive committee in April held separate meetings with representatives of the students and of the faculty.[56] Tensions flared about the same time, however, when feisty senior students, denied a request for time off to study for National Board examinations, presented the faculty with "an ultimatum to the effect that they would take ten days off regardless."[57] In June, the faculty's curriculum committee approved a modified "pass-fail-honors" grading system aimed at reducing student anxiety over examination scores.[58] In this still turbulent—though in some ways improving—environment the Committee on Admissions Policies presented its report to the board on 6 June 1969. It recommended that Woman's Medical College "should admit men in its undergraduate body," and that "in principle" coeducation should be achieved "by the *addition* of qualified male students rather than by the *supplanting* of women." Furthermore, "as rapidly as funds can be acquired . . . Woman's Medical College should substantially increase the size of its classes."[59]

Ironically, at the same meeting board president Louise Kaiser announced the recent death, on 27 May at the age of ninety-two, of
Catharine Macfarlane, zealous defender of the College and of its founding purpose. Kitty Mac had not lived to see the alteration of this purpose or loss of the name "Woman's Med" that she so venerated. At the
June meeting, Mrs. Kaiser indicated that she would distribute copies of
the report to the College community, and defer a vote by the board
until September.

The summer brought the College further tribulation. The state
tightened eligibility for its medical coverage of the indigent, while Philadelphia threatened to eliminate its payment for emergency department
care.[60] Board members probably had future eligibility for federal and
state funding much on their minds. At its meeting of 5 September 1969,
following discussion, the board approved the recommendation of the
Committee on Admissions Policies and endorsed the plan to "admit
sixty-six qualified first year women students for the current year" and
some men "only if they do not displace women." For the next two years,
resolved the board, the College would admit "a minimum of sixty qualified women" and "additional men . . . to the capacity of the first year
class."[61]

Twenty-two members voted for the resolutions, one abstained, and
seven opposed. The board of corporators, incessantly afflicted with fiscal shortfalls, and looking back on a year of discord and lamentation,
deemed coeducation a necessary, though not sufficient, answer to problems facing Woman's Medical College. In doing so, for better or worse,
the corporators of 1969 ended 120 years of unequivocal adherence to
the singular purpose which gripped the minds and souls of the first who
bore the duties of that office.

Implementing the Decision: An Addition of Men and Deletion of "Woman's"

The first men admitted to the medical classes of WMC apparently had
been waiting in the research wings.[62] Steven DeArmond, age twenty-
nine, was three years into graduate work in physiology at Woman's
Medical College when accepted into the first-year medical class as an
M.D.-Ph.D candidate. DeArmond was married to a fourth-year medi-

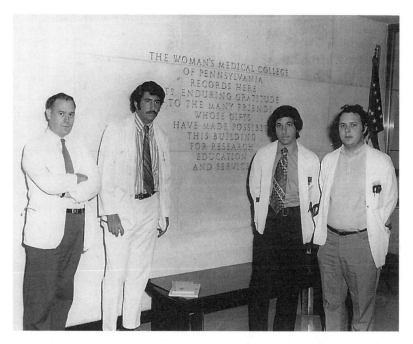

Figure 23. The first men to receive the M.D. graduated in 1972: Jay Ripka, Hardy Sorkin, Louis Rose, and Martin Schimmel.

cal student and active on College committees. Lewis Snitzer and Andrew Brenner, twenty-two-year-old bachelors who entered the first- and second-year classes respectively, also as combined M.D.-Ph.D students, attracted considerable attention. Distorted interviews with Snitzer and Brenner in the popular press focused on their social lives and dating opportunities rather than on academics. In an article from the *Philadelphia Inquirer Magazine* titled "A Tale of 239 Girls and Three Men," Snitzer is pictured seemingly gazing at several women medical students "in an unguarded moment." The three men together are said to have "reversed the blooming female revolution and injected themselves into the world of pediatrics, pathology, and petticoats at Woman's Medical College in East Falls."[63] If this portrayal of students at the Woman's Medical College appealed to readers of the *Philadelphia Inquirer*, it is clear that American women in medicine (or elsewhere) indeed had not yet won a full measure of professional respect by the time the Woman's Medical College went coeducational.

The first men to receive the M.D. from the College, in 1972, were

Jay Ripka, Louis Rose, Martin Schimmel, and Hardy Sorkin; they had entered as transfer students into the third year, and thus graduated before DeArmond, Brenner, and Snitzer.

Even students alarmed by the implications of the new admissions policy rarely directed their dissatisfaction toward male students, in particular or in general. Sophomore class president Rose Mohr remarked, "I have nothing against men in medicine, however, I think it is sad that Woman's admits men without the assurance that women interested in pursuing medicine as a career will be treated equally with men." Natalie Shemonsky, president of the junior class, stated that she was unhappy with the new policy "not because I doubt the positive influence that a coeducational environment would have" but because she was concerned with "the future disposition of women in my category—older, married, and already mothers. WMC has been our stronghold and I only hope that it will remain so."[64] Nor is there evidence or recollection of a pattern of ill-treatment of the new male students by even the most partisan of alumnae-faculty. Of course, women on the clinical faculty had been teaching men on the house staff for many years, while women scientists had supervised male graduate students.

Indeed, some of the first generation of male students quickly developed admiration and affection for alumnae faculty members such as Doris Bartuska, Boots Cooper, Jean Gowing, June Klinghoffer, Elizabeth Labovitz, Alma Morani, and others. An early male graduate, Lawrence Byrd (MCP, 1973), in a later interview recalled the "sensitizing" experience of being one of a handful of men in a class of women, "like going from white skin to dark overnight." He began to sense what a woman in medicine daily endured, even small things such as being mistaken for a nurse. He became respectfully aware that some of the senior women faculty had "carved out a career against odds" of the sort he would never need face.[65] Here is another irony: by becoming coeducational, Woman's Med could offer to some receptive men an unexpected new door of opportunity for personal growth.

Members of the faculty and board took satisfaction in learning in the fall of 1969, a month after the decision to admit men, that applications to the 1970 class were sharply ahead of those received at the same time in 1968 (298 vs. 113). Less than 15 percent were from men.[66]

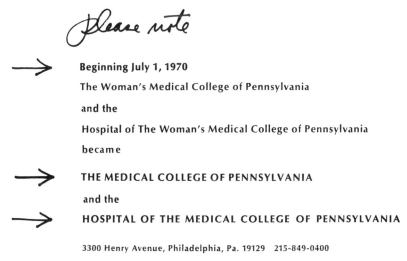

Figure 24. Alumnae and other persons connected to the College received this understated card announcing the name change, an outcome of the decision to admit men to the medical classes.

This surge in applications represented, however, at least in part the early phase of a national trend: over the 1970s, the number of American women seeking medical education rose nearly fivefold, while the number of men increased as well, but at a lesser rate. By 1974–75, 8,712 applications from women formed 20 percent of the total, and in the same year women occupied an unprecedented 22 percent of first-year places in United States medical schools.[67] During the 1970s and 1980s, as facilities allowed, the MCP class size rose from 68 to 120. Through the middle of the 1980s, the admissions committee yearly contrived to accept at least sixty to sixty-five women, in accordance with recommendations made in 1969. The perception in the 1970s that the country needed more doctors induced government to subsidize the enlargement of medical school enrollments. Thus MCP could add men without deleting places for women; the expansion thus made coeducation easier to accept. By the late 1980s, however, occasional entering classes showed a small preponderance of men, a trend reversed in the early 1990s.[68]

A dramatic outcome of the new admissions policy was a new College name, as recommended by the Committee on Admissions Policies.

In the December 1969 issue of *Woman's Medical College Today* Glen Leymaster requested suggestions for a name that would give "both women and men a sense of belonging" and "suggest an unlimited future, as well as to acknowledge our heritage."[69] No such divine name appeared, nor probably existed. "The Medical College of Pennsylvania" was not formally adopted until the following July. Though seemingly uncomplicated, the name change engendered bitter resentment among some of the College community. Phyllis Marciano, president of the Alumnae Association and clinical faculty member, summarized a good deal of alumnae sentiment when she declared that the name change "was premature, unwarranted, and stripped our college of its identity."[70]

Marciano organized alumnae protest against the new name based on the just argument that "the word *Woman* in the name need not necessarily reflect the nature of the student body but rather the original intent of its founders."[71] Changing the name represented a lack of nerve. If the new leaders of the College were going to succeed in achieving increased excellence, students and interns would come, regardless of the name. Furthermore, persons in the medical world with some knowledge of history would recognize not shame but honor in the name "Woman's Medical College" and what it stood for—opportunities once denied to half the nation's population. While admitting men may have accommodated the future, changing the name scorned the past and insulted women. Some alumnae came to perceive a larger loss: could the College, now so widely populated with men, continue to serve as a real and symbolic "homeland" for women physicians, as it had for 120 years? The name resection seemed to symbolize that the tradition was rapidly and irreversibly fading.[72]

It took many years before "Medical College of Pennsylvania" or the promoted short form, "MCP," linked to recognizable new attributes. Older Philadelphia patients in the College Hospital twenty years after the name change still answered "Woman's Med" to the standard orientation question ("where are we now?"), while semi-oriented Philadelphia cab drivers occasionally drove visiting speakers to the wrong medical school. No one proposed altering the engraved "WOMAN'S MEDICAL COLLEGE" atop the school's massive entrance portico.

In the Aftermath of Coeducation

In November of 1971 Congress adopted the Comprehensive Health Manpower Training Act, which forbade federal grants to health professions training institutions that discriminated on the basis of gender. Then in June of 1972, in response to rising feminist activism, came Title IX of the Education Amendments to the earlier Civil Rights law, which prohibited gender discrimination in most categories of educational institutions, including professional schools, though it allowed a six-year period of transition from single-sex status to coeducation.[73] Fearing the loss of federal funding, the board of corporators on 23 June 1973 authorized Bernard Sigel, then dean and president, to supply to the appropriate federal agencies a signed affirmation of compliance, effectively rescinding earlier commitments by the board to reserve a minimum number of places for women.[74] Unsuccessful in gaining an administrative exemption, the College leaders and several alumnae engaged the aid of Senator Richard Schweiker, who over the next several years attempted to effect a congressional deferment for MCP.[75]

Little more than a year after the decision to admit men, events had validated one of the rhetorical arguments used to support the radical change. Ironically, the institution that so long had assured opportunity for women seeking the medical degree now found it might not be able to legally do so without risking, in effect, charges of discrimination! Furthermore, this risk arose *after* the school decided to admit males to its medical classes. Those alumnae already bitter over the change in admissions policy and in the name now encountered another impediment to maintaining the College's traditional mission. (No known legal challenge arose, however, to the continued practice of usually admitting about 60 percent women, even when this proportion exceeded the proportion of women applicants.)

Still doubtful of MCP's commitment to women, leaders of the Alumnae Association in 1970 had formed a Special Trust Fund, independent of College administration, to further the education of women at MCP. The new legal threats of 1971 and 1972 seemed to underscore its need. That the trust fund entailed fund-raising in competition with the College itself painfully strained friendships between Marion Fay (serving as acting president of the College in 1971) and the fund's founding trustees such as Margaret Gray Wood (WMC, 1948) and

Phyllis Marciano. The trust fund had little trouble gathering contributions, and soon made grants to the College in aid of the new Center for Women in Medicine, a retraining program for inactive women physicians, and experiments in part-time residencies for women. It also would make funds available for loans and scholarships to women students. In later years, the fund supported programs within the College that enhanced education for women and men, and in 1998 would come to the aid of the historical Archives and Special Collections on Women in Medicine.[76]

Final Ironies

Although the decision to admit men to WMC ostensibly seems a product of the 1960s and Glen Leymaster's tenure, arguably the roots of the change reach back much further. The continuation of the exclusive admissions policy cannot be separated from the school's singular way of survival during much of the twentieth century. This survival, as we have seen, depended upon an often heroic alliance of alumnae, alumnae-faculty, other Philadelphia-bred faculty including men, and a very local philanthropy of lay women who both worked and gave money. This alliance began to weaken in the years after 1935, when loss of AMA approval led directly to the hiring of university-bred science faculty from outside Philadelphia and indirectly to the end of Sarah Logan Wister Starr's administration. The new faculty members created a dominantly feminine presence in the pre-clinical departments, but these women could not be expected to uniformly embrace the founding purpose and College saga: new perspectives could arise, even on issues of gender. Recall that as dean in 1949, Marion Fay, one of the 1935 recruits, in a report to the board casually suggested that so long as WMC remains a "good medical school," if the need for a women's medical school were to disappear (and she did not believe it had yet done so) "we can become a coeducational school."[77]

In the 1950s and early 1960s more and more chairmanships went to men as other criteria for appointment displaced gender, and most of these men were not Philadelphians or familiar with the historic background of WMC. Alumnae influence decreased as graduates no longer filled the deanship or chairs of large departments; and alumnae contributions, even when generous, became a smaller part of funding the budget. The consensus for single-sex education had eroded before Leymaster arrived, though certainly he was instrumental in bringing about coeducation. But the momentous alteration at Woman's Med in 1969–70 derived from historical, social, and economic shifts in addition to that in gender.

No one in the 1950s, however, could have predicted the extraordinary paradox that a rising national attempt to ensure equal rights to Americans long denied them would actually threaten the residual commitment to women of the remaining women's medical school. Or that the decision to admit men to Woman's Med occurred at the precise beginning of the new and multifaceted outpouring of feminism that transformed the United States in the late 1960s and 1970s. Indeed one strand of this new feminism advocated the unique possibilities of sisterhood, the advantages of women's community, and the creative power of women working together.[78] Of course, since its founding men always had been part of Woman's Medical. But the redefining acceptance of men *as students* at WMC/MCP came just as a new "Woman Movement" suggested the missed potential for becoming a greater center for women's medical education, conducted by and for women.

Chapter 12

Medical College of Pennsylvania

What Course Now?

With its founding purpose and familiar name altered, what course would Medical College of Pennsylvania pursue? How would this small medical school among many large ones find its place? Soon after deciding to admit men to the medical school classes, the board of corporators tried to answer this question by approving in 1971 a "Statement of Mission" drafted by an appointed committee:

> The Mission of the Medical College of Pennsylvania is twofold:
> —to teach men and women those arts and sciences related to the preservation of human health and the prevention and treatment of disease, and to advance the body of knowledge in these areas.
> —to continue its commitment to the education of women physicians and to develop and maintain programs which will expand the opportunities for women in the medical professions.[1]

The school succeeded with the first of these objectives but despite good intentions, the second proved more elusive. During the 1970s and 1980s the College attempted to become (as stated later in the mission document) "a health sciences university with a comprehensive medical center."[2] In the early 1970s virtually every medical school in the United States claimed to be or hoped to become an "academic medical center" carrying out laboratory research and technologically sophisticated hospital care. Society, through the mechanism of funding from government and medical insurers, rewarded these aspirations.

MCP showed remarkable progress in expanding its basic science and (to a lesser extent) clinical research programs, gradually attaining national prominence in several disciplines. Clinical capabilities of the College hospital accrued as well, but much more fitfully. The size of the budget, physical plant, and faculty soared. Yet at the very same time the College successfully nurtured and proclaimed its reputation as a small, "intimate" institution that functioned like a family. In growing larger, technologic, and more competitive while sustaining a milieu of intimacy and internal cooperation, MCP for many years pursued—with surprising success—seemingly disparate identities which might even be seen as culturally "masculine" and "feminine." Earnest efforts to create specific programs that would further the school's legacy of service to women physicians did not, however, find their place. More lasting were attempts, some of which grew out of experiments aimed at the needs of women, to make contributions in the realm of medical educational innovation.

This multifaceted program to change yet stay somehow the same, enlarge but remain in ambience small, progressed despite the impediments of administrative turmoil during the first MCP decade, and unceasing fiscal concerns. When Marion Fay came out of retirement in 1971 to serve for a year as acting president, she told an interviewer that she expected to spend her time fund-raising outside the institution and fostering communications within it—"The same old problems."[3]

The growth in all components of MCP beginning in the 1970s precludes, regrettably, citing in this chapter most faculty names, even those who made multiple contributions. Rather, we will focus largely on programs and their relationship to the development of MCP as a medical school almost undergoing rebirth.

A Sequence of Presidents

Dr. Fay returned to the presidency following Glen Leymaster's resignation while a search committee looked for a new administrative head. Irving H. Leopold, a prominent ophthalmologist, accepted the position in 1970, then—to the school's embarrassment—almost immediately changed his mind, perhaps as he learned more about the fiscal situation.[4] Marion Fay remained in office long enough to deal with a severe financial crisis and wage freeze,[5] then Dean Bernard Sigel became interim president. Academic pediatrician Robert Slater, former dean of the University of Vermont School of Medicine, assumed the presidency in 1974 (and also served as acting dean) but proved a disappointment and resigned in June of 1976.[6] Longtime board member Jeanne Brugger stepped in as interim president. An associate dean and professor of psychology and education at Drexel University, Mrs. Brugger proved an able leader during stressful times.

In its next presidential search, MCP again sought a prominent name. The ultimately unhappy result was the appointment in 1977 of Robert E. Cooke, another academic pediatrician, who had been vice chancellor for health sciences at the University of Wisconsin and previously pediatrician-in-chief at Johns Hopkins Hospital. Cooke owned a sharp intellect, a striking statesman-like presence, and fabled connections in Washington and to the Kennedy family. It was later learned, however, that considerable difficulties surrounded his tenure in Wisconsin.[7] Cooke's imperious and at times secretive manner in advancing his strategy for MCP led to strife unknown since the Tallant affair of 1923. But the threat revealed, as in years past, a resolve to defend the College felt by faculty and alumnae/i. Eventually, on 5 September 1979, the faculty passed an unprecedented vote of censure, accusing the president of such offenses as disregarding the actions and counsel of the faculty and medical staff of the hospital, abusing the office of the dean, attempting to "rush through" self-serving new corporate bylaws, and threatening retribution against faculty who attended a meeting at which these complaints were discussed. Despite support among some board members, the president was caused to resign, and the bruised College went on with its work. Rancor persisted, however, as the former president brought suit against three faculty members active in the opposition movement.[8]

What might have accounted for this series of presidential missteps? Almost certainly they were symptoms suffered by an institution still in the uncertain stages of transition from being small and local to assuming a more prominent place within academic medicine. Board members held differing views of what the College might be; search committees did not ask the right persons the right questions. In addition, despite its merits, MCP in the early and mid-1970s still lacked the standing to attract a major medical statesman (or woman) free of any flaws.

It was no surprise when Maurice Clifford, a familiar "insider," received appointment as interim president in 1979, then president in 1980 following a national search. A faculty member in the Department of Obstetrics and Gynecology since 1955, Clifford had been serving as vice president for clinical affairs.[9] Dr. Clifford *looked* like the sort of leader MCP needed at the moment: a large but graceful figure, he exuded a physical sense of intelligence, stability, even tranquility. With a solid background in literature and history, Maurice Clifford could speak with eloquence and a quiet moral passion, while quoting comfortably from the Bible or Tennyson. As a prominent African-American, he knew some of Philadelphia's ascending leadership and could plead with particular forcefulness concerning the needs of the largely poor clientele of MCP's emergency department and clinics.

In 1975, another Philadelphian, Alton I. Sutnick, became dean of MCP, a position he would hold until 1989. Dr. Sutnick, an internist by training, had worked in clinical and laboratory science as well as administration. When recruited by MCP, he held administrative posts at the Fox Chase Cancer Center in Philadelphia. Earlier, he had been a faculty member of the medical schools of Temple University and the University of Pennsylvania.[10] No doubt some alumnae would have preferred a woman dean: alumna and faculty member Doris Bartuska expressed this sentiment in 1977, while acknowledging that Dr. Sutnick seemed to be doing his job well.[11] Sutnick was, however, in part attracted to the deanship by the school's unique history, and borrowed a copy of Alsop's *History* from the library soon after arriving.[12] Alton Sutnick's fourteen-year tenure was remarkable for its time: the medical school dean of the 1970s and 1980s confronted a complex set of academic and business tasks with uncertain authority suspended between board and president above, and departmental chairs below. As professor of physiology and biochemistry Julian Marsh commented at the time of Dr. Sutnick's retirement, deans "get blamed for everything and have to share the credit."[13]

Dr. Sutnick maintained good relations with most department chairs, though the College's budgetary limits made his responses to requests often (in his words) "parsimonious." Some thought the dean perhaps *too* willing to hear all sides and too deliberative in arriving at certain decisions (this would have been sensed, no doubt, when a department chair hoped for a swift decision in his or her favor). Undoubtedly Dr. Sutnick's tenure and integrity lent needed stability to the College, and as will be seen, much was accomplished during the years he and Maurice Clifford held office. He suffered acutely during the Cooke years.

Becoming an Academic Medical Center: Research

Dean Sutnick deemed increasing research at the College a high priority; like Marion Fay's, his background included scientific work, which he viewed as essential for a medical school's intellectual integrity and for increasing revenues and faculty. On research more than anything else depends national reputation regardless of the excellence of clinical practice or teaching. During the 1970s and 1980s, basic science chairs such as Kurt Paucker and Page Morahan (microbiology), Jay Roberts (pharmacology), Julian Marsh and George Rothblatt (physiology/biochemistry), and Leonard Ross (anatomy) succeeded, despite limitations of space and resources, in attracting highly accomplished investigators. External research funding rose from about $1.5 million in 1971 to over $15 million in 1987.[14] Almost all the investigators also taught, and some emerged as compelling instructors. Students fed their "golden apple" awards to Nabil Abaza of pathology; Ann Barnes, Andrew Beasley, and Janet Smith of anatomy; Fred DeMartinis of physiology; Angelo Pinto of microbiology and immunology; and Charles Puglia of pharmacology. Several of these became educational program leaders and innovators.

In part through initial choices of faculty and in part as a way of gaining the most from limited space, MCP evolved a strategy of cultivating a limited number of research domains. The most important of these were neurosciences (including neural tissue repair), chemistry and disorders of lipids, and the biology of aging. This approach facilitated collaboration across science departments and between science and clinical departments.

All clinical departments also carried out research, but none with

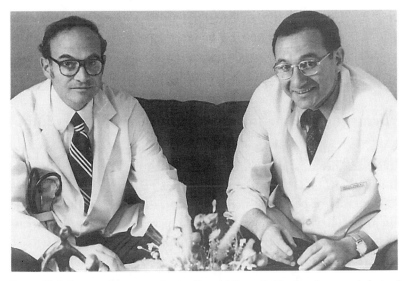

Figure 25. Infectious diseases authority Donald Kaye (left) as professor and chair of the Department of Medicine beginning in 1969 melded existing and new faculty into a strong department with a competitive residency; he became an influential figure at MCP. Gastroenterologist Walter Rubin (right) served as one of Kaye's lieutenants. Both brought enhanced research capability and NIH grants to the Department. *Iatrian,* 1977.

the sustained prominence seen in the basic sciences. Donald Kaye's Department of Medicine, which grew quickly in strength during the 1970s, focused on infectious diseases and geriatrics, though each of its divisions did some scholarly work. Under Robert Kaye in the 1980s, the small but vigorous Department of Pediatrics successfully entered the research realm. After MCP acquired the contract to manage the adjacent Eastern Pennsylvania Psychiatric Institute, or EPPI (a state facility), in 1981, and biological psychiatrist Wagner Bridger became chair of psychiatry in 1982, research took off in that department. The acquisition of EPPI counted, in fact, as a major coup for the medical school, not only bolstering programs in psychiatry but adding much needed space: the MCP complex with EPPI jumped from about eleven to thirty-three acres. The Departments of Anatomy and Pharmacology moved into unused space, allowing for their growth and for increased research in neurosciences and neuropharmacology.

No one at MCP conceived that it could or would become dominantly a research giant, but a formula was found to sustain more than enough serious work to provide a suitable academic environment and gain respectability. As noted before, funded research added faculty who would also teach, and the overhead payments which accompanied some research awards contributed to general revenues.

Becoming an Academic Medical Center: Tertiary Care

We noted earlier that the 1971 mission statement looked toward becoming a "health sciences university." An enthusiastic Alton Sutnick as newly appointed dean told the College's newsletter that he foresaw "opportunity to become a major tertiary care center in the area and also to develop new approaches to teaching in primary care."[15] Increasingly in the 1970s and 1980s progress in medicine meant sophisticated, technology-based diagnosis, and virtuosic interventional therapeutics, especially specialized surgery. Both governmental payers such as Medicare (initiated in 1966) and private insurers had come to pay maximally for surgery and procedures. Specialized surgery also helped fill hospital beds with paying patients. The needs of one activity, such as cardiac surgery, induced development in other areas, such as anesthesiology and intensive care. By the 1970s, most medical school hospitals wished to foster specialized, high-technology care.

In the early 1970s, nothing exemplified this direction and the "wonders" of medicine more than open-heart surgery (in which the heart is stilled, repaired, and started back up), usually preceded by diagnostic cardiac catheterization. In May of 1972, president and dean Bernard Sigel (himself a surgeon) pointed out to the board of corporators that "the College is the only medical school in Philadelphia without such a program [cardiac surgery], and possibly the only one in the Nation."[16] Hence, prestige was involved; but treasurer Edward Kane concluded that "this program was important to the College because it would generate new revenues and help change the mix of patients."[17] That is, such a program could attract new insured patients to help cover losses incurred through the large amount of indigent care the hospital provided.

Slowed by the sudden death (probably from heart disease) of the hospital's first cardiac surgeon soon after his arrival, the program nevertheless grew.[18] In the late 1970s, innovative MCP cardiologists became among the first in the Philadelphia region to employ angioplasty

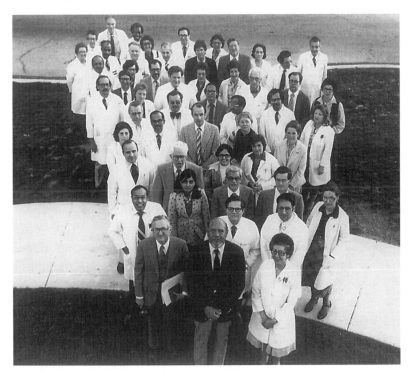

Figure 26. Between 1960 and 1980 the faculty—including full-time scientists and clinicians—had grown enormously. Some remembered to appear for this group portrait, also showing Dean Alton Sutnick and then acting-president Maurice Clifford (front row, left and center).

(dilatation of narrowed arteries using a catheter) in the care of coronary disease. The early 1980s brought the implantable automated defibrillator, an advanced and somewhat grotesque device to abort lethal cardiac rhythm disturbances.

The first computerized axial tomographic unit ("CAT scanner") came to MCP in 1979, but owing to lack of space (a persistent problem) dwelt at first in a trailer. New or expanded intensive care units—coronary, surgical, neurosurgical, and neonatal—appeared in the late 1970s and early 1980s.[19] A few endeavors, such as plasmapheresis and a hyperbaric chamber, did not succeed after considerable publicity.[20]

Despite these accomplishments, the Medical College Hospital never fully achieved the "feel" of a major downtown tertiary-care arena. The small East Falls facility seemed almost to resist transformation into a "medical mecca," as countless local patients, many indigent, continued to deliver through its doors their diabetic complications, pneumonias, asthma attacks, seizures, pregnancies, sickle cell crises, injuries, overdoses, and other daily miseries. Such patients and problems probably served the fundamental educational needs of medical students better than the insertion of defibrillators or the next allotment of intensive-care beds, but they did not win fame or bring in needed revenues.

MCP, like all American medical schools in the 1970s and 1980s, found itself subject to conflicting demands and signals from government and society. While financial reward went to sophisticated research and specialized surgical procedures, policy makers and advisors—responding to the rising expense of medical care—began in the 1970s to call on medical schools to encourage "primary care" and "generalism." Hence one heard statements such as Dr. Sutnick's (quoted at the beginning of this section) proclaiming the need to provide tertiary care and teach the primary version. Similarly, then acting-president Maurice Clifford in 1980 called upon MCP faculty to respond to the critique of medical schools and "exemplify generalism at its best."[21] Chair of Medicine Donald Kaye in 1978 created a "Primary Care Unit" within his enlarging department, which had been largely subspecialty-based. A Department of Family Medicine was not established at MCP until the 1990s. The Department of Pediatrics had long stressed outpatient work and the general care of children, though by the 1970s it contained subspecialists on the teaching staff.

As some educators in the departments and the Office of Medical Education turned their attention to "generalism" and the need to move medicine from the hospital to the office, a handsome expansion to the hospital opened in 1986, adding modern patient rooms and more space for intensive-care units, cardiac catheterization, and electrophysiology.[22] Medical schools at the time suffered widely from such seeming confusion of purpose; MCP was no exception, though it did eventually invest more than many schools in teaching basic clinical skills.

Still a Place for Women?

MCP had yet another, unique, purpose to acknowledge. Even before the change in admissions policy and name, Woman's Medical College initiated several specific programs aimed at medical women. Among the most enduring was the Retraining Program for Women Physicians. Begun in 1968, it provided a course of didactic and clinical work aimed at women who wished to resume practice after raising children—a situation assumed to be common in the 1960s. In fact some such women did enroll, as well as women and men hoping to reenter clinical work after careers in administration, public health, or research.[23] By 1974 the retraining class contained six women and four men.

Among the most welcome and forward-looking programs was the "Learning Center," a demonstration day-care facility established by the Department of Pediatrics with governmental and local funding; the chair of pediatrics at the time was a women (Doris Howell). Housed at a church property near MCP, the Center enrolled children of medical students and neighborhood families. It also participated in educational programs for medical students. It expired, a victim of finances, in 1983.[24] MCP was the first medical school in the United States to set up a training program (internship and later residency) in emergency medicine. It was initiated in 1971 in part to help create for women with family responsibilities a new form of medical career—that of the emergency department doctor—which could offer predictable, scheduled hours. But its charter class of trainees included three men and only one woman.[25] Later in the 1970s, a "Summer Health Policy Program" for women medical students was found to be in violation of the law: it could not exist only for women.[26] The irony was obvious and galling.

In 1972 the College created a part-time Office for Women in Medicine, then in 1973, with support by the National Board and the alumnae's Special Trust Fund, a Center for Women in Medicine (CWIM).[27] Nina Woodside (WMC, 1957), experienced in public health and administration and interested in women's issues, became the director of the CWIM in 1973. It assumed responsibility for the retraining program and for a summer program for college students contemplating medical careers and obtained grants to carry out a nationwide survey of inactive physicians. The CWIM also created a "Professional Development Experience for Women Faculty Members," forerunner to later successful advancement seminars for medical women sponsored by MCP into the 1990s, including "ELAM," the Executive Leadership in Academic Medicine Program.[28]

In 1976 Dr. Woodside resigned as CWIM director. In a letter to the dean, she stated that she could no longer sustain the commuting schedule (she lived in Virginia) and had decided to train in psychiatry, though she may also have been unhappy with some aspects of the Slater administration relating to the center.[29] Assistant dean for medical education Susan McLeer (WMC 1970) was appointed director of a renamed Division for Women in Medicine in 1977, but resigned in May of 1978 citing increasing demands of her primary duties and the limited resources and commitment she perceived as available to the initiatives for women.[30] In 1981, faculty physiologist Eva Ray became part-time director of "Programs for Women," but this reformulation also failed to take firm root.[31]

Clearly the well-intended efforts to find a structure for furthering the College's historic mission in the coeducational context ran aground of limited resources and a failure to agree on goals. Furthermore, most specific programs could not be offered only to women: this limitation diluted their real and symbolic impact. To some critics, a designated "Center" marginalized efforts on behalf of women: MCP should *be*, not *include*, a Center for Women in Medicine, they argued. They also counted with displeasure the few women in departmental chairs. Indeed, in 1977 the long lineage of women professors of obstetrics finally ended with the appointment of a man to this post.[32] In the original debates of the advisory committee on the CWIM, one consultant pointed out that in the early 1970s "the primary problem of women in medicine is . . . attitudes." How would specific programs of a Center address prejudicial perceptions?[33] While hardly insignificant, the structured "programs for women" did not prove the desired formula for embodying the College's founding mission in the new, MCP, context.

Yet for some women medical students at least, MCP remained meaningful—not so much because of programs it attempted on behalf of women, but because of what its women were doing on behalf of their careers, students, and College. In the mid-1980s approximately 33 percent of the full-time faculty were female, a minority but still about double the national figure of 17 percent.[34] Alumnae of the 1970s and 1980s (and some alumni as well) responding to a survey carried out in 1997 repeatedly cited as memorable aspects of their medical school years their interactions with women physicians on the faculty and house staff,

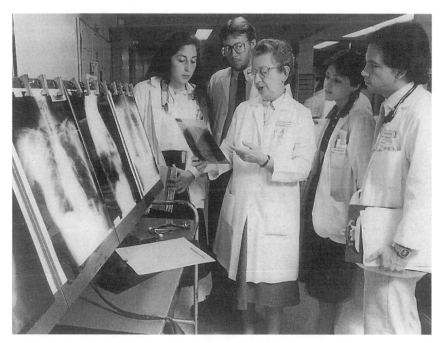

Figure 27. Professor of medicine June Klinghoffer (WMC, 1945) during her long tenure on the faculty came to serve as a link with the values and memories of Woman's Med, as well as teacher and mentor to generations of students.

particularly Ann Barnes, Boots Cooper, Lourdes Corman, Eva Fox, June Klinghoffer, and Elizabeth Labovitz.[35] Both medical and graduate students also had the opportunity to know women scientists such as Marie Diberardino, Nancy Berman, Jane Glick, Janet Smith, Paula Goldberg, Hazel Murphy, Donna Murasko, Denise Ferrier, and many others.

A woman graduate of 1977, responding to a survey, saw the school as "oriented to women & [it] had lots of women around"; another from the early 1980s appreciated the "many role models—women physicians who were skillfully and gracefully combining career and family." A graduate of 1991—twenty years after coeducation—still found value in "learning in an environment where being a woman was accepted and no big deal." At another hospital she found that women were yet "not accepted as equals." Several alumnae responding to the survey noted the satisfaction of experiencing a class environment where women were for once in the majority; for some, at least, this seemed perhaps more satisfying than a purely single-gender setting.[36]

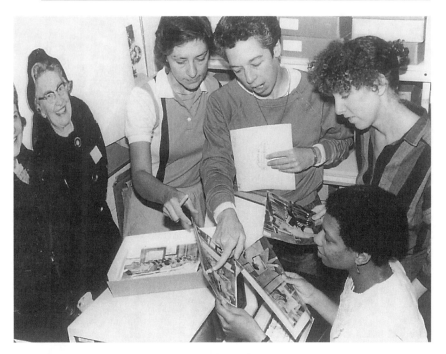

Figure 28. With funding from the National Endowment for the Humanities, the College organized its Archives and Special Collections on Women in Medicine in 1977. The "founding" staff included first director Sandra Chaff (center, holding pen), Jill Gates Smith (pointing), Margaret Jerrido (seated), and Barbara Malinsky (not shown). Archives assistant Linda Friedman is at the far right.

Three women who graduated in the early 1990s recalled in similar words a striking experience—discovering the gallery of College portraits: "It was when I walked down the hallway," wrote one, "that I knew I was in the right place. I passed large beautiful portraits of commanding appearing women—*all* women."[37] Actually, there *are* a few men in the collection, such as William Mullen and Hartwig Kuhlenbeck. But it is the women physicians' faces and hands, commanding indeed but also comforting, that dominate the gallery: Ann Preston, Emeline Horton Cleveland, Hannah Longshore, Catharine Macfarlane, Frieda Baumann, Katharine Sturgis, Virginia Alexander, and many others. Women students who needed to find forebears, found them—those daily seen working and teaching, those hallowing the College walls.

In 1976–77, the College undertook two valuable projects to further make known its past and the varied experiences of women physicians. With a grant from the National Endowment for the Humanities, a formal Archives and Special Collections on Women in Medicine was organized to make available the school's voluminous records and related materials (much of it affectionately protected over the previous three decades by the librarian Ida Draeger). An Oral History Project on Women in Medicine, carried out meticulously by the professional historian Regina Morantz-Sanchez, captured a wide range of memories and opinions, including those of several graduates and faculty of the College.[38] While the College and its women deans, as we have shown, long attended to its history, the Archives and Oral History Project represented something new. These academic and professional initiatives of the mid-1970s exemplified the awakening discovery of women's history in the United States; for WMC, they ironically demarcated a past that no longer felt seamlessly continuous with the present or future. Part of the saga of Woman's Med now dwelt, boxed and indexed, on the shelves of its archives.

"More Camaraderie than Competition"

But another part of the spirit of WMC was maintained, transformed, and categorically nurtured as what came to be referred to as the friendly, noncompetitive environment. As we have seen, cohesiveness and mutual support long characterized the small classes of Woman's Med, and even during the rigid years of the 1940s through the 1960s, students still might find help and collegiality from a faculty member or the dean's office. Students and everyone else came to know and rely upon long-time WMC and MCP employees such as Tessie Tricker the omniscient telephone operator, "Benny" Scola the grounds keeper (who announced spring's first crocus), and dean's assistant Ellen Harkins. They trusted old-order nurses Emma "Nick" Nicholson, "Johnny" Stotesbury, and operating room chief Norma Ciambella, who served and ruled her domain. Many longtime WMC and MCP employees lived in East Falls, and commonly more than one generation worked at the College or hospital. All this enhanced a sense of family.

Almost paradoxically, as the College grew larger and the classes more diverse during the MCP years, this sense of smallness and intimacy seemed to increase rather than dissipate. Respondents to the 1997 alumnae/i survey who graduated in the MCP years recalled again and again the eagerness of students to help one another, the aversion to competitive academic behavior, "the feeling of belonging and family," the "nurturing atmosphere," the "sensitivity of an institution dominated by a female touch," the "welcoming attitude from day 1," the "accessible faculty," and above all the sense of "camaraderie."[39] To their credit, students perpetuated these attitudes from year to year, while newer faculty, women and men, avoided the old, harsh, pedagogic styles. Institutional nurturing of the "nurturing atmosphere" did occur and can be assigned in good part to Mary Ellen Hartman and Andrew Beasley. These associate deans helped foster the supportive milieu through their role in the admissions process and by repeatedly themselves serving as friend and advisor to students.[40] They helped spread the word that MCP was such a place when meeting with premedical advisors.

The distinctive College environment was endorsed by upper-level administration as well: Alton Sutnick in an article in the alumnae magazine reported that despite the expansion of the 1980s, "we still retain the atmosphere of informality, friendliness, and cohesiveness—a family working together." In a report to the board, he listed the "intimate, rather informal" relationships as important in attracting students.[41] In his inaugural address of 1981, president Maurice Clifford referred to the "close, family atmosphere" and closed with the remarkable plea to "make our College and our Hospital above all others an excellent haven of respect and kindness and tranquility."[42] While no such ideal can be achieved in an institution made up of human beings, the author, as former house officer and faculty member since 1974, can attest that although discord was hardly unknown, the family-like milieu was no sham. As W. W. Keen had said about WMC a century earlier, MCP has been generally an "agreeable" place to work, teach, and learn. This milieu was a legacy of the best qualities of Woman's Med that, impossible to mandate, survived by its virtue and became a defining characteristic of MCP.

Also celebrated at MCP was openness to the nontraditional student, usually an older candidate who had worked in some other realm before choosing medicine. This attitude also had its roots in the Woman's Medical College; one need only recall that Ann Preston entered its first class at the age of thirty-seven! Alumnae/i who had come

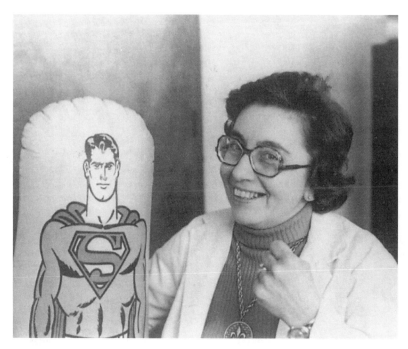

Figure 29. Anatomist and associate dean Mary Ellen Hartman was often the first representative of the College to meet with prospective students. She helped shape the attributes of the student population and encouraged minority and "nontraditional" students. *Iatrian,* 1978.

to MCP as nontraditional students expressed gratitude for their door of opportunity (some medical schools did not accept students over a specified age); while other graduates recalled with fondness the "older students with life experiences . . . shared lovingly."[43] Associate dean Mary Ellen Hartman probably more than anyone else promoted such diversity as she selected which applicants would be invited to interviews. Perceiving a need, in 1984 she obtained a grant from the Department of Health and Human Services to establish a minority student enrollment program at MCP; of this project she was most proud.[44]

Of course, medical school remained excessively arduous, and occasional faculty or house officers behaved in other than "nurturing" ways to students. The camaraderie within the diverse classes helped students deal with the work and pressure. Graduates of the 1970s and 1980s would remember exams, dissection, dull lectures, pathology slides, night

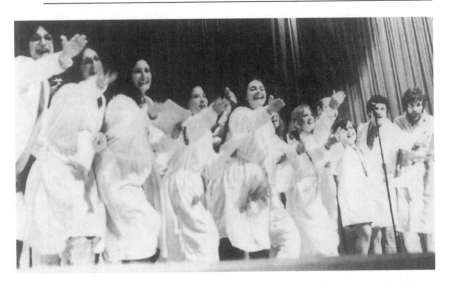

Figure 30. Students pointed out the foibles of faculty and displayed nonmedical talents at skit night; here a gowned, coeducational chorus performs in 1976. *Iatrian,* 1976.

call, surgery rounds at dawn, long operations, Dr. Kaye's professor's rounds, pediatrics clinics, admitting patients at three in the morning, figuring out "the V.A.," Jan Schneider's obstetrics lectures, evening ethics discussion groups, an oath at commencement; and, in union with their predecessors, old streets of East Falls, Wissahickon Park, shared meals and studies, "skit night."

Paying Attention to Education

As American medical schools in later twentieth century increasingly cultivated research and specialized clinical care, education itself often became an orphan, or at least third in line for recognition and funding. Unless motivated to do otherwise, busy faculty tended to do what had always been done, and the educational program of 1980 fundamentally differed little from that of the 1930s.

In part because of the open, cooperative milieu, and because research and clinical care never came to totally dominate MCP, the College gradually during the 1970s and beyond claimed a place as innovator in medical education. The first training program in emergency medicine has been mentioned already. In 1976 the College initiated a

"Teaching Program in Human Values in Medicine," later renamed the Medical Humanities Program, the first in the Philadelphia region and one of the earliest in the country. The program provided a required course in bioethics and an array of "medical humanities" elective courses, such as history of medicine, literature and medicine, and medicine and culture. It became a division within the Department of Community and Preventive Medicine and helped interest students in MCP.[45]

Many educational initiatives arose out of individual interests of faculty, encouraged by Gerald Kelliher and Gerald Escovitz, who held senior education posts in the dean's office. Dean Sutnick also welcomed such efforts, though he had to worry about paying for them. Informal use of "standardized patients" began in the early 1980s mainly in the second-year Introduction to Clinical Medicine Course. Standardized patients are lay persons trained to portray patients in a realistic setting for purposes of teaching or assessing such skills as medical interviewing, counseling, and physical diagnosis. The program expanded into all levels of clinical education at MCP and eventually occupied a sophisticated clinical skills training laboratory, another first among Philadelphia's medical schools.[46] The program and laboratory reflected a growing perception nationally that medical schools had not been adequately teaching rudimentary skills.

Courses or course segments were generated to address death and dying, human sexuality, and gerontology, subjects new to the formal medical curriculum. All worthy endeavors enthusiastically conceived, these new offerings sometimes reflected educational fashion and always threatened to overfill the teaching day. New courses and programs led to published research studies in medical education by MCP faculty and deans.

The utilization of the computer in medical education attracted the interest of adept faculty in several departments and in the Office of Medical Education. They created ingenious "computer-assisted instruction" programs with which students could simulate laboratory experiments, assess anemias, study problems in preventive medicine, "manage" cardiac arrest, interpret laboratory data, or auscultate breath sounds under the direct computer-generated guidance of the stethoscope's inventor, Theophile Laennec.[47] Some of these programs were displayed at national meetings.

Scattered use of case-based learning (as opposed to purely didactic lecturing) occurred in some basic science courses at MCP in the 1980s. In 1990, the dean (then Leonard Ross, former chair of anatomy) and a group of faculty studied the possibility of creating a "problem-based track" similar to ones in use at several progressive medical schools such as those of the University of New Mexico and McMaster University. In the problem-based format most conventional lectures are eliminated; instead students in largely self-directed small groups explore the necessary basic-science knowledge using extended clinical cases written for this purpose. A faculty facilitator works with each group. Headed by pharmacologist Charles Puglia, already an acclaimed educator at MCP, this alternative track was offered for the first time in 1992 under the name "Program in Integrated Learning" (PIL); it was perhaps the most radical and ambitious educational innovation yet seen, and again in advance of other schools in the region.

Of course, not all students praised all new ideas (often in the role of guinea pigs, they had little say in their implementation), and some clinical faculty particularly expressed skepticism. Also, few of these initiatives addressed the clinical work of the third and fourth years, which—as in most medical schools—remained under the control of departments and episodically revealed vagaries and deficiencies. But relatively few schools nationally or regionally emphasized educational methodology or innovation. Here was a domain in which recognition could be—and was—achieved relatively quickly by a school in search of identity and of ways to make itself better known. Of equal importance, innovative educational programs helped distinguish MCP in the minds of prospective students judging the relative merits of medical schools.

Yet, Somehow Not Enough

During the 1970s and 1980s, Medical College of Pennsylvania pursued progress in ways both conventional and unusual for an American medical school. It greatly increased laboratory research; expanded its hospital and faculty; and sought ways to make the educational process more effective, interesting, and humane. MCP cultivated a refreshing "family-like" milieu for students and even managed, as a coeducational school, to retain considerable gendered meaning for some of its students and faculty, though not particularly through special programs for women. MCP still contained much that had been of worth in WMC.[48] The College hospital was less successful in moving to tertiary care, but certainly offered a wider range of medical and surgical services than previously imagined. Fundamentally, it took care of the sick and helped train new doctors and nurses.

By most criteria the MCP of the 1980s was a "success." Despite its flaws, its leaders, faculty, and students largely felt confidence in its daily work and integrity and considered MCP a unique and even superior medical school slowly gaining the recognition it deserved. Yet somehow, all this did not suffice. As in the long history of WMC, economic well-being did not reward merit or accomplishment. In his presidential inaugural address of 1981 Maurice Clifford tempered optimism with the report of an estimated three-million-dollar loss in the hospital.[49] Addressing the board in June of 1985 as he began his *last* year in the presidency, Clifford reviewed accomplishments and disappointments, predicted that "MCP will continue to thrive," but added: "Dare I say, too, that we need an angel." And he urged the board to seek one.[50]

The reasons why MCP in 1985 still needed an angel are complex and can only be summarized here in the most basic terms. The hospital remained too small to achieve economies of scale, and despite Medicare and Medicaid suffered a large burden of unreimbursed care not offset by lucrative specialty practice. The College and its hospital always took care of the poor: it sought the poor in the slums of south Philadelphia in the 1890s, fled in fear when poverty overtook North College Avenue, but served the indigent again from Henry Avenue. Of course, MCP was not the only urban medical school subject to losses from indigent care in its hospital, but it enjoyed little economic buffering. The College budget was easier to predict and manage, but the comparatively small class size of 100 to 120 limited tuition income, though few desired a larger class. By the early 1980s federal capitation support for medical education had been largely eliminated. And finally, even as late as 1987 MCP owned a small endowment of only nine million dollars; at larger and more prominent medical schools at this time the figure was often several *hundred* million dollars.[51]

Smallness had been one solidifying attribute that allowed WMC students of the 1930s to enjoy "practically individual instruction," and MCP students of the 1980s to feel part of a family; but it was also the legacy of smallness that brought with it too few beds and too little endowment. So, with a desperate hope of preserving the cherished values of its smallness, the MCP sought further enlargement and fiscal stability through a merger or partnership. In June of 1983 the College explored merger with three hospitals in the Philadelphia region.[52] No agreement emerged. Securing a merger or alliance became the primary charge to D. Walter Cohen, D.D.S, who succeeded Maurice Clifford as president in 1986. Cohen, a dental scientist and practitioner, as dean of the University of Pennsylvania School of Dentistry had successfully carried out a major reform program. He had also proved highly effective as an ambassador for his school and as a fund-raiser. By early 1987, Cohen and a Merger Committee had been discussing a relationship with Mayo Clinic, Cleveland Clinic, and Allegheny Health Systems, Inc. (AHSI), parent corporation of Allegheny General Hospital in Pittsburgh.[53]

Allegheny General Hospital served Pittsburgh as a large and extremely successful (over eight hundred beds) tertiary care center emphasizing specialized surgery such as orthopedics, neurosurgery, heart surgery, and transplantation. It desired a firm medical school affiliation to meet certain accreditation requirements for its residency programs, and to compete in prestige with the University of Pittsburgh's medical center. Furthermore, as a nonprofit entity Allegheny's actual large profits could prove embarrassing; investing in a medical school might solve this dilemma. By May of 1987, discussions with Allegheny had become serious. Boards of both MCP and Allegheny perceived "a great deal of compatibility" in their needs and missions.[54] Following nearly a year of intensive negotiations, an affiliation agreement was concluded on 24 December 1987. Readers of the Medical College of Pennsylvania *Annual Report* for 1987 were assured that "we will stay in Philadelphia, our mission will remain unchanged and our identity will stay strong." Hearing this message at meetings and seeing it in print, the MCP family hoped it would be so.

Afterword

The Collapse of Allegheny

Although documents and publicity called the association with AHSI an "affiliation" and referred to a separate MCP corporation, the true relationship seemed apparent. Allegheny agreed to provide annual stipends to the College and to match funds raised for endowments. William P. Snyder III, chair of the AHSI board, would become chair of MCP's board of corporators, whose members would eventually be selected by AHSI. AHSI would become the sole "member" of the MCP corporation, which technically became a subsidiary of the Pittsburgh institution.[1] Soon after conclusion of the agreement, Allegheny effected a change in the MCP deanship.

On the other hand, the "clinical campus" established at Allegheny General Hospital proved popular with MCP students, who could elect to do some of their rotations under that hospital's highly qualified staff (some of whom became MCP faculty). The infusion of AHSI money to MCP stabilized the shaky financial picture and in 1990 allowed for the purchase and renovation of a building near the Henry Avenue campus to serve as the location for first- and second-year instruction.[2] Another major effort backed by Allegheny led to the creation, for the first time at MCP, of endowed professorships; several honored WMC alumnae. Despite the loss of autonomy, many faculty and students felt optimism. Applications to the medical school rose and outpaced the average for northeast medical schools.[3]

In late 1989 and early 1990 Allegheny entered discussions with Hahnemann University (Philadelphia's former Hahnemann Medical College and Hospital) about a merger with MCP. Most MCP faculty and students vehemently opposed such a further loss of identity, though some recognized potential economic and clinical advantages. Talks terminated suddenly, though whether local MCP opposition played a role is unclear.[4] In 1993, however, a merger of MCP and Hahnemann was announced by Allegheny president Sherif S. Abdelhak as a *fait accompli*. The remnant name and identity of MCP would limp on within the "MCP♦Hahnemann School of Medicine" of the newly-fashioned "Allegheny University of the Health Sciences." Everyone within the system received strict orders to use the new names and ungainly logo.[5]

Meanwhile, Allegheny (renamed the Allegheny Health, Education and Research Foundation, AHERF, in 1992) had commenced an expansion program that led to the purchase in 1991 of United Hospitals, Inc., a local group that included the prestigious St. Christopher's Hospital for Children. Allegheny also acquired numerous physicians' practices in the Delaware Valley and in 1996 took over the debt-ridden Graduate Health System, which included a large general hospital only a few city blocks from Hahnemann Hospital.[6] The addition of Graduate seemed folly to some observers and suggested that a plausible strategy of expansion and consolidation in response to a competitive "health care" environment had mutated into almost imperial ambition.

In early 1997 the *Philadelphia Inquirer* revealed salaries of area health-care senior administrators showing Allegheny leaders among the top; the income figures amazed and appalled MCP faculty, staff, and students.[7] Later that year saw the revelation of profound financial problems within the Allegheny system. Allegations also spewed forth in the newspapers of greed, chicanery, and mismanagement by senior Allegheny officials. By early 1998 Allegheny was seeking a buyer for its Philadelphia area hospitals, and on 20 July 1998, Allegheny Health Education and Research Foundation, then one of the largest health-care networks in the country, announced bankruptcy for its Philadelphia area operations, including the university, medical school, and hospitals.[8] The careful old Quaker merchants who sustained the early Woman's Medical College no doubt shuddered in their graves that day.

On 29 May 1998, the last "independent" class of Medical College of Pennsylvania (that is, the class before the first merged class) received degrees at the Academy of Music. Professor of medicine June Klinghoffer (WMC, 1945), though recently ill, led the procession, ceremonial mace in hand.

With Allegheny in bankruptcy and in withdrawal from Philadelphia, the medical school became an academic orphan that would need two stepparents. After a harrowing period of negotiations which eventually involved senior political figures, the again renamed "MCP Hahnemann University" emerged as a new nonprofit entity under the management of Philadelphia's Drexel University; and most of the former Allegheny hospitals in the Philadelphia region, including MCP Hospital, were purchased by Tenet Healthcare, a national for-profit corporation.[9]

The above skeletal sketch of the rise and fall of the Allegheny conglomerate—a story that will no doubt become the subject of one or more books—does not hint at the disruption, mass anxiety, anger, and strife which ensued as the system disintegrated. Thousands of persons suddenly lost their jobs, and students went to class uncertain if their school would be open in a year or a month. Millions of dollars of trust funds, endowments, and research accounts vanished into the Allegheny rubble. Many valued faculty members fled to more secure situations and census dipped at the system's hospitals. That the medical school survived the fiasco recalls the Phoenix-like recoveries of WMC.

A Long Sequence of Survivals: WMC and MCP

As part of Allegheny, the once small and independent MCP found itself within a few years forced into an unwanted academic marriage, then submerged within a giant medical amalgamation. Then came a bitter and monstrously trivial moral demonstration: small no longer works in modern America, but get too big and the structure can crash into dust.

How did the Female Medical College . . . Woman's Medical College . . . MCP, whose doors of opportunity opened in 1850, even survive into the era of corporate medicine; and why was it the first medical school taken over by another medical corporation—with bizarre and calamitous result? While this book has already addressed these questions, let us conclude by summarizing and elaborating upon some answers, keeping issues of gender necessarily in mind.

Woman's Medical as a college only for women students outlived the other regular women's medical colleges not by a few years, but by five decades. Strong sister schools in Baltimore, Chicago, and New York City had closed between 1899 and 1910 when unable to pay for new expectations of reformed medical education, or in favor of coeducation, as when Cornell agreed to accept students from the Woman's Medical College of the New York Infirmary.[10] As the oldest of the women's medical schools, by 1900 WMC had enjoyed the most time in which to create its foundational and sustaining saga, the meaning and power of which have been described earlier in this work. In 1875, when the regular women's medical schools in New York and Chicago were but a few years old, WMC alumnae had already formed their association. Though not all alumnae stayed loyal to the College or single-sex education, a segment of graduates would always tenaciously defend at least the former. Through much of its history, the majority of women faculty at WMC were alumnae. The alumna/faculty member perhaps more vigorously than anyone else upheld the school. She did so ideologically, perhaps nostalgically, and surely out of sound self-interest, since until relatively recently few medical schools (as we have seen) appointed women to senior teaching positions. That Philadelphia's other medical colleges proved remarkably slow to accept women students (or faculty) also probably motivated the supporters of WMC to stay open.[11] On the other hand, the long succession of liberal men who taught at WMC and became part of it helped maintain the school's credibility and access to certain teaching opportunities, such as those at Philadelphia General Hospital. Woman's Med was never a separatist enclave; male-female collaboration served it well through much of its history.

We have referred in several chapters to the local support enjoyed by WMC and MCP—from the founding Quaker doctors and William Mullen, from Anna Jeanes and other Quaker Women, from Margaret Kelly and Louise Kaiser, whose families were associated with the College's East Falls neighborhood. The numerous nineteenth-century newspaper clippings in the Archives and Special Collections suggest as well that Philadelphians of that time looked favorably on the experiment and the young "hen medics" in their city. More generally, we have pointed out that Philadelphia nurtures a fondness for its historic or quaint institutions and shows a proclivity to keep them around. Woman's Medical College was a gendered and medical example of this phenomenon.

Finally, just as being the first women's medical college favored its survival, WMC recognized the implications of being the *last* to stay open, and this recognition no doubt fostered further efforts to keep going. As early as 1915, when every other regular women's medical school had closed, a College publication proclaimed (with discernible meaning though dubious logic) "our unique position." Woman's Medical College of Pennsylvania is not "in any sense an opponent of co-education," but its continuation serves all medical women: "The existence of even one high grade college for the separate instruction of women in medicine protects the interests of all women medical students and all women practitioners in medicine, in that it constitutes a safeguard against possible restriction of women's opportunities in co-educational institutions."[12]

Schools such as Cornell University and Northwestern University had indeed drawn back on their welcome to women after the women's schools in New York City and Chicago closed.[13] Later in the twentieth century, few would imagine that coeducational medical schools would revert to only taking men, but other forms of discrimination persisted: many schools accepted only a quota of women, certain specialties limited access to women, and, again, until recent decades senior women medical faculty remained scarce. Thus, as the last women's school, the College still enjoyed symbolic and potential meaning for some women doctors: it was the "stockade for protecting their rights" in the words of Bertha Van Hoosen's telegram of 1946 opposing merger into Jefferson Medical College (chapter 9), and June Klinghoffer's image of a medical women's "homeland." The College provided female medical mentors and well into the MCP years assembled classes in which women formed the majority. Admittedly, these gender attributes did not matter to all women students or graduates, but they held deep meaning for many. Even in 1999 the author has met women students who chose the successor MCP Hahnemann School of Medicine in part because of the heritage it encompasses.

Why then could the College not survive independently beyond the 1980s, even as a much modified and limited women's place of medical study and practice? By this period, few independent urban medical schools had an easy time of it as governmental support declined and changes in the medical economy such as managed care reduced income. MCP lived long enough to find itself in a city overcrowded with medical schools and hospitals while losing population and jobs. But why was MCP the first to seek refuge in what became an ill-fated "buyout"? Our chapters have already suggested some answers relating to gender. It was not by chance that WMC/MCP was the smallest and poorest of Philadelphia's five regular medical schools, with the smallest hospital. Since relatively few women entered medical careers until the 1970s, and WMC competed with both other women's schools and coeducational schools, the College and the number of its alumnae remained small. Furthermore, women long were excluded from the most lucrative specialties of medicine. Thus, those alumnae faithful to the alma mater could not build a major endowment. Never, as we have noted, did the medical training of women emerge as an object of American women's philanthropy, nor did the College as the sole survivor attract much financial aid from female physicians who were not alumnae. Abraham Flexner channeled none of the foundation aid he controlled to WMC, but neither did it go to any other Philadelphia schools once it became clear that they would not form one university-based medical program. In any such arrangement, however, the small women's college would have been swallowed up, not bolstered.[14]

Another reason WMC did not win wide support was that in certain periods it was seen by many men and women as second-rate. Certainly it was late in embracing research, suffered at times from parochial, if devoted, leadership, and lagged in embracing high-technology medicine and surgery. And we have pointed out the regrettable effect of the strained institutional atmosphere of the 1950s and 1960s. Yet the worth of its clinical training and the superior ability of many faculty members were often overlooked: graduates rarely felt ill-prepared when as interns they matched their skills with those of colleagues from other schools. We would contend that in part the College was seen as second-tiered for so long because it was a women's institution. The entrenched and even unaware assumption that an institution staffed or run by women could not be first rate probably limited support (including even from some alumnae), and contributed, as we have seen, to the decision to become coeducational and drop "Woman's" from the name. It is difficult to determine to what extent lack of resources or inadequate ambition prevented WMC from transforming itself in a different direction—becoming the "center for the medical education of women" that some loyalists envisioned. Even the limited women's programs at MCP in the 1970s made clear, however, that the era of equal rights would make dedicated activities aimed solely at women difficult to implement. So MCP entered an economically strenuous time for academic medicine with too little endowment, too small a hospital, an inadequate substrate of constituencies, and a diluted sense of mission.

As this afterword is being written, students, faculty, and staff of the MCP Hahnemann School of Medicine and Medical College of Pennsylvania Hospital live in the grace of reprieve from dissolution—a reprieve which all hope will be permanent. Most persons at the institution who situate themselves within the traditions of Woman's Med and MCP have been too anxious, too distracted, and too busy working toward a future to concern themselves with the sesquicentennial in 2000 of the founding of the College in 1850. Woman's Medical College of Pennsylvania and even the Medical College of Pennsylvania seem to recede farther into the past, their identities obscured by change and mergers, their names mocked by a series of inelegant transformations. Indeed, whether alumnae/i and persons who work and study at the current MCP Hahnemann School of Medicine can accept that it somehow perpetuates MCP, much less WMC, has become a matter of individual perspective and need. In no case, however, can the contributions and meanings of the College, for women and for men, be diluted or appropriated. As this book opened with words of Ann Preston, so it can close by recalling some others. In a moment of despair, when Dr. Preston in 1861 thought her College and the "new and untried course" it offered would end prematurely, she had to remind herself that even should such occur, "thy work has been no failure, and the Everlasting will preserve it, and attest it forever."[15]

Notes

Unless otherwise specified, all unpublished sources cited in the notes are in the Archives and Special Collections on Women in Medicine (ASCWM) of MCP Hahnemann University, 3200 Henry Avenue, Philadelphia, Pennsylvania. All published materials of WMC and MCP, such as annual announcements and proceedings of the Alumnae/i Association, are available at ASCWM, although some may also be found in other collections.

The following abbreviations have been adopted for frequently cited sources:

MBC Minutes of meetings of the Board of Corporators
MECBC Minutes of meetings of the Executive Committee of the Board of Corporators
MF   Minutes of meetings of the faculty

Preface

1. Naomi Rogers, An Alternative Path: *The Making and Remaking of Hahnemann Medical College and Hospital of Philadelphia* (New Brunswick: Rutgers University Press, 1998).

Chapter 1 *"A New and Untried Course"*

1. "The Female Medical College," *The Pennsylvanian*, 31 December 1851.
2. For the first commencement, also see MF, December 1851 or early January 1852 (date not indicated); Gulielma Fell Alsop, *History of the Woman's Medical College, Philadelphia, Pennsylvania, 1850–1950* (Philadelphia: Lippincott, 1950), pp. 33–36; "Female Medical College," *North American and United States Gazette*, 31 December 1851; Pauline Poole Foster, "Ann Preston, M.D. (1813–1872): A Biography. The Struggle to Obtain Training and Acceptance for Women Physicians in Mid-Nineteenth-Century America" (Ph.D. dissertation, University of Pennsylvania, 1984), pp. 174–177. The description of Musical Fund Hall is from R. A. Smith, *Philadelphia as It Is in 1952: Being a Correct Guide* (Philadelphia: Lindsay and Blakiston, 1852), pp. 81–83. The building, considerably modified, still stands.
3. "The Female Medical College."
4. Joseph S. Longshore, *Valedictory Address Delivered before the Graduating Class at the First Annual Commencement of the Female Medical College of Pennsylvania* (Philadelphia, 1852), p. 4.

5. J. Longshore, *Valedictory Address*, pp. 10, 12.

6. *Philadelphia Public Ledger*, 31 December 1851.

7. "The Female Medical College."

8. The attendance figures of two thousand total and five hundred medical students is found in the description in MF, but these numbers are clearly written over earlier entries.

9. For accounts of this period, see Alice Felt Tyler, *Freedom's Ferment* (New York: Harper and Row, 1962; originally published 1944); Steven Mintz, *Moralists and Modernists: America's Pre–Civil War Reformers* (Baltimore: Johns Hopkins University Press, 1995).

10. There is of course a vast literature on the history of American feminism and women's rights. I have used primarily Catherine Clinton, *The Other Civil War: American Women in the Nineteenth Century* (New York: Hill and Wang, 1984); Sara M. Evans, *Born for Liberty: A History of Women in America* (New York: The Free Press, 1989); Mintz (especially pp. 142–146 and bibliographic essay pp. 169–170); Janet Zollinger Giele, *Two Paths to Women's Equality: Temperance, Suffrage, and the Origins of Modern Feminism* (New York: Twayne Publishers, 1995). The role of rural Quaker women is discussed by Nancy Hewitt in "Feminist Friends: Agrarian Quakers and the Emergence of Woman's Rights in America," in Nancy Cott, ed., *History of Women in the United States* (Munich: K. G. Sauer, 1994), v. 20, pp. 3–25 (originally published in 1986 in *Feminist Studies*).

11. For the entry of women into medical schools in the United States, the best general sources are Regina Morantz-Sanchez, *Sympathy and Science* (New York and Oxford: Oxford University Press, 1985); Thomas Neville Bonner, *To the Ends of the Earth: Women's Search for Education in Medicine* (Cambridge, Mass.: Harvard University Press, 1992); Virginia Drachman, *Hospital with a Heart: Women Doctors and the Paradox of Separatism at the New England Hospital, 1862–1969* (Ithaca, N.Y.: Cornell University Press, 1984). There exists a large amount of journal literature in clinical and historical periodicals on individual women physicians and themes. See Sandra L. Chaff et al., eds., *Women in Medicine: A Bibliography of the Literature on Women Physicians* (Metuchen, N.J.: Scarecrow Press, 1977).

12. See Elizabeth Blackwell, *Pioneer Work in Opening the Medical Profession to Women* (New York: Schocken Books, 1977; first published in the United States in 1914), pp. 58–64; MBC, 23 May 1853.

13. See Morantz-Sanchez, *Sympathy and Science*, pp. 28–44, 49–51; Bonner, *To the Ends of the Earth*, pp. 6–10; Clinton, *Other Civil War*, 141–146; arguments in favor of women physicians appear, in varying length, in the annual announcements of the College. The *First Annual Announcement of the Female Medical College of Pennsylvania* is reprinted in Alsop, *History of the Woman's Medical College*, pp. 15–22.

14. Thomas Longshore, "History of the Female Medical College of Pennsylvania," manuscript, Longshore Papers; Deborah Jean Warner, *Graceanna Lewis: Scientist and Humanitarian* (Washington, D.C.: Smithsonian Institution Press, 1979); see also Brooke Hindle, "The Quaker Background and Science in Colonial Philadelphia," *Isis* 46 (1955): 243–250.

15. See discussion on the opposition to women physicians in Morantz-Sanchez, *Sympathy and Science*; Bonner, *To the Ends of the Earth*, especially pp. 10–12; Richard H. Shryock, "Women in American Medicine," in *Medicine in America: Historical Essays* (Baltimore: Johns Hopkins University Press, 1966), pp. 177–199.

16. See J. Collins Warren, *The Social Side of Student Life* (Boston, 1912; reprinted from *Boston Medical and Surgical Journal*, 13 June 1912); Thomas Neville Bonner, *Becoming a Physician: Medical Education in Great Britain, France, Germany, and the United States, 1750–1945* (New York and Oxford: Oxford University Press, 1995), pp. 74–75, 215–217.

17. Ann Preston, *Valedictory Address to the Graduating Class of the Woman's Medical College of Pennsylvania at the Eighteenth Annual Commencement, March 12, 1870* (Philadelphia, 1870).

18. Regina Morantz-Sanchez, "The 'Connecting Link': The Case for the Woman Doctor in 19th-Century America," in Judith Walzer Leavitt and Ronald L. Numbers, eds., *Sickness and Health in America*, 2d ed. (Madison: University of Wisconsin Press, 1985), pp. 161–172.

19. Morantz-Sanchez, *Sympathy and Science*, p. 119; Mary Roth Walsh, *Doctors Wanted, No Women Need Apply: Sexual Barriers in the Medical Profession, 1835–1975* (New Haven, Conn.: Yale University Press, 1977), pp. 133–138.

20. From the *Boston Medical and Surgical Journal* 40 (1849): 1, quoted in Bonner, *Becoming a Physician*, p. 209.

21. T. Longshore, "History"; Clara Marshall, *The Woman's Medical College of Pennsylvania: An Historical Outline* (Philadelphia: Blakiston, 1897); Alsop, *History of the Woman's Medical College*.

22. Clara Marshall, "History Proper," manuscript, undated but 1900 or after, Marshall Papers, quote from p. 6. The story of the meeting at the Fussell home also appears in R. C. Smedley, *History of the Underground Railroad in Chester and Neighboring Counties of Pennsylvania* (Lancaster, Pa.: 1883), pp. 267–268.

23. The faculty minutes record that at the meeting of 16 February 1857 someone proposed that Bartholomew Fussell be appointed "Emeritus Professor of Practice of Medicine," though he does not appear as such in subsequent catalogs.

24. T. Longshore, "History"; "Constitution of the American Female Medical Education Society" and "Appeal," in "Orphans" box.

25. For information on Mullen, see *Biographical Encyclopedia of Pennsylvania in the Nineteenth Century* (Philadelphia: Galaxy Publishers, 1874), pp. 399–401; Negley K. Teeters, *They Were in Prison: A History of the Pennsylvania Prison Society* (Chicago and Philadelphia: Winston's, 1937). The Pennsylvania Prison Society had been the Philadelphia Society for Alleviating the Miseries of Public Prisons, of which Mullen was member then employee; William J. Mullen, *Thirteenth Annual Report of William J. Mullen, Prison Agent* (Philadelphia, 1867), and other such reports at Historical Society of Pennsylvania; miscellaneous materials in Mullen folder, Vertical Files.

26. *Laws of the General Assembly of the Commonwealth of Pennsylvania Passed at the Session of 1850* (Harrisburg, Pa.: 1851), Act 148, p. 171. Those listed with "their associates" as "incorporated under the name, style and title of 'The Female Medical College of Pennsylvania'" were Mullen; Frederick A. Fickard, M.D.; Henry Gibbons, M.D.; Joseph S. Longshore, M.D.; Ferdinand Dreer; William J. Birkey, M.D.; R. P. Kane; and John Longstreth.

27. See MBC, e.g., 10 June 1853, undated passages late 1857 or early 1858; MF, 20 April 1852, 25 October 1852. There are many other brief references to pecuniary perils. The building in the rear lot of 229 Arch Street may have been chosen because it had recently briefly housed the Homeopathic Medical College, a predecessor of Hahnemann Medical College; thus it may have already been modified for instructional use. Also, the location was in a Quaker district near several meetinghouses.

28. By comparison (local but extreme), at the University of Pennsylvania's medical school, which graduated huge classes of well over one hundred students in the 1840s, faculty income from lecture fees amounted to over four thousand dollars annually! See Thomas S. Huddle, "Competition and Reform at the Medical Department of the University of Pennsylvania," *Journal of the History of Medicine and Allied Sciences* 51 (1996): 251–292.

29. Of the faculty during the first five years, none appears in Howard A. Kelly and Walter L. Burrage's *Dictionary of American Medical Biography* (Boston: Milford House, 1971; facsimile republication of the 1928 edition). Some information was obtained through Lisabeth Holloway's useful *Medical Obituaries: American Physicians' Biographical Notices in Selected Medical Journals before 1907* (Boone, N.C.: by the author, 1995; also available on CD-ROM).

30. MF, 18 November 1850; MBC, 5 December 1850, 28 May 1852. Thomas Longshore later accused the nonposting member of inebriety—if true, intolerable to temperance zealots William Mullen and Joseph Longshore.

31. Preston to Hannah Darlington, 4 January 1851, Preston Papers.

32. See T. Longshore, "History"; Kristin Bunin, "Proclaiming a Truth in Advance of His Age: Joseph Longshore and the Female Medical College of Pennsylvania, 1850–1853," HSHM Senior Essay, Yale University, 1996 (copy at ASCWM); Harold J. Abrahams, *Extinct Medical Schools of Nineteenth-Century Philadelphia* (Philadelphia: University of Pennsylvania Press, 1966), pp. 176–231. In his *Valedictory Address*, Joseph Longshore endorsed regular medicine as containing more "truth and philosophy than is possessed by any other [system] claiming the attention of the Medical Student," but declared it far from perfect, and urged his listeners to "reject nothing as worthless, until you have proved it to be so" (p. 11).

33. Eclecticism claimed to "pick and choose from what its adherents considered the best components of the other therapies." It also drew away from massive dosing, and at least in its early period favored the use of native plant remedies. See James H. Cassedy, *Medicine in America: A Short History* (Baltimore: Johns Hopkins University Press, 1991), pp. 38–39.

34. *J. S. Longshore vs. the Female Medical College of Pennsylvania*, Appearance Docket, Court of Common Pleas for the County of Philadelphia, June Session 1854, case 197, p. 60, at Philadelphia City Archives.

35. For disputing medical faculties in the nineteenth century, see Kenneth M. Ludmerer, *Learning to Heal: The Development of American Medical Education* (New York: Basic Books, 1985), especially p. 15; and Henry Burnell Shafer, *The American Medical Profession* (New York: AMS Press, 1968; originally published 1938), pp. 81–86.

36. MBC, 28 September 1852.

37. MBC, 25 February 1853.

38. MBC, 10 May 1853. Martha Mowry returned to her practice in Providence, enjoying a long and productive life. Like many women physicians of the nineteenth century, she participated in the suffrage campaigns and numerous women's clubs; see Seebert J. Goldowsky, "Rhode Island's First Woman Physician," *Rhode Island Medical Journal* 54 (1971): 546–549.

39. MBC, 19 May 1858. The board of lady managers no doubt was conceived in part to aid in fund-raising, but also probably to bring a larger presence of women to the conduct of the College. It also linked with Ann Preston's work at the time to establish a hospital run by and for women, discussed in chapter 2.

40. For general sources on the history of medical education in the United States,

including curriculum, see Ludmerer, *Learning to Heal*; Martin Kaufman, *American Medical Education: The Formative Years* (Westport, Conn.: Greenwood Press, 1976); Bonner, *Becoming a Physician*. For some discussion of the lecture question, see Steven J. Peitzman, "Lecturing in American Medical Schools," *Archives of Internal Medicine* 143 (1983): 1593–1596.

41. MF, 24 October 1850; 22 September 1857. In 1857 some courses were reduced from four to three hours per week.
42. Smith, *Philadelphia as It Is*, p. 181.
43. Female Medical College of Pennsylvania, day-book from outpatient clinic, 1856–1858; MF, 17 September 1850.
44. MF, 25 February 1859.
45. Annie Sturges Daniel, "'A Cautious Experiment': The History of the New York Infirmary for Women and Children and the Woman's Medical College of the New York Infirmary," *Medical Woman's Journal* (September 1939): 235 and (October 1939): 299.
46. The theses and a loose-leaf list of writers and topics by year are held at the ASCWM. The typical comments on the quality of dissertations are from MF, 16 February 1857.
47. This section is based on materials in Deceased Alumnae Folders; and for Emily Varney-Brownell (FMC, 1855), John King and Caroline King, "Early Women Physicians in Vermont," *Bulletin of the History of Medicine* 25 (1951): 429–441. The several well-known graduates of the first decades who became leaders of the WMC, such as Ann Preston and Emeline Horton Cleveland, will be discussed in more detail later in this book; they also have entries in Edward T. James, ed., *Notable American Women 1607–1950* (Cambridge, Mass.: Harvard University Press, 1971).
48. Teachers were Cleveland, Preston, Susanne Hayhurst (1857), and Chloe Buckel (1858); daughters, wives, or sisters of physicians included Longshore-Potts, Elizabeth Bates (1854), Lucinda Brown (1854), Samantha Nivison (1855), and Orie Moon-Andrews (1857).
49. Associated with health spas were Angenette Hunt (1852), Longshore-Potts (1852), and Nivison (1855).
50. My overall conclusions about the early graduates of the Female Medical College fit nicely with Thomas Bonner's generalizations about pioneering women medical graduates in *To the Ends of the Earth*.
51. Preston to Hannah Darlington, 4 January 1851, Preston Papers.
52. A few of these lecture books survive from the nineteenth-century Woman's Medical College: those of Emma Rogers from 1881 (at ASCWM) and of Anna McAllister from 1872 to 1873 (McAllister Family Papers, Historical Society of Pennsylvania, Philadelphia). Examples from male medical students may be found at large medical-historical libraries, such as the College of Physicians of Philadelphia.
53. MBC, 10 March 1856; see also MBC, 8 February 1858.
54. See Russell F. Weigley, ed., *Philadelphia: A 300–Year History* (New York: Norton, 1982), pp. 385–394; Sam Bass Warner Jr., *The Private City: Philadelphia in Three Periods of Its Growth*, 2d ed. (Philadelphia: University of Pennsylvania Press, 1987), esp. pp. 130–137. Maryland and Delaware, to the immediate south of Philadelphia, were slave states, which made the Chester County Underground Railroad, for which the Preston and Fussell families worked, so crucial.
55. MF, undated entry, late 1857 or early 1858; MBC, 21 February 1859.
56. MBC, 8 July 1861.

57. MF, 10 October and 17 October 1861.
58. Cited in Eliza E. Judson, *Address in Memory of Ann Preston, M.D. Delivered by Request of the Corporators and Faculty of the Woman's Medical College of Pennsylvania* (Philadelphia, 1873), p. 19. This is a printed pamphlet, in the Preston Papers. The actual journal of Dr. Preston has been, lamentably, long lost. Preston's reference to her "disabled mother" reflects that during this period she was spending considerable amount of time in Chester County looking after her ailing parent.

Chapter 2 **Building Within, Opposition Without**

1. I am using the term "professionalization" slightly more loosely than is done in much of current sociological and historical literature, which tends to stress expertise-based authority, control of entry, and division of expertise.
2. Quotations are from Eliza E. Judson, *Address in Memory of Ann Preston, M.D., Delivered by Request of the Corporators and Faculty of the Woman's Medical College of Pennsylvania* (Philadelphia, 1873), p. 18. For the founding of Woman's Hospital of Philadelphia, see also Gulielma Fell Alsop, *History of the Woman's Medical College, Philadelphia, Pennsylvania* (Philadelphia: Lippincott, 1950), pp. 45–52.
3. Girard College, opened in 1848, was built with a bequest from Stephen Girard (1750–1831), a famous Philadelphia businessman and financier of the Federal period. The original building, now called Founders' Hall, is a massive and stately Greek temple.
4. The hospital agreed to rent "the first story and the back room of the fourth story of the East Building" initially for five years.
5. *An Act Incorporating the Woman's Hospital of Philadelphia* (Philadelphia, 1861), p. 6.
6. For American hospitals in this period and their role in education, see Charles E. Rosenberg, *The Care of Strangers: The Rise of America's Hospital System* (New York: Basic Books, 1987).
7. A fine overview of "the first 100 years" of professional nursing is Susan M. Reverby's *Ordered to Care: The Dilemma of American Nursing, 1850–1945* (Cambridge and New York: Cambridge University Press, 1987).
8. For the rise of gynecological surgery and its relationships with women, see Regina Morantz-Sanchez, *Conduct Unbecoming a Woman: Medicine on Trial in Turn-of-the-century Brooklyn* (New York and Oxford: Oxford University Press, 1999).
9. Woman's Hospital of Philadelphia, Minutes of the Board of Managers, 19 December 1861, 3 April 1862.
10. *Fifteenth Annual Report of the Board of Managers of the Woman's Hospital of Philadelphia* (Philadelphia, 1876; for 1875); Minutes of the Board of Managers of the Woman's Hospital of Philadelphia, 1 April 1869.
11. Report of Mary Scarlett-Dixon, Chief Resident, in Minutes of the Board of Managers of Woman's Hospital of Philadelphia, 1 April 1869. ("Appeals for the admission of unfortunates come so frequently, that without presuming to know what is right in the case, I would ask the managers to consider carefully whether good might not be done in exceptional cases by protecting young unmarried mothers in their hour of trial? Not the abandoned—but the weak, who need sympathizing care to prevent a further fall.")
12. [Emeline Horton Cleveland, "reported by one of her lady pupils"], "Successful

Ovariotomy at the Woman's Hospital of Philadelphia," *The Clinic* (Cincinnati) 9 (1875): 100–102. The other case report describing Cleveland's difficult repair of a vesico-vaginal fistula is "Complicated Case of Vesico-Vaginal Fistula," *Transactions of the Philadelphia Obstetrical Society* 5 (1877): 62–64. Since no women then were allowed membership in this society, the paper was read by Albert H. Smith, an obstetrician and friend to women doctors in Philadelphia.

13. Mary Putnam Jacobi, "Women in Medicine," in Annie Nathan Meyer, ed., *Women's Work in America* (New York: Henry Holt and Co., 1891), p. 152; Sarah R. Munro, letter "To the Alumnae," *Report of Proceedings of the Alumnae Association of the WMC* (1889): 21. For accounts of Cleveland, see *Papers Read at the Memorial Hour Commemorative of the Late Prof. Emeline H. Cleveland, M.D. March 12, 1879* (Philadelphia, 1879), especially Rachel Bodley's "Tribute"; see also Patricia Spain Ward's article in *Notable American Women*, vol. 1 (Cambridge, Mass.: Belknap Press of Harvard University Press, 1971), pp. 349–350.

14. *Eighteenth Annual Announcement of the Woman's Medical College of Pennsylvania, 1867–68* (Philadelphia, 1867), p. 6.

15. For Hale's interest in Vassar and its name, see Edward R. Linner, *Vassar: The Remarkable Growth of a Man and His College, 1855–1865*, ed. Elizabeth A. Daniels (Poughkeepsie, N.Y.: Vassar College, 1984), pp. 120–129. Quote is on p. 126.

16. See *Godey's Lady's Book*, January 1864, p. 95.

17. The faculty minutes books for 1865–1874 are missing, and there is no "dean's correspondence" from that period to document which initiatives were Preston's. Similarly, Preston's personal journal, cited by nineteenth-century writers, was long ago lost. In a relatively small community with strong Quaker influences, probably many decisions of board and faculty arose out of discussion and attempt at consensus.

18. The Minutes of the Board of Corporators state (20 December 1865) that Fussell had agreed to stay on, that Matthew Semple had resigned from the chair of chemistry, and that Rachel Bodley was appointed to the latter.

19. *Historical Record of the Polytechnic College of the State of Pennsylvania, 1853–1890, by a Committee of the Alumni Association* (Philadelphia, 1890). See also James McGivern, "Polytechnic College of Pennsylvania (a Forgotten College)," *Journal of Engineering Education* 52 (1961): 106–112. This extinct school was part of a movement to offer teaching in science and engineering for the industrializing country.

20. For a biography of Bodley, see Hannah Croasdale, "Tribute from the Faculty of the Woman's Medical College," in *Papers Read at the Memorial Hour Commemorative of the Late Prof. Rachel L. Bodley, M.D.* (Philadelphia, 1888); Gulielma Fell Alsop, "Rachel Bodley, 1831–1888. Chemist-scientist, Third Woman Dean of the Woman's Medical College," *Journal of the American Medical Women's Association* 4 (1949): 534–536; the entry by Alsop in *Notable American Women*, 1:186–187; and miscellaneous reprints and materials in Bodley folder, Vertical Files. Her entry into sociology was a study of the status, income, etc., of WMC graduates, one of the first such surveys of professional women, published as *The College Story. Valedictory Address to the Twenty-ninth Graduating Class of the Woman's Medical College of Pennsylvania* (Philadelphia, 1881), discussed in chapter 4. Bodley's M.D. was an honorary degree awarded by WMC in 1879.

21. Rachel Bodley, *Introductory Lecture to the Class of the Woman's Medical College of Pennsylvania, Delivered at the Opening of the Nineteenth Annual Session, October 15, 1868* (Philadelphia, 1868), p. 13.

22. See Margaret W. Rossiter, *Women Scientists in America: Struggle and Strategies to 1940* (Baltimore: Johns Hopkins University Press, 1982), pp. 7, 75, 78; Nancy Slack, "Nineteenth-Century American Women Botanists: Wives, Widows, and Work," in Pnina G. Abir-Am and Dorinda Outram, eds., *Uneasy Careers and Intimate Lives: Women in Science, 1789–1979* (New Brunswick, N.J.: Rutgers University Press, 1987), pp. 77–103. According to John W. Harshberger's *The Botanists of Philadelphia* (Philadelphia, 1899), p. 285, Bodley presented a lecture series in 1867–1868 on "Cryptogamous Plants of Land and Sea" and wrote botanical articles for the *Public Ledger*.

23. The characterization was by WMC board of corporators' member and secretary C. Newlin Peirce on the occasion of the presentation to the College of portraits of Emeline Horton Cleveland and Rachel Bodley, in "Dr. Peirce's Reply," *Report of Proceedings of the Seventeenth Annual Meeting of the Alumnae Association of the Woman's Medical College of Pennsylvania* (1892): 168.

24. For a biography of Hartshorne, see the "Biographical Sketch of Henry Hartshorne, M.D., L.L.D" by James Darrach in the *Transactions and Studies of the College of Physicians of Philadelphia* 3d ser., 19 (1897): lxv–lxxvi, and the introduction and finding aid to the collection of Hartshorne Papers at the Library of the College of Physicians of Philadelphia. Another important set of Hartshorne materials is held at the Quaker Collections, Haverford College Library, Haverford, Pennsylvania.

25. Henry Hartshorne, *A Conspectus of the Medical Sciences* (Philadelphia: Lea, in print from 1867 through at least 1874); idem., *Essentials of the Principles and Practice of Medicine: A Handbook for Students and Practitioners* (Philadelphia: Lea, in print from 1867 through at least 1881).

26. The contemporary was the famous surgeon Samuel Gross, quoted in Thomas S. Huddle, "Competition and Reform at the Medical Department of the University of Pennsylvania, 1847–1877," *Journal of the History of Medicine and Allied Sciences* 51 (1996): 251–292, p. 275.

27. Burton Konkle and Frederick P. Henry, *Standard History of the Medical Profession of Philadelphia*, second edition enlarged and corrected by Lisabeth Holloway (New York: AMS Press, 1977; original edition Chicago: Goodspeed Brothers, 1897), p. 337.

28. Whitfield Bell, "Doctors of the Old School," *Transactions and Studies of the College of Physicians of Philadelphia*, 5th ser., 17 (1995): 146–163.

29. Actually, the two went in 1870 (to Washington, D.C.), and Thomas in 1871 (to San Francisco). They attended, but were not actually accepted as registered delegates because the AMA did not yet sanction the medical education of women. See Marshall, *Woman's Medical College*, pp. 55–58.

30. MBC, 25 November 1870.

31. *Twenty-second Annual Announcement of the Woman's Medical College of Pennsylvania, 1871–1872* (Philadelphia, 1871), p. 5. Hunt and two colleagues in 1876 published a monthly series of *Photographs in Histology, Normal and Pathological*.

32. MBC, 13 March 1872. For Hunt, see Howard A. Kelly and Walter L. Burrage, *Dictionary of American Medical Biography* (Boston: Milford House, 1971; reprint of the 1928 edition), p. 619. Hunt served on the WMC board for some years. Three of his daughters became physicians, two of whom were likely WMC graduates (Lydia Hunt, 1880, and Rebecca Hunt, 1881).

33. For the early history of the medical societies, see Henry Burness Shafer, *The American Medical Profession, 1783–1850* (New York: AMS Press, 1968; reprint of original 1936 edition), pp. 200–240; and James H. Cassedy, *Medicine in America: A Short History* (Baltimore: Johns Hopkins University Press, 1991), pp. 32–33, 90–91.

34. The story of the struggles with the medical societies is extremely complex, since events occurred at the county, state, and even national level. I have not attempted a full account. For more information, see Hiram Corson, *A Brief History of Proceedings in the Medical Society of Pennsylvania in the Years 1859, '60, '66, '67, '68, '70 and '71 to Procure the Recognition of Women Physicians by the Medical Profession of the State* (Norristown, Pa.: 1894), pp. 5, 11. Other useful sources include Martin Kaufman, "The Admission of Women to Nineteenth-Century American Medical Societies," *Bulletin of the History of Medicine* 50 (1976): 251–260; Marshall, *The Woman's Medical College*, pp. 40–66; and Alsop, *History of the Woman's Medical College*, pp. 60–74.

35. The circular is quoted in its egregious entirety in "Medical Societies. Philadelphia County Medical Society," *Medical and Surgical Reporter* 16 (1867): 285–287.

36. See MBC, 19 April 1867.

37. Quoted in Alsop, *History of the Woman's Medical College*, pp. 66–67. It was adopted at the meeting of 20 March 1867; see "Medical Societies," p. 287.

38. See Eleanor Flexner, *Century of Struggle: The Woman's Rights Movement in the United States* (New York: Athenaeum, 1974), pp. 146–147.

39. Lilian Welsh, a WMC graduate of 1889, when recalling her participation in suffrage activities, drew an analogy between "educational freedom for women" and "political freedom"; see her autobiography, *Reminiscences of Thirty Years in Baltimore* (Baltimore: Norman, Remington Co., 1925), p. 112.

40. See Steven J. Peitzman, "The Quiet Life of a Philadelphia Medical Woman: Mary Willits (1855–1902)," *Journal of the American Medical Women's Association* 34 (1979): 443–446, 448, 450, 454–457, 460.

41. *Philadelphia Bulletin*, 6 November 1869.

42. "The Other Side. Special Telegraph to the *New York Tribune*, 9 November 1869," reprinted in *The Press* [Philadelphia?], 13 November 1869, in Scrapbook, Eliza Wood-Armitage Deceased Alumna folder. The accuracy of any one account cannot be assumed.

43. Ibid.

44. "Our Philadelphia Correspondence," 7 November 1869; clipping marked "Anti-Slavery Standard," in Eliza Wood-Armitage Scrapbook.

45. "Disgraceful," clipping, source not identifiable, in College Clippings Collection, leaf 19.

46. This statement is based on reviews of the numerous clippings gathered in several scrapbooks and in the College Clippings Collection, leafs 1–77.

47. Sarah A. Hibbard, Manuscript Drafts of Lectures and Sermons, folder 1.

48. In *Transactions of the Thirty-first Annual Meeting of the Alumnae Association of the Woman's Medical College of Pennsylvania* (1906), p. 36.

49. "Current Topics of the Town. A Pioneer in the Medical Education of Women Describes Student Battles Once Waged about Them." Clipping, source not indicated, "1926" written at top, in Broomall's Deceased Alumna folder.

50. Minutes of the Board of Managers of the Pennsylvania Hospital, 13 November 1996, Library of the Pennsylvania Hospital, Philadelphia.

51. "City Bulletin," unidentified clipping, and "The students. A Quiet Clinic at

the Pennsylvania Hospital," also unidentified but dated 16 November 1869; both in College Clippings Collection, leaf 15.

52. Minutes of the Board of Managers of the Pennsylvania Hospital, 29 November, 6 December, 27 December, 1869; 5 May, 23 May, 30 May, 26 September, 1870; 29 May 1871, Library of the Pennsylvania Hospital, Philadelphia.

53. See, e.g., Flexner, *Century of Struggle*, pp. 120–123; Carroll Smith-Rosenberg, *Disorderly Conduct: Visions of Gender in Victorian America* (New York: Knopf, 1985), pp. 249–253. Smith-Rosenberg describes the treatment afforded some early college coeds by male students, which included mostly stares, ostracism, and private mockery.

54. Smith-Rosenberg, *Disorderly Conduct*, p. 250.

55. "The Other Side," signed "R.W.M," clipping headed "Ed. New Republic," no date indicated, in College Clippings Collection, leafs 33 and 34.

56. Quoted in Regina Morantz-Sanchez, *Sympathy and Science* (New York and Oxford: Oxford University Press, 1985), p. 70.

57. E. Anthony Rotundo, *American Manhood: Transformations in Masculinity from the Revolution to the Modern Era* (New York: Basic Books, 1993), pp. 31–55, 255–257. Rotundo quotes a headmaster named Henry Coit as declaring (p. 255) that boys were "possessed, in a greater or lesser degree, by the devil."

58. See Robert A. Nye, "Medicine and Science as Masculine 'Fields of Honor,'" *Osiris* 12 (1997): 60–79.

59. "The Other Side."

60. See Mark C. Carnes, *Secret Ritual and Manhood in Victorian America* (New Haven, Conn.: Yale University Press, 1989).

61. It may be worth noting, partly in fairness to Philadelphia men of that long-ago time, that similar events occurred at the Edinburgh Royal Infirmary, Queen's University in Kingston, Ontario, and at the University of Michigan (the latter concerning an organic chemistry class, of all things). See Thomas Bonner, *To the Ends of the Earth: Women's Search for Education in Medicine* (Cambridge, Mass.: Harvard University Press, 1992), pp. 127–128, 145–146; Morantz-Sanchez, *Sympathy and Science*, p. 113.

62. Welsh, *Reminiscences of Thirty Years in Baltimore*, p. 112; Alsop, *History of the Woman's Medical College*, p. 54 (her full account of the event occupies pp. 54–59). Marshall reviews it on pp. 17–30 of her *Woman's Medical College of Pennsylvania*.

63. *Twentieth Annual Announcement of the Woman's Medical College of Pennsylvania, 1869–70* (Philadelphia, 1869), p. 6. The term "progressive" in the context used to identify this curricular reform in medical education should not be confused with the later use of the phrase "progressive education," a set of ideas formulated most cogently by Thomas Dewey. Progressive education stressed adaptive and lifelong learning, experiential instruction and observation, and denounced mere memorization.

64. Ibid., pp. 6–7.

65. Thomas S. Huddle, "Competition and Reform at the Medical Department of the University of Pennsylvania, 1847–1877," *Journal of the History of Medicine and Allied Science* 51 (1996): 286–291.

66. WMC, Registration Book of Matriculants, 1852–1890, session of 1872–1873 (no pagination).

67. MBC, 7 February 1871.

68. In 1865 a faculty member, George B. Wood, endowed an "auxiliary faculty" at the University of Pennsylvania to offer lectures on special topics during a spring

course; see Huddle, "Competition and Reform," pp. 279–280. WMC clearly kept her eye on the University of Pennsylvania, not as a direct competitor (since it would long turn away women students), but rather as a sort of medical education benchmark.

69. *Twenty-third Annual Announcement of the Woman's Medical College of Pennsylvania, 1872–73* (Philadelphia, 1872), p. 8.

70. The College acknowledged that it was still trying to improve the spring course to "justify this extension of their collegiate instruction" in the *Twenty-fourth Annual Announcement of the Woman's Medical College of Pennsylvania, 1873–74* (Philadelphia, 1873), p. 7.

71. See the section on "progressive medical education" in Kenneth Ludmerer's *Learning to Heal: The Development of American Medical Education* (New York: Basic Books, 1985), pp. 65–71.

72. Notes in the Registration Book indicate that students occasionally withdrew for financial reasons (three in 1876). Two sisters from New York State dropped out in 1876 and went to the New England Female Medical College in Boston "because the College w[oul]d not abbreviate their time of study as they desired." See "Registration Book of Matriculants" for years cited.

73. The other schools were New England Female Medical College, Boston; New York Medical College and Hospital for Women (homeopathic), New York City; Woman's Medical College of the New York Infirmary, New York City; Homeopathic Medical College for Women, Cleveland (expired in 1870); Woman's Medical College of Chicago. Others sprouted up in the 1880s and 1890s, most of them short-lived. See a detailed list in Esther Pohl Lovejoy, *Women Doctors of the World* (New York: Macmillan, 1957), p. 120.

74. Woman's Hospital of Philadelphia, Board of Managers Minutes, 6 April 1871.

75. The same concern, amplified enormously, would erupt in the 1890s when relations between the Woman's Hospital and WMC deteriorated further.

76. E.g., MBC, 2 March 1874.

77. Bodley, *Introductory Lecture to the Class of the Woman's Medical College of Pennsylvania, Delivered at the Opening of the Nineteenth Annual Session, October 15, 1868.* In this address, Bodley condemns the rarity of endowments for women's colleges as a whole.

78. MBC, 29 December 1871, 3 November 1873. The price for the lot was $15,000.

79. See MBC, 3 November 1873, 4 March 1874, 8 April 1874, 7 May 1874, 29 June 1874.

80. Ibid., 11 August 1874.

81. *Twenty-fifth Annual Announcement of the Woman's Medical College of Pennsylvania, 1874–75* (Philadelphia, 1874), p. 15.

82. Ibid.

83. Ibid., p. 19.

84. Harriet Belcher to Elizabeth Johnson, 22 October 1875, quoted in "Dr. Harriet G. Belcher's Letters," *Noticias: Quarterly Bulletin of the Santa Barbara Historical Society* 25 (1979): 18.

85. Description of the building is based on floor plans and other information published in the *Twenty-sixth Annual Announcement of the Woman's Medical College of Pennsylvania, 1875–76* (Philadelphia, 1875) and in subsequent announcements; also newspaper accounts of the formal opening in College Clippings Collection, leafs 139–140; and from inspection of numerous exterior and interior photographs both in Photograph Collection at ASCWM and those published in the *Annual Announcements* beginning in the 1890s.

86. MBC, 13 March 1876.

87. For the WMC offering at the Centennial Exhibition, I used the account in John Francis Marion, "Voices Past and Present," unpublished short history of the WMC, 1980, pp. VI–8 to VI–10.

88. *Twenty-fifth Annual Announcement of the Woman's Medical College of Pennsylvania, 1874–75* (Philadelphia, 1874), p. 20. Bodley bid her listeners to "speak the word of encouragement, supply the means, and send them hither without delay," the "them" being "these daughters and sisters and friends of yours in this city, and throughout the land."

89. Figures are from the Registration Book. It includes occasional nondegree students and those who found the need to drop out.

90. Emeline Horton Cleveland to "Dear Friend Richardson" (probably Hannah Richardson), 27 October 1874, Josiah White Papers, Special Collections, Haverford College Library.

Chapter 3   Ann Preston, M.D.: An Excursus

1. The most comprehensive study of Ann Preston is the Ph.D. dissertation of Pauline Poole Foster, "Ann Preston, M.D. (1813–1872): A Biography. The Struggle to Obtain Training and Acceptance for Women Physicians in Mid-Nineteenth-Century America" (University of Pennsylvania, 1984); it has unfortunately not been published. Also invaluable, though not easily secured, is Eliza E. Judson's printed *Address in Memory of Ann Preston, M.D., Delivered by Request of the Corporators and Faculty of the Woman's Medical College of Pennsylvania, March 11, 1873* (Philadelphia, 1873), copies at ASCWM. An entry by Gulielma F. Alsop appears in *Notable American Women, 1607–1950*, vol. 3 (Cambridge, Mass.: Harvard University Press, 1971), pp. 96–97. Gulielma Fell Alsop also discussed Preston at length in her *History of the Woman's Medical College, Philadelphia, Pennsylvania, 1850–1950* (Philadelphia: Lippincott, 1950), pp. 45–59, 75–94.

2. Newspaper clipping, "From Philadelphia—Female Medical College," exact date not indicated but by internal evidence from 1870, unknown writer, probably a student at the College, newspaper name not indicated, in box labeled "Fragile Newspaper Clippings, Bibliography Files."

3. Preston to Hannah Darlington, 4 January 1851, Preston Papers.

4. Ann Preston, *Valedictory Address to the Graduating Class of the Female Medical College of Pennsylvania, 1864* (Philadelphia, 1864), p. 10.

5. Ann Preston, *Introductory Lecture to the Course of Instruction in the Female Medical College of Pennsylvania for the Session 1855–56* (Philadelphia, 1855). The phrase "by diet and regimen" is on page 11, in quotation marks, so may not be her own.

6. Quoted in Foster, *Ann Preston, M.D.*, p. 232.

7. Judson, *Address in Memory*, p. 20.

8. The kind of treatment Preston would have received at the Pennsylvania Hospital for the Insane is described in Nancy Tomes, *A Generous Confidence: Thomas Story Kirkbride and the Art of Asylum-Keeping, 1840–1883* (Cambridge and New York: Cambridge University Press, 1984); see p. 190 for statement about male physicians as patients.

9. There has been some doubt that Preston actually practiced medicine, but there is convincing evidence that she did; see Foster, *Ann Preston, M.D.*, p. 373; Judson, *Address in Memory*, p. 16; and obituaries in the *Philadelphia Press*, 20

April 1872, and *Philadelphia Evening Bulletin*, 19 April 1872, in College Clippings Collection, leaves 58, 59. A recently discovered manuscript in the ASCWM, "Women Physicians in Philadelphia," appears to be the handwritten text for an article, by content and style most likely from the late 1850s or 1860s. The anonymous writer says that "Miss Preston's taste and talent as a teacher has [sic] induced her to turn her attention in that direction more particularly than to practice, yet she has some practice & probably as much as she can attend to." She was for some years Lucretia Mott's doctor.

10. Judson, *Address in Memory*, p. 24; for more on Preston's home life, see Foster, "Ann Preston, M.D.," pp. 370–372.

11. Comments of C. Newlin Peirce, secretary of the board of corporators, *Report of Proceedings of the Seventeenth Annual Meeting of the Alumnae Association of the Woman's Medical College of Pennsylvania* (Philadelphia, 1892), p. 169.

12. Judson, *Address in Memory*, p. 12.

13. For rhetoric and writing in the nineteenth century, I used Nan Johnson, *Nineteenth-Century Rhetoric* (Carbondale: Southern Illinois University Press, 1982), especially pp. 173–19; James A. Berlin, *Writing Instruction in Nineteenth-Century American Colleges* (Carbondale: Southern Illinois University Press, 1984); and Charlotte Downey's "Introduction" to Samuel Phillips Newman, *A Practical System of Rhetoric, or the Principles and Rules of Style* (Delmar, N.Y.: Scholars' Facsimiles and Reprints, 1995; reproduction of 1835 edition), pp. 9–21. I am indebted to Susan Wells, Ph.D., of Temple University, for her guidance concerning nineteenth-century rhetoric and gender differences.

14. Ann Preston, *Valedictory Address to the Graduating Class of the Female Medical College of Pennsylvania, for the Session 1857–58* (Philadelphia, 1858), p. 10.

15. Preston, *Valedictory Address to the Graduating Class of the Female Medical College of Pennsylvania, 1864*, pp. 7–8.

16. Preston to Hannah Monaghan, 21 October 1832, Preston Papers.

17. Judson, *Address in Memory*, p. 5.

18. Ann Preston, *Nursing the Sick and the Training of Nurses. An Address Delivered at the Request of the Board of Managers of the Woman's Hospital, At Philadelphia* (Philadelphia: James B. Rodgers, 1874), p. 16.

19. Preston's "Reply" appeared first in the journal *Medical and Surgical Reporter*, 4 May 1867, and has been reproduced in Clara Marshall's *The Woman's Medical College of Pennsylvania: An Historical Outline* (Philadelphia: Blakiston, 1897), pp. 45–53, and (with some few deletions) in Alsop's *History of the Woman's Medical College*, pp. 68–70.

Chapter 4   *Approaching a Golden Age*

1. Estimate by Jon Kingsdale, quoted in William G. Rothstein, *American Medical Schools and the Practice of Medicine: A History* (New York and Oxford: Oxford University Press, 1987), p. 78.

2. An immense literature addresses medicine and medical education in later nineteenth-century America. Examples include James H. Cassedy, *Medicine in America: A Short History* (Baltimore: Johns Hopkins University Press, 1992); Thomas Neville Bonner, *Becoming a Physician: Medical Education in Great Britain, France, Germany, and the United States 1750–1945* (New York and Oxford: Oxford University Press, 1995); Ronald Numbers, ed., *The Education of American Physicians: Historical Essays* (Berkeley and Los Angeles: University of California Press, 1980), especially the essay on pathology by Russell C.

Maulitz; Kenneth Ludmerer, *Learning to Heal: The Development of American Medical Education* (New York: Basic Books, 1985).

3. See statistics in Mary Roth Walsh, *Doctors Wanted, No Women Need Apply: Sexual Barriers in the Medical Profession, 1835–1975* (New Haven, Conn.: Yale University Press, 1977), p. 186.

4. My main sources for women's activities in the late nineteenth century were Catherine Clinton, *The Other Civil War: American Women in the Nineteenth Century* (New York: Hill and Wang, 1984); Eleanor Flexner, *Century of Struggle: The Woman's Rights Movement in the United States* (New York: Athenaeum, 1974); and Sara M. Evans, *Born for Liberty: A History of Women in America* (New York: Free Press, 1989).

5. For Philadelphia history and institutions in this and other periods, I relied on Russell F. Weigley, ed., *Philadelphia: A 300–Year History* (New York: Norton, 1982); John Lukacs, *Philadelphia Patricians and Philistines, 1900–1950* (New York: Farrar Strauss Giroux, 1981), pp. 3–47; Jean Barth Toll and Mildred S. Gillam, eds., *Invisible Philadelphia: Community through Voluntary Organizations* (Philadelphia: Atwater Kent Museum, 1995); Sam Bass Warner, *The Private City: Philadelphia in Three Periods of Its Growth*, 2d ed. (Philadelphia: University of Pennsylvania Press, 1987).

6. For the early women's clubs of Philadelphia, see Toll and Gillam, eds., *Invisible Philadelphia*, pp. 350–356, including the excellent account of the Civic Club by Julie Johnson.

7. For the Alumnae Association, see Gulielma Fell Alsop, *History of the Woman's Medical College, Philadelphia, Pennsylvania, 1850–1950* (Philadelphia: Lippincott, 1950), pp. 119–120; Elizabeth Keller, "The History of the Alumnae Association," *Transactions of the Twenty-fifth Annual Meeting of the Alumnae Association of the Woman's Medical College of Pennsylvania* (1900): 35–37. The association published annual transactions of its meeting from 1876 through 1939. A collection of association papers, directories, and other materials is housed at ASCWM. For early women's medical societies in the United States, see Cora Bagley Marrett, "On the Evolution of Women's Medical Societies," *Bulletin of the History of Medicine* 53 (1979): 434–448.

8. Rachel L. Bodley, *The College Story. Valedictory Address to the Twenty-ninth Graduating Class of the Woman's Medical College of Pennsylvania* (Philadelphia, 1881). There is also a good synopsis in Alsop, *History of the Woman's Medical College*, pp. 127–134. For sources on the life of Rachel Bodley, see note 20 of chapter 2.

9. Bodley, *The College Story*, p. 4.

10. Ibid., p. 5.

11. Ibid., p. 7.

12. Ibid., pp. 8, 9.

13. Ibid., p. 9.

14. Most of the senior faculty women and deans of the nineteenth-century WMC did not marry (Ann Preston, Rachel Bodley, Clara Marshall, Frances Emily White, Anna Broomall), though several did (Emeline Horton Cleveland, Mary Scarlett-Dixon, and Hannah Croasdale).

15. Bodley, *The College Story*, p. 10.

16. Bodley, *The College Story*, pp. 10, 11. Regina Morantz-Sanchez in *Sympathy and Science* (New York and Oxford: Oxford University Press, 1985), pp. 138–142, cites other examples of supportive husbands, several of whom were themselves physicians.

17. Bodley, *The College Story*, p. 11.
18. See Clinton, *The Other Civil War*, pp. 42–44, for a brief overview of the role of women in religion, and of religion in women, in nineteenth-century America.
19. This figure is cited in Patricia R. Hill, *The World Their Household: The American Woman's Foreign Mission Movement and Cultural Transformation, 1870–1920* (Ann Arbor: University of Michigan Press, 1985), p. 3. I have relied on this source for understanding the scope and context of the women's missionary enthusiasm.
20. Mrs. J. T. Gracey, *Medical Work of the Woman's Foreign Missionary Society of the Methodist Episcopal Church* (Boston, 1888), p. 92.
21. There exists an extensive literature on female medical missionaries, including many autobiographies. See the section on "Missionary Activity" in Sandra Chaff et al., *Women in Medicine: A Bibliography of the Literature on Women Physicians* (Metuchen, N.J.: Scarecrow Press, 1977), pp. 581–609; the chapter on "Pioneer Women Missionaries of the Woman's Medical College," in Alsop, *History of the Woman's Medical College*, pp. 135–144; Marion Fay, "Alumnae Service as Medical Missionaries in Many Parts of the World," *Medical College of Pennsylvania Alumnae-i News* 26 (1975): 16–17; Bodley, *The College Story*, pp. 14–15.
22. Gracey, *Medical Work*.
23. For night clinics see Lilian Welsh, *Reminiscences of Thirty Years in Baltimore* (Baltimore: Norman Remington Co., 1925), pp. 49–62; *Report of Proceedings of the Twelfth Annual Meeting of the Alumnae Association of the Woman's Medical College of Pennsylvania* (1887): 43–44.
24. Alsop, *History of the Woman's Medical College*, p. 139.
25. Ibid., p. 142.
26. The Society for Ethical Culture, of which the Philadelphia Ethical Society (founded in 1885) was the third such group in the United States, raised ethical behavior to primacy in its religion, and discounted ritual, liturgy, and much of the supernatural. Some members, however, also belonged to traditional congregations. WMC faculty who were members included Frances Emily White (a materialist and fervid student of evolution), C. Newlin Peirce (longtime board member and professor of dental subjects), and Henry Leffmann.
27. "Concerning Foreign Missions," *Bulletin of the Woman's Medical College of Pennsylvania* 66 (December 1915): 16.
28. Kate Campbell Hurd-Mead, "Forty Years of Medical Progress: Reminiscences and Comparisons," in *Seventy-fifth Anniversary Volume of the Woman's Medical College of Pennsylvania* (Philadelphia, 1925), pp. 172–173. Anandibai Joshee graduated in 1886, Kei Okami and Susan LaFlesche in 1889, and Sabat Islambooly in 1890.
29. Bodley to Jane Addams, 11 July 1885, Jane Addams Papers, microfilm, reel 2, frames 78–81 (the author used the set at the Peace Collection, Library of Swarthmore College, Swarthmore, Pennsylvania). Addams attended WMC during the 1881–82 term, but left early owing to illness, then changed her mind about studying medicine.
30. For biographical information on Marshall, see entry by Steven J. Peitzman in Martin Kaufman, Stuart Galishoff, and Todd L. Savitt, eds., *Dictionary of American Medical Biography* vol. 2 (Westport, Conn.: Greenwood Press, 1984), p. 497; materials in Marshall's Deceased Alumna Folder, including obituary in the *Public Ledger*, 14 March 1931; and chapters on Marshall in Alsop, *History*

of the Woman's Medical College. An incomplete collection of her official papers as dean is housed at ASCWM.

31. MF, 18 and 20 March 1876.
32. *Professional Directory of Physicians & Druggists of Philadelphia* (Philadelphia, 1912); her hours were "10–12 and 7 p.m." Most of her publications were clinical cases, with emphasis on obstetrics and gynecology.
33. The Board of Corporators Minutes for 25 February 1853 contain a formal resolution to seek qualified female physicians for the faculty. Of course the Marshall episode came over twenty years later, though there were five board members from 1853 still on it in 1876.
34. Class of 1897 Minutes Book, in Edith Flower Wheeler Papers.
35. Clara Marshall, *The Woman's Medical College of Pennsylvania: An Historical Outline* (Philadelphia: Blakiston, 1897), pp. 34–39 and 84–88 (appointments), and pp. 89–142 (bibliography). Many of the cited articles are case reports (the staple of medical literature then). The largest number of cited papers are those of Mary Putnam Jacobi (1842–1906), a graduate of 1864 who became nineteenth-century America's most renowned woman physician and medical scientist.
36. See "Women Candidates Plan for Church and Parlor Campaign," *Philadelphia North American*, 27 January 1902 (found in College Clippings Collection, leaf 318); *Third Annual Address of Mrs. Cornelius Stevenson, President of the Civic Club. Annual Meeting, January 8, 1897* (Philadelphia, 1897); *Nineteenth Annual Report of the New Century Club of Philadelphia, 1896* (membership lists show WMC faculty members Marshall, Hannah Croasdale, Anna Broomall, and Frances Emily White; associate members [men] included WMC board members C. N. Peirce, Warner Redwood, and Enoch Lewis). While the campaign for state and national suffrage moved in fits and starts, a parallel effort aimed at "school suffrage," which meant the right of women to vote in school-board contests, gained considerable success, and represented another mechanism for women transforming a domestic concern into a public presence.

Chapter 5 Curriculum, Clinics, and Coeducation

1. For curricular extension and reform in this period, I used Kenneth M. Ludmerer, *Learning to Heal: The Development of American Medical Education* (New York: Basic Books, 1985), pp. 47–101; Lester S. King, *American Medicine Comes of Age, 1840–1920* (Chicago: American Medical Association, 1984), pp. 83–87; and William G. Rothstein, *American Medical Schools and the Practice of Medicine: A History* (New York and Oxford: Oxford University Press, 1987), pp. 89–116.
2. Harold Alderfer, "Legislative History of Medical Licensure in Pennsylvania," *Pennsylvania Medical Journal* 64 (1961): 1605–1609. This did not necessarily mean four years of structured course work in one medical school: "study" might still mean apprenticeship, a year accomplished previously at another school, etc.
3. See Ludmerer, *Learning to Heal*, especially chapters 2, 3, and 4.
4. Ludmerer, *Learning to Heal*, especially pp. 139–151.
5. A treasurer's report in the Board of Corporators Minutes for 1 March 1897 shows $283,072.64 of "investments."
6. E.g., James Tyson [dean of the University of Pennsylvania School of Medicine] to Marshall, 29 January 1891, Marshall Papers.

7. Blackwell to Marshall, 23 January 1892, in Emily Blackwell folder, "Individuals" Collection.
8. MF, 21 November 1891; Alfred Jones to faculty of WMC, 11 December 1891, in Marshall Papers.
9. "Medical Education in the United States," *JAMA* 22 (1894): 393–394.
10. *Forty-fourth Annual Announcement of the Woman's Medical College of Pennsylvania, 1893–1894* (Philadelphia, 1893), p. 12.
11. [Emma Billstein], "Report on Histology and Embryology [for the session of 1897–98]," in box 4 of Board of Corporator Minutes.
12. For White's efforts concerning gymnastics, see *Report of Proceedings of the Thirteenth Annual Meeting of the Alumnae Association of the Woman's Medical College of Pennsylvania* (Philadelphia, 1888), p. 22; also MF, 17 November 1888.
13. MF, 13 September 1879. This trip was paid for by White's close friend Elizabeth Keller, a WMC graduate of 1871 and a successful surgeon in Boston.
14. *Thirty-third Annual Announcement of the Woman's Medical College of Pennsylvania, 1882–1883* (Philadelphia, 1882), p. 9.
15. Diary of Mary Theodora McGavran ("My Life and Work"), typescript from holograph, first volume of two, p. 23. Excerpts from this diary (but not including these cited passages) have been published with an introductory essay: Robert M. Kaiser, Sandra L. Chaff, and Steven J. Peitzman, "A Philadelphia Medical Student of the 1890s: The Diary of Mary Theodora McGavran," *Pennsylvania Magazine of History and Biography* 108 (1984): 217–236.
16. For an excellent account of Rabinowitsch's years at WMC, see Lori R. Walsh and James A. Poupard, "Lydia Rabinowitsch, Ph.D., and the Emergence of Clinical Pathology in Late 19th-Century America," *Archives of Pathology and Laboratory Medicine* 113 (1989): 1303–1308.
17. MF, 21 December 1895.
18. Catherine Macfarlane, Typescript Autobiography, p. 21, in Macfarlane Papers, ASCWM, and a copy is also in the Macfarlane Papers at the Library of the College of Physicians of Philadelphia.
19. Ibid., p. 123.
20. In fairness to the board, it went out of its way to salvage the relationship, sending three wires to Germany during the fall of 1898, bidding her return. She did not appear to reply; MF, 15 October 1898.
21. MBC, 7 February 1898. Of course, the total income of senior clinical faculty was much higher than this, most of it derived from practice. Like Rachel Bodley before her, Rabinowitsch as a non-physician of course had no such additional source of remuneration.
22. For clinical teaching of medical students in the late nineteenth and early twentieth centuries, see Edward Atwater, "'Making Fewer Mistakes': a History of Students and Patients," *Bulletin of the History of Medicine* 57 (1983): 165–187; Ludmerer, *Learning to Heal*, esp. pp. 152–165; William G. Rothstein, *American Medical Schools*, esp. pp. 107–115; the essays on clinical departments in Ronald Numbers, ed., *The Education of American Physicians: Historical Essays* (Berkeley and Los Angeles: University of California Press, 1980); Thomas Neville Bonner, *Becoming a Physician: Medical Education in Great Britain, France, Germany, and the United States, 1750–1945* (New York and Oxford: Oxford University Press, 1995), esp. pp. 318–324; Thomas S. Huddle and Jack Ende, "Osler's Clinical Clerkship: Origins and Interpretations," *Journal of the History of Medicine and Allied Science* 49 (1994): 483–503. For an excellent account of the hospital's stance in the pressure for clinical instruction, see Charles E.

Rosenberg, *The Care of Strangers: The Rise of America's Hospital System* (New York: Basic Books, 1987), esp. pp. 190–211.

23. Later known as Lankenau Hospital.

24. The hospital in the 1880s had committees on "graduates" (the interns) and of course a committee on the nursing school. The minutes of the board of managers of the hospital throughout the 1880s rarely mention medical students.

25. MF, 15 October 1887.

26. MF, 26 January 1889 and 19 January 1895.

27. For Broomall's life, see Martin Kaufman et al., *Dictionary of American Medical Biography*, vol. 1 (Westport, Conn.: Greenwood Press, 1984), p. 98; Mary Griscom, "Pioneering Medical Women—a Beloved Physician [Anna Broomall]," reprinted from *Medical Woman's Journal*, July 1931; and materials in her Deceased Alumna Folder. For prenatal care (though the word was not used in the 1890s), see Lida Stewart-Cogill, "'Prenatal care' as conducted in the Woman's Hospital and the West Philadelphia Hospital for Women," *Transactions of the Forty-first Annual Meeting of the Alumnae Association of the Woman's Medical College of Pennsylvania* (Philadelphia, 1916), pp. 123–125. For comparison of Broomall's methods with those taught in Germany, see letters by her protégé Anna Fullerton to Rebecca White, 5 April and 8 June 1884, in Josiah White Papers, Quaker Collections, Haverford College Library, Haverford, Pennsylvania; and Kate Campbell Hurd-Mead, "Forty Years of Medical Progress Reminiscences and Comparisons," in *Seventy-fifth Anniversary Volume of the Woman's Medical College of Pennsylvania* (Philadelphia, 1925), pp. 175–176.

28. For practical teaching of obstetrics in American medical schools of the nineteenth century, see Lawrence Longo, "Obstetrics and Gynecology," in Numbers, *Education of American Physicians*, esp. pp. 216–221; Rothstein, *American Medical Schools*, p. 114; and Charlotte Borst, *Catching Babies: The Professionalization of Childbirth, 1870–1920* (Cambridge, Mass.: Harvard University Press, 1995), pp. 90–101.

29. MF, 20 February 1892.

30. Professor of surgery John B. Roberts, a highly concerned faculty member, in a letter of January 1892, offered what seems like a sensible little plan (with sketch) to construct a sort of appendage to the Woman's Hospital, of sixteen to twenty beds, run by the College faculty for teaching purposes, with the hospital contracted to supply nursing and dietary service. Roberts to Marshall, 24 January 1892, Marshall Papers.

31. MF, 1 October 1892. The College agreed to pay five hundred dollars for these "clinical advantages."

32. *Report of Proceedings of the Twentieth Annual Meeting of the Alumnae Association of the Woman's Medical College of Pennsylvania* (Philadelphia, 1895), pp. 50–53.

33. Report by Gertrude Walker to the Board of Corporators, MBC, 17 May 1897.

34. Ibid.

35. See Bonnie Blustein, *Educating for Health and Prevention: A History of the Department of Community and Preventive Medicine of the (Woman's) Medical College of Pennsylvania* (Canton, Mass.: Science History Publications, 1993); Regina Morantz-Sanchez, *Sympathy and Science: Women Physicians in American Medicine* (New York and Oxford: Oxford University Press, 1985), esp. pp. 215–216, 283. See also Anna I. von Sholly, "Women in Preventive Medicine," *Columbia University Quarterly* 17 (1915): 236–240.

36. *Report of Proceedings of the Twelfth Annual Meeting of the Alumnae Association of the Woman's Medical College of Pennsylvania* (Philadelphia, 1887), pp. 4–51.

37. *Report of Proceedings of the Thirteenth Annual Meeting of the Alumnae Association of the Woman's Medical College of Pennsylvania* (Philadelphia, 1888), pp. 22–24; MF, 17 November 1888.

38. See Helen Lefkowitz Horowitz, *Alma Mater: Design and Experience in the Women's Colleges from Their Nineteenth-Century Beginnings to the 1930s* (New York: Knopf, 1984), p. 169. Certainly men's colleges did the same.

39. *Report of Proceedings of the Sixteenth Annual Meeting of the Alumnae Association of the Woman's Medical College of Pennsylvania* (Philadelphia, 1891), p. 31.

40. Ibid.; *Report of Proceedings of the Seventeenth Annual Meeting of the Alumnae Association of the Woman's Medical College of Pennsylvania* (Philadelphia, 1892), pp. 32–34.

41. Kaiser, "A Philadelphia Medical Student," p. 230; Hurd-Mead, "Forty Years," p. 17. Broomall read several languages, traveled to China in 1890 with Dr. Elizabeth Reifsnyder (WMC, 1881), a medical missionary on leave, to visit and teach former pupils, and devoted her retirement years to regional history of Delaware County, Pennsylvania.

42. Kaiser, "A Philadelphia Medical Student," p. 230; Macfarlane, Autobiography, p. 34 (other comments about Broomall appear on p. 23).

43. Macfarlane, Autobiography, p. 28.

44. Anna Fullerton to Rebecca White, 5 April 1884, Josiah White Papers, Quaker Collection, Haverford College Library, Haverford, Pennsylvania. Fullerton indicates her fervid hope of working as assistant to Broomall in another letter to White, 8 June 1884. Fullerton was born to missionary parents in India, and after her service at the Woman's Hospital and WMC returned there in 1910.

45. Grace Schermerhorn to Marion Fay, 19 December 1945, in Schermerhorn Deceased Alumna Folder.

46. Information on Croasdale is from the small amount of material in her Deceased Alumna Folder; an obituary in *Transactions of the Thirty-seventh Annual Meeting of the Alumnae Association of the Woman's Medical College of Pennsylvania* (Philadelphia, 1912), pp. 39–41; Hurd-Mead, "Forty Years," pp. 176–177; Macfarlane, Autobiography, pp. 21–22; Wheeler, Autobiography, pp. 112–113; Schermerhorn to Fay, 19 December 1945; Rosalie Slaughter Morton, *A Woman Surgeon* (New York: Grosset and Dunlop, 1937), p. 20.

47. Macfarlane, Autobiography, p. 20; Hurd-Mead, "Forty Years," pp. 172–173; Lydia Hunt King to Clara Marshall, 8 July 1891, Marshall Papers; Grace Schermerhorn to Marion Fay, 19 December 1945, Schermerhorn Deceased Alumna Folder.

48. For White's difficulties, see MF, 27 January 1877 and 1 February 1877, and letter of Henry Hartshorne to White 1 February 1877 in Hartshorne Papers, Quaker Collections, Haverford College Library, Haverford, Pennsylvania.

49. For Sherwood, see the interesting little volume by her close friend and co-worker Lilian Welsh (WMC, 1889), *Reminiscences of Thirty Years in Baltimore* (Baltimore: Norman, Remington, 1925).

50. See "Fifty Years Ago—Dr. Marie Formad," *Medical Woman's Journal* 45 (1936): 132–133.

51. Hurd-Mead, "Forty Years," p. 174.

52. MF, 18 May 1889.

53. Hurd-Mead, "Forty Years," pp. 174, 181; MF, 16 May 1891.

54. MF, 16 May 1891. For a brief account of Henry's career, see his "Memoir" by

Francis X. Dercum in the *Transactions and Studies of the College of Physicians of Philadelphia*, ser. 3, 41 (1920): lvii–lxi.

55. Macfarlane, Autobiography, p. 23.

56. Still in use is Burton Konkle, *Standard History of the Medical Profession of Phila-delphia*, Frederick P. Henry, ed., enlarged and corrected, 1973–1974, by Lisabeth M. Holloway (New York: AMS Press, 1977). See Holloway's "Editor's Note" for the history of the book's authorship, and the "Preface" for references to WMC faculty who assisted Henry.

57. For information about Leffmann, see his *Outline Autobiography* (Philadelphia, 1905), which contains his compilation of publications until that time; Joseph S. Hepburn, "Medical Annals of Central High School of Philadelphia," *Barnwell Bulletin* 18 (1940): 31–32; Charles LaWall, "American Contempo-raries: Henry Leffmann, A.M., M.D.," *Industrial and Engineering Chemistry* 18 (1926): 648–651; [No author], "Dr. Henry Leffmann," reprint from *Journal of the Franklin Institute, 1931*, and other obituaries and materials in the Leffmann folder in Vertical Files. Unfortunately, no collection of Leffmann's professional or private correspondence has been located.

58. Kaiser, "A Philadelphia Medical Student," pp. 231, 235.

59. For Roberts's life and work, only thinly sketched here, see his "Memoir" by William Robertson in the *Transactions and Studies of the College of Physicians of Philadelphia*, ser. 3, 49 (1927): lxxvii–lxxxii; Whitfield J. Bell Jr., *The College of Physicians of Philadelphia* (Canton, Mass.: Science History Publications, 1987), pp. 240–241; entry in Howard A. Kelly and Walter L. Burrage, *Dictionary of American Medical Biography* (Boston: Milford House, 1971; reprint of the 1928 edition), p. 1042; for the Committee of Seventy and Roberts's work with it, see Russell F. Weigley, ed., *Philadelphia: A 300–Year History* (New York: Norton, 1982), p. 540 (chapter by Lloyd Abernethy); letters of Roberts to Clara Marshall, 24 January 1892 and 18 May 1897, Marshall Papers.

60. Student Association Minutes, 16 May 1898; Truman G. Schnabel, "Memoir of Arthur A. Stevens," *Transactions and Studies of the College of Physicians of Phila-delphia*, ser. 4, 13 (1945–46): 88–90. *The Scalpel*, 1911 (WMCP yearbook), p. 132.

61. See Steven J. Peitzman, "'Thoroughly Practical': America's Polyclinic Medi-cal Schools," *Bulletin of the History of Medicine* 54 (1980): 166–187. The poly-clinics also supplemented the woefully meager clinical experience available in the typical M.D.-granting college of nineteenth-century America. The Phila-delphia Polyclinic freely admitted women to its classes and appointed many WMC graduates to posts as teaching assistants. Roberts even tried to arrange for the Polyclinic to instruct WMC students as part of strenuous efforts to shore up clinical instruction in the newly required fourth year.

62. Weigley, ed. *Philadelphia: A 300–Year History*, p. 340. Central had authority to award the bachelor of arts degree since 1849.

63. MF, 17 October 1885.

64. Alsop, *History of the Woman's Medical College*, p. 190.

65. MF, 8 November 1883.

66. MF, 25 March 1882, 13 January 1883. The author has been unable to recon-struct the actual charges from available minutes and other documents, nor learn much about Benjamin Wilson.

67. Mary Scarlett [later Scarlett-Dixon] to Edwin Fussell, 15 June 1869, Scarlett-Dixon Deceased Alumna Folder.

68. White to Hartshorne, 30 August 1876, and Hartshorne to White, 1 February 1877, in Hartshorne Papers, Quaker Collections, Haverford College Library.

69. Keen to Marshall, 21 May 1889, Marshall Papers.
70. MF, 20 April 1889.
71. James B. Walker to the faculty of the Woman's Medical College of Pennsylvania, undated, but would have been written sometime in May 1891, in Clara Marshall Papers.
72. MF, 9 December 1878.
73. MF, 25 November 1882.
74. *Report of Proceedings of the Twelfth Annual Meeting of the Alumnae Association of the Woman's Medical College of Pennsylvania* (Philadelphia, 1887), pp. 43–44; *Report of Proceedings of the Seventeenth Annual Meeting of the Alumnae Association of the Woman's Medical College of Pennsylvania* (Philadelphia, 1892), p. 116.
75. *Philadelphia Public Ledger*, 1 May 1896, and *Philadelphia Evening Bulletin*, 7 May 1896, clippings in College Clippings Collection, leaf 250.
76. Dentistry was sometimes part of the medical school curriculum in the nineteenth century. The WMC building opened in 1875 included a dental suite. Some dental skills would have well served doctors in isolated regions and perhaps women medical missionaries.
77. Caroline Katzenstein, *Lifting the Curtain: The State and National Woman Suffrage Campaigns in Pennsylvania as I Saw Them* (Philadelphia: Dorrance & Co., 1955), p. 20.
78. Ibid., p. 21. For another account of Charlotte Woodward's attendance at the Seneca Falls Convention, see Eleanor Flexner, *Century of Struggle: The Woman's Rights Movement in the United States* (New York: Athenaeum, 1974), pp. 76–77. According to Flexner's sources, Woodward had the ambition to become a typesetter and work in a print shop. Some secondary sources refer to the Declaration of Principles rather than Declaration of Sentiments; the latter term is certainly used in the first volume of the *History of Woman Suffrage* by Elizabeth Cady Stanton, Susan B. Anthony, and Matilda Joslyn Gage (Rochester, N.Y., 1887), pp. 70–71.

Chapter 6   *Student Life at the Mature "Woman's Med"*

1. Statements in this paragraph are based mainly on inspection of lists of matriculants in the *Annual Announcements* from 1885 through 1900; also materials cited in note 2 below.
2. The McGavran diary and a transcript of it are in the McGavran Collection, ASCWM. Excerpts may be found in Robert M. Kaiser, Sandra L. Chaff, and Steven J. Peitzman, "A Philadelphia Medical Student of the 1890s: The Diary of Mary Theodora McGavran," *Pennsylvania Magazine of History and Biography* 108 (1984): 217–236 (hereafter "Kaiser/McGavran"). A typescript of Wheeler's autobiography (hereafter "Wheeler"), which she tentatively titled "She Saunters into her Past," is in her collection of papers at ASCWM. Her recollections of student years are based on letters to her father written at the time, so do not depend only on memory. Both McGavran and Wheeler enjoyed wit and some ability with words, so are good companions. Other sources for this chapter include the minutes of the Student Association from 1895 through 1910 (in Students Collection), the minutes of the Class of 1897 (in the Wheeler collection), and other reminiscences as noted.
3. Wheeler, p. 100.
4. Kaiser/McGavran, pp. 229–230.

5. Wheeler, p. 86.

6. [Anon], *North of Market Street: Being the Adventures of a New York Woman in Philadelphia* (Philadelphia, 1896), p. 11; quoted in Jill Gates Smith, "'I have some college pictures you *might* like . . .': The Photograph Album of a Nineteenth Century Woman Medical Student" (Master's thesis in history, Temple University, 1987). Jill Gates Smith was an archivist at ASCWM.

7. Ibid., p. 83.

8. Anne Walter Fearn, *My Days of Strength: An American Woman Doctor's Forty Years in China* (New York: Harper & Brothers, 1939), p. 14.

9. Kaiser/McGavran, pp. 227, 230.

10. Wheeler, p. 108.

11. McGavran diary, typescript, pp. 23–24.

12. The two extracts are from Kaiser/McGavran, pp. 232, 233. Lawrence Wolff (1845–1901) attended at German Hospital and held the title of clinical professor of medicine at WMC; John B. Deaver (1855–1931), on the surgical staff at the German, was among Philadelphia's leading surgeons and surgical teachers.

13. Wheeler, p. 99.

14. Another grisly description of a clinic by Catharine Macfarlane, an 1898 graduate and later luminary of the College, details Hannah Croasdale's operation for "complete prolapse of the rectum" (in her Typescript Autobiography, p. 22, Macfarlane Papers, ASCWM; another copy is at the Library of the College of Physicians of Philadelphia).

15. Rosalie Slaughter Morton, *A Woman Surgeon* (New York: Grosset and Dunlap, 1937), p. 36.

16. Wheeler, pp. 106–107.

17. Ibid., pp. 121–122.

18. Morton, *A Woman Surgeon*, p. 43.

19. The casebooks consulted are in the collection "Clinics and Hospitals" at the ASCWM: Hospital and Dispensary of the Alumnae of the Woman's Medical College of Pennsylvania, casebooks ("Children's Clinic 1895–98," "L. N. Tappan Book 1 1895–97," "Out Practice 1896–97").

20. Kaiser/McGavran, p. 232.

21. MF, 21 November 1896, 19 December 1896, 15 January 1898, 16 April 1898, 18 February 1899.

22. MF, 21 November 1891.

23. Student Association Minutes, 13 March 1896; copy of letter tipped in MBC, dated 17 March 1896.

24. For faculty response, see MF, 21 March 1896, 28 March 1896, 18 April 1896.

25. MF, 16 November 1900.

26. Student Association Minutes, 26 March 1900; see also other reports of the Committee on Hospitals, 1 December 1898, 12 March 1904.

27. Student Association Minutes, 2 October 1895; this is the first mention of the reception, but it was held yearly. The references to decorating for the reception recall the dances and other activities women students held in women's colleges; see Helen Lefkowitz Horowitz, *Alma Mater: Design and Experience in the Women's Colleges from Their Nineteenth-Century Beginnings to the 1930s* (New York: Knopf, 1984), p. 169.

28. Discussion of the cap and gown appear in MF, 19 January 1889, 15 November 1890, 21 February 1891, 21 March 1891, 18 November 1893 (discussion of cap and gown "indefinitely postponed"); in Student Association Minutes, 2 October 1895; there is also discussion in the Class of 1897 Minutes, 1 November 1893.

29. Student Association Minutes, 25 February 1897, 15 December 1899, 23 April 1903.

30. Class of 1897 Minutes, 1 November 1893, 13 March 1894.

31. Student Association Minutes, 15 December 1895; MF 18 December 1897, 16 December 1899.

32. Wheeler, pp. 102–103.

33. Lilian Welsh, *Reminiscences of Thirty Years in Baltimore* (Baltimore: Norman, Remington, 1925), p. 100. "Dr. Welsh was one of the great pioneers of suffrage, one of the old war horses, as Mary Agnes Hamilton has recently called them." (Margaret Shove Morriss, *A Tribute to Lilian Welsh* [Baltimore: Goucher College, 1938], p. 35.)

34. Barbara Miller Solomon, *In the Company of Educated Women: A History of Women and Higher Education in America* (New Haven, Conn.: Yale University Press, 1985), pp. 111–114.

35. Class of 1897 Minutes, 13 December 1893 and passim.

36. Kaiser/McGavran, p. 232; McGavran Diary, p. 9. For typhoid fever in Philadelphia in the 1890s, see Michael P. McCarthy, *Typhoid and the Politics of Public Health in Nineteenth-Century Philadelphia* (Philadelphia: American Philosophical Society, 1987).

37. Macfarlane, Autobiography, p. 33.

38. Ibid.

39. See MF, 21 November 1891, and 15 April 1893. The faculty contributed to the bed fund.

40. *Report of Proceedings of the Sixteenth Annual Meeting of the Alumnae Association of the Woman's Medical College of Pennsylvania* (Philadelphia, 1891), pp. 21, 32.

41. Student Association Minutes, 27 January 1896.

42. *Daughters of Aesculapius: Stories Written by Alumnae and Students of the Woman's Medical College of Pennsylvania and Edited by a Committee Appointed by the Students' Association of the College* (Philadelphia: George Jacobs, 1897). The phrase "life aware of itself" is from the short story "The Other Margaret" by Lionel Trilling in *Of This Time and That Place and Other Stories* (New York: Harcourt Brace Jovanovich, 1979).

43. Shirley Marchalonis, *College Girls: A Century in Fiction* (New Brunswick, N.J.: Rutgers University Press, 1995), pp. 50–51.

44. For friendship among medical women, see Regina Morantz-Sanchez, *Sympathy and Science: Women Physicians in American Medicine* (New York and Oxford: Oxford University Press, 1985), pp. 132–133; Smith, "I Have Some College Pictures," pp. 4–5.

45. Alice Seabrook, "The Home Side," in *Daughters of Aesculapius*, pp. 150–155. Ann Walter Fearn, an 1893 graduate, referred to doing "light housekeeping" with her classmate and best friend, Sarah Poindexter (Fearn, *My Days of Strength*, p. 15).

46. Wheeler, e.g., pp. 85, 110, 113.

47. Louise Ashby to Clara Marshall, 31 August 1891, Marshall Papers.

48. Eliza Grier to the "President or Proprietor of the Woman's Medical College, Philadelphia, Pa.," 6 December 1890, in her Deceased Alumna Folder.

49. Kaiser/McGavran, p. 229.

50. McGavran Diary, pp. 20, 76 (reservoir), 78–79, 84 (croquet, tennis).

51. Kaiser/McGavran, p. 234. A "tallyho" is a four-in-hand carriage used mainly for pleasure outings.

52. Kaiser/McGavran, pp. 224–225.

53. Wheeler, pp. 83–84. Ignaz (Jan) Paderewsi was a celebrated Polish piano solo-ist, composer, and patriot, who made several American tours in the 1890s. Adelina Patti was the renowned Italian-Spanish-American coloratura soprano.

54. McGavran Diary, pp. 17, 63. The "German Symphony" might have been Philadelphia's Germania Orchestra, a partly amateur group that to some ex-tent prefigured the Philadelphia Orchestra, founded in 1900.

55. Wheeler, p. 89. The main building, now called Founders Hall, is one of America's greatest Greek revival structures, designed by Thomas U. Walter after the Parthenon and completed in 1847.

56. Macfarlane, Autobiography, p. 35. The Sparks Shot Tower, not far from the Washington Avenue location of Broomall's maternity building, was built in 1808 and is still a neighborhood landmark.

57. Reported for the class of 1898 as "Weird Rites. Woman's Medical College Stu-dents Chant Around a Funeral Pyre," clipping from unidentified newspaper, possibly the *Philadelphia Public Ledger*, in College Clippings Collection, leaf 265.

58. For full accounts of student life at women's colleges in the nineteenth cen-tury, see Solomon, *In the Company*, pp. 94–114; Horowitz, *Alma Mater*, pp. 147–178.

59. I do not know to what extent the same applied to the other women's medical schools.

60. Horowitz, *Alma Mater*, pp. 174, 172.

61. Not the same as Musical Fund Hall, where the first graduation of the Female Medical College took place in 1852.

62. "Weird Rites," note 59 above.

63. Typed page of verse for commencement rites, found in Laura Heath Hills Col-lection. The reference to soldiers and quinine indicates that the class of 1898 briefly helped look after some soldiers of the Spanish-American War who were treated at the Woman's Hospital of Philadelphia.

64. Burton Clark, *The Academic Life: Small Worlds, Different Worlds* (Princeton, N.J.: Carnegie Foundation, 1987), p. 7.

65. Though it must be noted that reading the numerous discussions in the Alum-nae Association Transactions during the 1910s and 1920s reveals that by no means did all members oppose coeducation. Also, only a minority of alumnae joined the Association—less than 25 percent, for example, were members in 1911; see Eleanor Jones, "Address of the President," *Transactions of the Thirty-sixth Annual Meeting of the Alumnae Association of the Woman's Medical College of Pennsylvania* (Philadelphia, 1911), p. 78.

66. Printed note to "My dear fellow alumna" from Eleanor C. Jones, copy in Catharine Macfarlane Scrapbook, 1913–1918.

67. These events will be described in chapter 7.

68. Compiled for the author by Kristin Bunin when a medical student at MCP Hahnemann School of Medicine. Biographical information cited is from obitu-aries and other materials in these alumnae folders except where otherwise noted.

69. "Geographical Distribution of Alumnae," *Bulletin of the Woman's Medical Col-lege of Pennsylvania* 65 (1914): 18.

70. See also Alsop, *History of the Woman's Medical College*, pp. 150–151.

71. See entry (as Lillian Herreld South) in Martin Kaufman, Stuart Galishoff, and Todd L. Savitt, eds., *Dictionary of American Medical Biography*, vol. 2 (Westport, Conn.: Greenwood Press, 1984), 706–707.

72. Dilip Ramchandani and Steven Peitzman, "Alice Bennett: Doctor or Lady?" *Psychiatric News*, 3 November 1995, pp. 16, 25.

73. Of course, the fullest folders tend to be those with the longest, most visible careers, so the sample is biased. Some who practiced for fifty or more years include Anna Littlefield (1895; general practice in Connecticut), Mary L. Montgomery-Marsh (1895; fifty-eight years of general practice in Mount Pleasant, Pennsylvania), Mary Loog (1896), Laura Heath Hills (1896; general medicine), Caroline Marshall (1899; general practice in Homewood, Pennsylvania), Olive B. Steinmetz (1900; general practice in Homestead, Pennsylvania), Elsie Treichler Reedy (1901; general medicine in Philadelphia).

74. Sources for this section include obituaries and other materials in their Deceased Alumna Folders and in the created "Black Women Physicians Collections" at ASCWM. See also Darlene Clark Hine, "Co-Laborers in the Work of the Lord: Nineteenth-Century Black Women Physicians," in Ruth J. Abram, ed., *"Send Us a Lady Physician": Women Doctors in America, 1835–1920* (New York: Norton, 1985).

75. Clara Marshall used the phrase "door of opportunity" in "Our Point of View," a reprint of the toast she gave at the Anniversary Dinner of WMC, 4 May 1915, in Clara Marshall Papers, "Additions" box. Though African-Americans were certainly admitted to WMC, we have no way of knowing if others were turned away. While the association of Friends with abolition and service to freedmen is unquestioned, racial prejudice was not unknown to Philadelphia Quakers. Haverford and Swarthmore Colleges, Friends schools near Philadelphia, did not admit African-Americans during the nineteenth century; see Philip Benjamin, *The Philadelphia Quakers in the Industrial Age, 1865–1920* (Philadelphia: Temple University Press, 1976), esp. pp. 145–147.

76. Darlene Clark Hine, "Co-Laborers in the Work of the Lord," p. 15.

77. Halle Tanner Dillon [not yet Johnson] to Clara Marshall, 3 October 1891, copy in Halle Tanner Dillon Johnson folder, Black Women Physicians Collection.

78. Halle Tanner Dillon Johnson, "The La Fayette Dispensary," *Report of Proceedings of the Nineteenth Annual Meeting of the Alumnae Association of the Woman's Medical College of Pennsylvania* (Philadelphia, 1894), pp. 106–107.

79. *Report of Proceedings of the Thirteenth Annual Meeting of the Alumnae Association of the Woman's Medical College of Pennsylvania* (Philadelphia, 1888), pp. 33–34.

80. Eliza Anna Grier to Susan B. Anthony, 7 March 1901, copy in Grier folder, Black Women Physicians Collection.

81. Russell F. Weigley, ed., *Philadelphia: A 300-Year History* (New York: Norton, 1982), pp. 491–494.

82. Class of 1897 Minutes Book, entries for 9 January 1896 and ? April 1896.

83. Irene Gates, *Any Hope, Doctor?* (London: Blandford Press, 1954), pp. 47–48.

Chapter 7 *The Age of Educational Reform*

1. Regina Morantz-Sanchez's section on the College's early struggles in the twentieth century in *Sympathy and Science: Women Physicians in American Medicine* (New York and Oxford: Oxford University Press, 1985) has served this current author as an invaluable guide to thinking about WMC in the period discussed in this chapter; see esp. pp. 255–261, 268–274.

2. The last regular women's medical school to survive, other than WMC, was the Woman's Medical College of Baltimore, which closed in 1910 in part owing

to lack of funds. The homeopathic New York Medical College and Hospital for Women survived until 1918.

3. For reform of medical education and standards during the first two decades of the twentieth century, see Kenneth Ludmerer, *Learning to Heal: The Development of American Medical Education* (New York: Basic Books, 1985), esp. pp. 166–190, 234–254, and Martin Kaufman, *American Medical Education: The Formative Years, 1765–1910* (Westport, Conn.: Greenwood Press, 1976), pp. 154–182.

4. The Carnegie Foundation was established in 1905; its first major function was the establishment of a pension plan for teachers, but its activities expanded under the leadership of its first president, Henry Pritchett.

5. For discussion of the impact of the "Flexner Report," see Ludmerer, *Learning to Heal*, pp. 168–190; Robert P. Hudson, "Abraham Flexner in Perspective," *Bulletin of the History of Medicine* 46 (1972): 545–561; Thomas Neville Bonner, "Abraham Flexner and the Historians," *Journal of the History of Medicine and Allied Sciences* 45 (1990): 3–10. For Flexner's later role as manager of philanthropy to medical schools, see Steven C. Wheatley, *The Politics of Philanthropy: Abraham Flexner and Medical Education* (Madison: University of Wisconsin Press, 1988). The standard citation for the "Report" is Abraham Flexner, *Medical Education in the United States and Canada: A Report to the Carnegie Foundation for the Advancement of Teaching* (New York: Carnegie Foundation, 1910); it was technically the Foundation's *Bulletin Number Four.*

6. The report on WMC is on p. 296, Flexner's discussion of what medical education in Pennsylvania ought to look like on pp. 298–300, and his discussion of "The Medical Education of Women" on pp. 178–179, all in Flexner, *Medical Education*.

7. It is still not historically clear why the number of American women seeking medical education declined after 1900; for a full discussion of this question, see Morantz-Sanchez, *Sympathy and Science*, pp. 232–265. See also Stephen Cole, "Sex Discrimination and Admission to Medical School, 1929–1984," *American Journal of Sociology* 92 (1986): 549–567.

8. A summary of the value of WMC property and investment funds from 1898 through June of 1902 is found in the MECBC, 5 January 1903.

9. MECBC, 18 May 1903.

10. Clara Marshall to Abraham Flexner, 2 June 1909 (letter showing total enrollment at WMC 1900 through 1909) in Marshall Papers.

11. Quoted in Wheatly, *Politics of Philanthropy*, p. 16.

12. Quoted in Morantz-Sanchez, *Sympathy and Science*, p. 78.

13. Quoted in Philip Benjamin, *The Philadelphia Quakers in the Industrial Age, 1865–1920* (Philadelphia: Temple University Press, 1976), p. 105.

14. Benjamin, *Philadelphia Quakers*, pp. 146–147.

15. Ludmerer, *Learning to Heal*, p. 148.

16. For lack of alumnae capacity to make large gifts, see Clara M. Hammond-McGuigan, in "Discussion," *Transactions of the Thirty-Eighth Annual Meeting of the Alumnae Association of the Woman's Medical College of Pennsylvania* (Philadelphia, 1913), p. 132; the discussion followed a paper by Catharine Macfarlane, "Presentation of a Plan Whereby the Alumnae May Assist the College" (pp. 125–128) in which she discussed the Graduate Council of Princeton University, which achieved a significant role in raising funds and managing that school.

17. In April of 1896, the physician-in-chief of Woman's Hospital, Anna Fuller-

ton, who looked after much of the educational program for medical students, resigned amidst a storm of internal discord. (Minutes of the Board of Managers of Woman's Hospital of Philadelphia, 27 April 1896.)

18. For the deterioration of relations between WMC and the Woman's Hospital of Philadelphia, and efforts by the College to compensate, see Morantz-Sanchez, *Sympathy and Science*, pp. 257–259; Gulielma FellAlsop, *History of the Woman's Medical College, Philadelphia, Pennsylvania* (Philadelphia: Lippincott, 1950), pp. 159–161. Primary materials in the minutes and correspondence of the institutions are numerous, including MF, 18 April 1896, 13 October 1898, 21 January 1899; George Hay Materials, folders 13 and 14 (correspondence and reports relating to the dispute).

19. Note of Croasdale's resignation appears in the MF, 21 March 1902 and Broomall's, 26 May 1902. At learning of Broomall's resignation, the Student Association dispatched a petition to the board and the faculty urging that she not be lost to the institution (Student Association Minutes, 23 May 1902, in Students Collection). An inquiry by C. N. Peirce found that "the want of much needed rest seemed to be the main cause of retiring at this time" and that Broomall "still has the deepest interest" in the College. Broomall did stay on for another year while a replacement was sought (MECBC, 29 May 1902; MF, 17 September 1902). There is, however, a suggestion surrounding these events of some discord between Broomall and the College. Ella Everitt proved a popular teacher but died young in an automobile accident.

20. E. F. Halloway to C. N. Peirce, 13 May 1903, pasted in MBC following p. 186 of volume 1899–1907. Rodman (1858–1916) was professor of surgery from 1901 until 1909. A well-known figure both as a surgeon and authority on breast cancer, he was instrumental in founding the National Board of Medical Examiners.

21. In an extraordinary letter the president and secretary of the board of the College proposed a complete reconciliation through merger. They offered to allow the hospital to name to the board of the proposed new merged institution "two thirds of the members thereof from its Board of Managers and at the same time select the remaining third from the Corporators of the College." (Mary Mumford and C. N. Peirce to Board of Managers of Woman's Hospital of Philadelphia, 18 May 1903, pasted in MECBC following p. 8 of volume for 1903–1907.) The hospital declined the merger, leaving the College in need of its own clinical facility.

22. E. F. Halloway to Board of Corporators of WMC, 1 April 1903, pasted in MBC, after p. 176 of volume 1899–1907.

23. Ibid.

24. Rosenberg, *Care of Strangers*, pp. 147–150, 246–248.

25. Catharine Macfarlane, Typescript Autobiography, p. 52, in Macfarlane Papers at ASCWM and another copy at the Library of the College of Physicians of Philadelphia.

26. J[ohn] P[rice] Crozer Griffith to Henry S. Cattell, 9 December 1901, in George Hay Materials, box 1, folder 14. Griffith was a prominent Philadelphia physician who tried to mediate the dispute.

27. Years later, some reconciliation occurred and WMC students once again spent valuable time at the Woman's Hospital, especially in outpatient work and pediatrics.

28. The report, undated and without a title, is found in the George Hay Materials, box 1, folder 13.

29. Dean William Pepper of Penn's medical school expressed a belief that the school should become coeducational "provided a way seems open to our obtaining some distinct financial or material benefit therefrom"; see George Corner, *Two Centuries of Medicine: A History of the School of Medicine of the University of Pennsylvania* (Philadelphia: Lippincott, 1965), pp. 248–249.

30. That this was so is amply documented as late as 1938 in a series of responses of senior students to a survey conducted by then professor of gynecology Catharine Macfarlane, found in her Deceased Alumna Folder and discussed in a later chapter.

31. Pleas for a hospital occur in the MF, 20 February 1892, 18 April 1896, 12 June 1897, 16 October 1897, 15 October 1898, 5 April 1899, 27 October 1900, 19 December 1902, and 8 July 1903.

32. Pasted into the MBC volume for 1899–1907 after page 200 is the "Decree by Court of Common Pleas Number 1 for the City and County of Philadelphia," declaring the corporate merger of the College and the Hospital and Dispensary of the Alumnae.

33. Letter from Holstein DeHaven Bright to Samuel M. Vauclain, 8 September 1904, in MBC, volume for 1899–1904, after page 210. The expenditures at this point were $6,946.74. The total costs were $9,759 as noted in the First Report of the Hospital of the Woman's Medical College of Pennsylvania (Philadelphia, 1905), p. 10. Vauclain during this period was among the most devoted and hard-working members of the board. He was supervisor (and later president) of Philadelphia's mighty Baldwin Locomotive Works.

34. *First Report of the Hospital of the Woman's Medical College of Pennsylvania* (Philadelphia, 1905), pp. 14–16.

35. Pennsylvania was one of few states that supported general hospitals. Philadelphia's other medical schools had been successfully and repeatedly to the trough for amounts totalling in the hundreds of thousands of dollars; see Rosemary Stevens, "Sweet Charity: State Aid to Hospitals in Pennsylvania, 1870–1910," *Bulletin of the History of Medicine* 58 (1984): 287–214, 474–495; see table of appropriations to 1898 and to 1910 on p. 300.

36. Documented in the detailed financial reports in each *Annual Report* of the hospital. The state grant is noted in MECBC, 15 May 1905, the Carnegie grant in the *Bulletin of the Woman's Medical College of Pennsylvania* 65 (December 1914): 23–25.

37. Entrance requirements were, of course, listed in each *Annual Announcement*. The added expectation for inorganic chemistry began in 1911. A joint faculty-board committee had reviewed the whole subject of admission standards in early 1910 (MF, 18 February 1910).

38. N. P. Colwell to Dr. Annie W. Bosworth, 14 February 1913, in Marshall Papers. Bosworth was Dean Marshall's assistant.

39. *Transactions of the Thirty-sixth Annual Meeting of the Alumnae Association of the Woman's Medical College of Pennsylvania* (Philadelphia, 1911), pp. 34–43. In 1913, under the impetus of Catharine Macfarlane, the association formed a "Graduate Council" which undertook to both raise funds and aid the College in other ways (*Transactions of the Thirty-eighth Annual Meeting of the Alumnae Association of the Woman's Medical College of Pennsylvania* (Philadelphia, 1913), pp. 125–136.

40. E.g., in *Transactions of the Thirty-eighth Annual Meeting of the Alumnae Association of the Woman's Medical College of Pennsylvania*, p. 136.

41. *An Appeal for Increased Endowment of the Woman's Medical College of Pennsyl-*

vania. Issued by the Alumnae [1911], in collection referred to as "Finances and Published Materials 1904–1975," accession 75.

42. Gertrude Walker, "Report of the Publicity Committee," *Transactions of the Thirty-ninth Annual Meeting of the Alumnae Association of the Woman's Medical College of Pennsylvania* (Philadelphia, 1914), pp. 40–41. The following year, the College engaged the American Publicity Bureau, to which it paid $125 a month, no small amount.

43. See Gertrude Walker, "Report of the Representative of the Publicity Committee," *Transactions of the Fortieth Annual Meeting of the Alumnae Association of the Woman's Medical College of Pennsylvania* (Philadelphia, 1915), pp. 50–51. The College Clippings Collections contain numerous newspaper articles about the motion pictures, e.g., "Fair Crowds to View Local College in Film," *Philadelphia Record*, 11 April 1915 (leaf 375). Lamentably, the film does not survive.

44. Mimeographed letter, Gertrude Walker to "DEAR FELLOW ALUMNA," 1 November 1914, in Macfarlane Scrapbook.

45. The Alumnae Association president in 1917, Frances Van Gasken, reported that by 1916 the alumnae "with the aid of friends" had added over $150,000 to endowment; see *Transactions of the Forty-second Annual Meeting of the Alumnae Association of the Woman's Medical College of Pennsylvania* (Philadelphia, 1917), p. 50.

46. Enrollment figures are from the *Annual Announcements*.

47. "Cash Statement of General Expenses and Income 6/1/17 to 2/1/18," in MECBC volume for 1912–1919, pasted after p. 152; and "Income Account June 1, 1917 to May 31, 1918," ibid., p. 175. Berta Benson and Ellen C. Potter to Hilda Justice, 28 December 1918, in MECBC volume for 1912–1919, pasted on page 183. Soon after, alumna and faculty member Frances Van Gasken turned over a check from the Campaign Committee for four thousand dollars, which was used to pay bills.

48. Edgar Fah Smith to James M. Baldy, 28 June 1916, Marshall Papers. Baldy, head of Pennsylvania's Bureau of Medical Education and Licensure, was sympathetic to WMC so sent the letter to Marshall.

49. MBC, 14 June 1920, 10 May 1921, 13 June 1921, 7 October 1921, 8 November 1921.

50. Mary Mumford was a woman of wide accomplishment: early in life she had been a writer and editor, later a founder of Philadelphia's Civic Club and staunch battler for suffrage, good government, and municipal betterment. Women on the board of corporators, pressing for more status, with the aid of some male allies managed to elect Mumford as the first female president of the board in 1893. The affair was genteel and polite. See MBC, 6 March 1893; for Mary Mumford, see her entry in Edward T. James et al., eds., *Notable American Women*, vol. 2 (Cambridge, Mass.: Harvard University Press, 1971), 598–599. Mrs. Starr became the third woman president and the first to actually manage the College as an executive.

51. MBC, 10 June 1921.

52. *Transactions of the Forty-sixth Annual Meeting of the Alumnae Association of the Woman's Medical College of Pennsylvania* (Philadelphia, 1921), pp. 28–33. A recently discovered "Emergency Loan Fund" ledger for the 1921 campaign is now at ASCWM. Within are various receipts and notes signed by Mrs. Starr.

53. *Bulletin of the Woman's Medical College of Pennsylvania* 71 (March 1921): 2.

54. Sources for the fiscal crisis and reorganization include MBC, 13 June 1921, 17

June 1921, 19 September 1921, 7 October 1921, 25 October 1921, 8 November 1921; also Sarah Logan Wister Starr, "To the Alumnae of the Woman's Medical College of Pennsylvania" in the June 1932 "Special Bulletin" (*Bulletin of the Woman's Medical College of Pennsylvania* 73 [June 1923]: 1–3). The phrase "centralized, executive control" appears here.

55. Starr, "To the Alumnae," p. 2.

56. To some extent, the notions of centralized management derive from the famous work of Frederick W. Taylor, who was, coincidentally, like Sarah Logan Wister Starr a resident of the Germantown section of Philadelphia. His book *The Principles of Scientific Management* appeared in 1911.

57. Lathrop served on the faculty from 1892 to 1923, first in subsidiary posts then as professor of physiology from 1904; she had been White's assistant. Peckham was professor of bacteriology from 1899—when she replaced the eloped Lydia Rabinowitsch—until she retired in 1919.

58. MF, 20 April 1917.

59. MF, 2 March 1917.

60. MF, 30 March 1917.

61. Van Gasken is much noted in student publications from 1911 through 1915, and in one extant yearbook from that period, the 1911 *Iatrian*. She apparently was nicknamed "Dr. Can Askem" for her capacity to generate questions on rounds or at a quiz class.

62. For curriculum in this period, see, e.g., *Sixty-sixth Annual Announcement of the Woman's Medical College of Pennsylvania and its Hospital for session of 1915–1916* (Philadelphia, 1915), pp. 26–43. Quote on frogs is from *The Scalpel*, 1911, p. 79. This was the first WMC yearbook.

63. MF, 19 March 1915.

64. *Sixty-sixth Annual Announcement*, p. 36.

65. *The Scalpel*, 1911, p. 84.

66. Ibid., p. 118.

67. Robert H. Wiebe, *The Search for Order, 1877–1920* (New York: Hill and Wang, 1967), p. 169. This is one of the most enduring brief histories of the Progressive Era.

68. MF, 21 October 1904. Material concerning the life of Eleanor Jones may be found in her Deceased Alumna Folder and in an obituary in *Transactions of the Fiftieth Annual Meeting of the Alumnae Association of the Woman's Medical College of Pennsylvania* (Philadelphia, 1925), pp. 19–21. Her interest in "baby saving" is revealed in a report to the Alumnae Association, "Baby Saving Campaign of 1918," *Transactions of the Forty-third Annual Meeting of the Alumnae Association of the Woman's Medical College of Pennsylvania* (Philadelphia, 1918), pp. 43–47. Professor of obstetrics Alice Weld Tallant was also devoted to reducing infant mortality.

69. MF, 20 March 1918, 17 April 1918.

70. Margaret P. Saunders to Martha Tracy, 11 May 1918, copied in MF, 22 May 1918.

71. MF, 19 March 1919.

72. Ibid.

73. Morantz-Sanchez, *Sympathy and Science*, pp. 282–283.

74. *Sixty-fourth Annual Announcement of the Woman's Medical College of Pennsylvania, Session of 1913–1914*, p. 26. For a detailed history of the development of preventive medicine at WMC and Medical College of Pennsylvania, see Bonnie Ellen Blustein, *Educating for Health and Prevention: A History of the De-*

partment of Community and Preventive Medicine of the (Woman's) Medical College of Pennsylvania (Canton, Mass.: Science History Publications, 1993).

75. This course was planned by professor of obstetrics Alice Weld Tallant and professor of physiology Ruth Webster Lathrop (MF, 17 March 1916) and is described in the *Sixty-seventh Annual Announcement of the Woman's Medical College of Pennsylvania for the Session 1916–1917* (Philadelphia, 1916), p. 46.

76. Blustein, *Educating for Health*, pp. 21–22.

77. *Eighty-third Annual Announcement of the Woman's Medical College of Pennsylvania, Session of 1932–1933* (Philadelphia, 1932), p. 42. A brochure aimed at the Philadelphia medical profession announcing the availability of the screening examinations is found in the Vertical File, folder "W/MCP: Anna Howard Shaw Health Clinic."

78. Several graduates of the 1940s in conversations with the author distinctly recalled these field trips.

79. Blustein, *Educating for Health*, pp. 27–41; author's interview with Doris Willig, 9 September 1997, Philadelphia. Sarah Morris counts as another of the lesser-known heroines of WMC, particularly for her supportive attitude toward medical students and her persistence in trying to understand and reduce the tuberculosis problem among them.

80. Blustein, *Educating for Health*, pp. 33–37.

81. Much information on student life from 1910 to 1914 is available in issues of the student magazine published during these years. It was first called the *Esculapian*, then the name was changed to *Iatrian* in October 1911.

82. It was called *The Scalpel*, though subsequent WMC yearbooks have carried the title *Iatrian*.

83. *Iatrian*, January 1912, pp. 4–5.

84. Rita S. Finkler, "Good Morning Doctor," typescript autobiography, 1964(?), p. 69.

85. *Esculapian*, December, 1910, p. 11.

86. *Scalpel*, 1911; *Iatrian*, 1914.

87. "F.P.M" (Frances Petty Manship), "Our Evening In," *Iatrian*, June 1912, pp. 7–8. The indications for the "C-Section" were central placenta praevia, with two days of persistent bleeding, and unfavorable pelvic measurements.

88. It has proved difficult to learn much about Frances Petty Manship. News clippings show that she was resident physician at the Barton Dispensary in the early 1920s. She appeared in the newspapers in January of 1920 protesting the lack of adequate refuse collection and deplorable inattention of city services in the poor district.

89. The quoted phrase is from Russell F. Weigley, ed., *Philadelphia: A 300–Year History* (New York: Norton, 1982), p. 527.

90. Elizabeth Clark to Ada Peirce McCormick, 3 January 1909, in Ada Peirce McCormick papers.

91. Irene Gates, *Any Hope Doctor?* (London: Blandford Press, 1954), p. 50.

92. This and the following quotes are from Frances Petty Manship, "Ten Cases," *Iatrian*, June 1912, pp. 1–4. For a contemporary published description of the outdoor maternity work, see Mary W. Griscom, "Report of the Maternity Hospital of the Woman's Medical College of Pennsylvania from January, 1888, to May, 1903," *American Medicine* 7 (1904): 7–9.

93. The bags contained "the usual obstetric armamentarium, excepting forceps and ether," which the students were not expected to apply on their own (Griscom, "Report").

94. The two adjuncts referred to were the outpatient maternity and the nearby Barton Dispensary, the continuation of the Alumnae Dispensary, renamed for its founder.
95. *Scalpel*, 1911, pp. 118–119.
96. Interview with Lillian Seitsiv, Class of 1931, 23 May 1997, Philadelphia; group interview with members of the Class of 1947, 24 May 1997, Philadelphia. By the 1930s, the students went to poor districts closer to the College, not south Philadelphia. The home delivery program seems to have ended around 1948.
97. A newspaper article from 1911 noted that "as these foreigners are accustomed to employ midwives, and prefer the care of women, this quarter of the city offers a particularly wide scope for the work of the hospital [but refers to outpatient maternity practice], which has been from the first carried on exclusively by women." *Philadelphia Public Ledger*, 18 February 1911, clipping pasted in front of MECBC, v. 5, 1907–1911. Chief of the service Alice Weld Tallant referred to one woman who came to the College maternity for all of her twenty-one pregnancies ("Annual Report of the Maternity Department," in *Annual Report of the Hospital of the Woman's Medical College of Pennsylvania* (Phiadephia, 1911). She also asserted that the mothers referred affectionately to the "little lady doctors."
98. Manship, "Ten Cases," p. 3.
99. *The Scalpel*, 1911, p. 119.

Chapter 8 **The Troubled 1920s and the Tallant Affair**

1. See Regina Morantz-Sanchez, *Sympathy and Science: Women Physicians in American Medicine* (New York and Oxford: Oxford University Press, 1985), pp. 312–328.
2. "To the Alumnae of the Woman's Medical College of Pennsylvania," *Bulletin of the Woman's Medical College of Pennsylvania* 73 (June 1923, "Special Bulletin"): 1–12, p. 4.
3. From *Documentary Evidence in the Present Crisis of the Woman's Medical College of Pennsylvania*, undated pamphlet indicating no author or editor, but obviously published by a group of alumnae of WMC, 1923, p. 11, in Walter Sheppard Papers, folder 185.
4. *Documentary Evidence*, p. 3.
5. Information about Mrs. Starr's personality is based on a telephone interview with her grandson, Daniel Blain, on 26 June 1997, and on a collection of newspaper clippings filed under her name in the Clippings Collections of the *Philadelphia Bulletin*, at the Urban Archives, Library of Temple University, Philadelphia.
6. "Special Report of the Executive Committee," in MF, 13 April 1923.
7. Ibid.
8. MF, 9 March 1923.
9. "Documentary Evidence," pp. 6–7.
10. Van Gasken to Noble, 6 May 1923, Sheppard Papers, folder 189.
11. MF, 12 April 1923. The junior class sent a similar letter. That students did attempt to transfer is documented in a letter from William Pepper, dean of the University of Pennsylvania School of Medicine, who complained to Martha Tracy about "all these visits and these applications from your students." (Letter from juniors in MF, 12 April 1923; letter from William Pepper to Martha

Tracy, 14 May 1923, in Sheppard Papers folder 192.) Most students stayed at WMC, but the next entering class showed a small enrollment.

12. They did not sever forever all ties to the College. For example, Clara Marshall, Henry Leffmann, and Marie Formad sat with the "reunioning" class of 1896 at the Alumnae dinner of 1926, where Leffmann entertained with "anecdotes of the old days." (*Transactions of the Fifty-first Meeting of the Alumnae Association of the Woman's Medical College of Pennsylvania* [Philadelphia, 1926], p. 32.)

13. For Macfarlane's indifference to Tallant, see her Typescript Autobiography, p. 65, in Macfarlane Papers at ASCWM and another copy at the Library of the College of Physicians of Philadelphia.

14. For biographical information on Alice Weld Tallant, see obituary in *Philadelphia Inquirer*, 3 June 1958, article "Woman Physician Reminisces about World War I Exploits," *Germantown Courier*, 4 July 1957, and information sheet kindly supplied by the Sophia Smith Collection, Smith College.

15. She became a member of the Executive Committee and Board of Directors of the American Association for the Study and Prevention of Infant Mortality (AASPIM), and chair of its Section on Prenatal and Maternal Care. See Jeffrey P. Brosco, "Sin of Folly: Child and Community Health in Philadelphia, 1900–1930" (Ph.D dissertation, University of Pennsylvania, 1994), p. 141; Phillip Van Ingen, *The Story of the American Child Health Association* (New York: American Child Health Association, 1936).

16. Alice Weld Tallant, *Textbook of Obstetrical Nursing* (Philadelphia: Lea and Febiger, 1922).

17. "To the Alumnae," pp. 8–9.

18. Typed copies of unsigned, undated notes; typed undated notes signed by Mary Spears; typed letter from Anne Thomas dated 4 April 1923, in Sheppard Papers, folder 182.

19. See Grant R. Grissom, "Philadelphia House of Refuge (Glen Mills School for Boys, Sleighton Farm School)," in Jean Barth Toll and Mildred S. Gillam, eds., *Invisible Philadelphia: Community Through Voluntary Organizations* (Philadelphia: Atwater Kent Museum, 1995), pp. 642–645. The school still exists as this is written. The House of Refuge was an outgrowth of the Philadelphia Society for Alleviating the Miseries of Public Prisons, which long before had employed the College's first president, William J. Mullen.

20. Information on Stewart-Cogill is from obituaries in her Deceased Alumna Folder, e.g., "Dr. Lida S. Cogill Dies at Age of 74," *Philadelphia Evening Bulletin*, 19 April 1943.

21. See author's entry on Maude Abbott in Martin Kaufman, Stuart Galishoff, and Todd L. Savitt, eds., *Dictionary of American Medical Biography* (Westport, Conn.: Greenwood Press, 1984), I:3–4.

22. Quoted in H. E. MacDermot, *Maude Abbott: A Memoir* (Toronto: Macmillan, 1941), p. 166.

23. Maude Abbott was an "Oslerian," a student and admirer of the great Canadian-American clinician, pathologist, bedside teacher, historian, and essayist William Osler. In 1939 Abbott published a definitive *Classified and Annotated Bibliography of Sir William Osler's Publications*. While at WMC, she gave several talks to alumnae and students about Osler.

24. "Report of the Executive Committee May 9, 1923," in Sheppard Papers, folder 195.

25. Vida Hunt Francis was another remarkable woman. A Smith College graduate, she did social work in Philadelphia then later served as co-principal of

the Hillside School in Norwalk, Connecticut. She was active in the child labor campaigns and in Philadelphia circles promoting good government. She
was also a photographer and illustrator (information from several clippings in
her packet at the *Philadelphia Bulletin* clippings collection, Urban Archives, Library of Temple University, Philadelphia).

26. Interview with Marion Fay conducted by Regina Morantz-Sanchez, 11 July
1977, Oral History Project on Women in Medicine, p. 7.

27. Jennifer Georgia, *Legacy and Challenge: The Story of Dr. Ida B. Scudder* (Sa-
line, MI: McNaughton & Gunn, 1994), p. 26.

28. The statement about Dr. Macfarlane is based mainly on conversations with
persons who knew her, including alumnae of the 1930s, 1940s, and 1950s.

29. Rose Hirschler, "Report of the Senior Alumnae Representative on the Board
of Corporators," *Transactions of the Fifty-First Annual Meeting of the Alumnae
Association of the Woman's Medical College of Pennsylvania* (Philadelphia, 1926),
p. 38. Hirschler's report was assembled with the help of the Board's secretary,
Vida Hunt Francis.

30. "Twenty-one Reasons for Giving the Woman's Medical College of Pennsylvania Your Support," in collection titled Finances and Miscellaneous Published
Material, folder 5.

31. For the Great Migration and Philadelphia, see Lloyd M. Abernethy, "Progressivism: 1905–1919," in Russell F. Weigley, ed., *Philadelphia: A 300-Year History* (New York: Norton, 1982), pp. 530–532.

32. "The Greater Woman's Medical College Finds a Site," *Bulletin of the Woman's
Medical College of Pennsylvania* 76 (June 1926): 3–4.

33. Various brochures, invitations, and letters related to the campaign for the
Greater Woman's Medical College can be found in an unlabeled scrapbook,
accession number 123.

34. Buildings by Ritter and Shay in Philadelphia include the striking One East
Penn Square Building, with Mayan inspired Art Deco ornament, the magiste-
rial Drake Hotel, and the subdued Art Deco Custom House.

35. *Transactions of the Fifty-second Annual Meeting of the Alumnae Association of the
Woman's Medical College of Pennsylvania* (Philadelphia, 1927), p. 41.

36. *Transactions of the Fifty-sixth Annual Meeting of the Alumnae Association of the
Woman's Medical College of Pennsylvania* (Philadelphia, 1931), p. 24.

37. The Kelly family of East Falls, of whom Grace Kelly was of course the most
celebrated, would become loyal friends of the College beginning in the 1940s.

38. In 1930, virtually all municipal planning and expenditure in Philadelphia for
improvement of services, the business environment, and transportation looked
to the downtown, not the neighborhoods. See Sam Bass Warner Jr., *The Private City: Philadelphia in Three Periods of Its Growth*, 2d ed. (Philadelphia: University of Pennsylvania Press, 1987), esp. pp. 205–208.

39. Figures are from the annual announcements of the College and Martha Tracy's
annual reports to the alumnae published in their Association's annual *Transactions*. A significant error that slipped into the works of Regina Morantz-
Sanchez and Mary Roth Walsh states that during the period when it was the
only remaining women's medical school WMC graduated "between 120 and
200 women each year." These figures actually indicate the *maximum total enrollment* for all four classes during this period, not the number graduating. WMC
never graduated 120 women in any year. The number for the period 1920
through 1970 ranged generally from the twenties to the sixties.

40. For women's higher education in the 1920s, see Barbara Miller Solomon, *In the Company of Educated Women: A History of Women and Higher Education in America* (New Haven, Conn.: Yale University Press, 1985), esp. pp. 141–167. For attitudes and choices of American women in the 1920s, see Sarah Evans, *Born for Liberty: A History of Women in America* (New York: Free Press, 1989), pp. 175–196, and Peter G. Filene, *Him/Her/Self: Sex Roles in Modern America,* 2d ed. (Baltimore: Johns Hopkins University Press, 1986), pp. 120–126.

41. "Future Doctors—Girls from Four Countries who are First-year Students at the Woman's Medical College Here," *Philadelphia Record,* 4 October 1927, in College Clippings Collection leaf 882y.

42. Mark P. Solomon and Mark S. Granick, "Alma Dea Morani, MD: A Pioneer in Plastic Surgery," *Annals of Plastic Surgery* 38 (1997): 431–436. See also excerpts from her oral history in Regina Markell Morantz, Cynthia Stodola Pomerleau, and Carol Hansen Fenichel, *In Her Own Words: Oral Histories of Women Physicians* (Westport, Conn.: Greenwood Press, 1982), pp. 73–98.

43. See Solomon, *In the Company,* p. 143.

44. MF, 11 March 1927.

45. For Sarah Cohen-May, see Ruth Abram, ed., *"Send Us a Lady Physician": Women Doctors in America, 1835–1920* (New York: Norton, 1985), pp.,134, 157–158, 185–188. For Rebecca Fleisher, see materials in her Deceased Alumna Folder, including a compilation of her activity at Alumnae Association meetings by former ASCWM archivist Terry Taylor. For Cornelia Kahn, see Fanny B. Hoffman, *Dr. Cornelia Kahn: A Memoir* (privately printed pamphlet, 1931), in Kahn's Deceased Alumna Folder); also, other materials in the folder, including a letter from Fanny B. Hoffman (Kahn's sister, who cared for Cornelia before her death) to The Dean of the Woman's Medical College, 22 May 1946, and clippings about Ramabai maintained by Dr. Kahn and later sent to the WMC collections with other mementos by her sister.

46. "The Woman's Medical College of Pennsylvania. Negro Graduates 1867–1962," dated 26 June 1962; and Registrar to Dr. Sara W. Brown, 21 May 1923, reporting number of "colored students" enrolled and graduating in that year, both in Black Medical Women's Collection, Box 1.

47. See Vanessa Northington Gamble, "Taking a History: The Life of Dr. Virginia Alexander. The Fielding H. Garrison Lecture of the American Association for the History of Medicine," Toronto, Canada, May 1998; copy kindly provided to the author by Dr. Gamble. See also biographical materials and correspondence in Alexander's Deceased Alumnae File. Despite the racism she encountered, including refusal of an internship in the College's hospital, Alexander later joined the Alumnae Association and even helped Dean Marion Fay defend the College's record in training African-American women in 1948; see MF, 21 April 1948.

48. MF, 7 January 1938.

49. From *Eighty-seventh Annual Announcement of the Woman's Medical College of Pennsylvania, Session of 1936–1937* (Philadelphia, 1936), pp. 72–73.

50. Mabel Emery to Martha Tracy, 5 March 1938, in Emery's Deceased Alumna Folder.

51. The school's new location in East Falls is virtually on the edge of the Wissahickon Creek Valley portion of Philadelphia's Fairmount Park.

52. Mollie Geiss (1886–1966) was an M.D. graduate of the University of Texas Medical Branch at Galveston. She joined the WMC faculty in 1923; she taught

first pharmacology, then pathology, and finally in the radiology department in the 1950s! A folder of biographical material is found under her name in the "Vertical Files" of the ASCWM.

53. Mary Bruins Allison, *Doctor Mary in Arabia: Memoirs by Mary Bruins Allison*, edited by Sandra Shaw (Austin: University of Texas Press, 1994), pp. 13–17.

54. MBC, 18 March 1931.

Chapter 9 **As One Hundred Years Approached**

1. For Philadelphia in the Depression, see Margaret B. Tinkcom, "Depression and War: 1929–1946," in Russell F. Weigley, ed., *Philadelphia: A 300–Year History* (New York: Norton, 1982), pp. 601–613.

2. By the mid-1930s, for which data has been located, income from endowment was about $25,000, from student fees $44,000, and from the Commonwealth of Pennsylvania grants, between $40,000 and $50,000. Gifts and other sources added variable amounts. Interest on mortgages was between $17,000 and $18,000. Total income for 1936–1937 was $127,269, and expenditures $127,335. From "Woman's Medical College. Annual Receipts and Disbursements for the Year Ending May 31, 1937 and Estimate of Receipts and Expenditures for the Year Ending May 31, 1938," in Student Affairs Papers, box 1, AMA Survey 1935, folder 3.

3. For the failed initiative with the Federated Women's Clubs, see William M. David to Fred C. Zapffe, 22 December 1937, in Student Affairs Papers, box 1, AMA Survey 1935, folder 3. David was treasurer of the College, Zapffe secretary of the Association of American Medical Colleges.

4. *Transactions of the Fifty-seventh Annual Meeting of the Alumnae Association of the Woman's Medical College of Pennsylvania* (Philadelphia, 1932), p. 22.

5. Ibid., p. 21.

6. Author's interview with Lillian Seitsiv, 23 May 1997.

7. Interview with Alma Dea Morani, Conducted by Regina Morantz-Sanchez, 19 and 21 January 1977, p. 27, in Oral History Project on Women in Medicine.

8. Author's interview with Angie Connor, 23 May 1997.

9. Morani Interview, p. 32.

10. *Transactions of the Fifty-eighth Annual Meeting of the Alumnae Association of the Woman's Medical College of Pennsylvania* (Philadelphia, 1933), pp. 29–34.

11. Ibid., p. 34. See also MBC, 21 June 1933 reporting the cut in hospital appropriations from the Welfare Federation, and the failure of the Philadelphia Company for Guaranteeing Mortgages. Mrs. Starr reported that there would be further cuts in faculty salaries.

12. *Transactions of the Fifty-eighth Annual Meeting of the Alumnae Association of the Woman's Medical College of Pennsylvania*, p. 35.

13. Martha Tracy, "Medical Education in the United States," document prepared for board of corporators, written in 1934 but dated for board of corporators meeting of 16 January 1935, Tracy Papers, folder 42.

14. Rosemary Stevens, *American Medicine and the Public Interest* (New Haven, Conn.: Yale University Press, 1971), pp. 176–178.

15. The historical literature dealing with the AMA is considerable. It is discussed throughout Stevens's *American Medicine and the Public Interest* and Paul Starr's *The Social Transformation of American Medicine* (New York: Basic Books, 1982). Starr discusses the AMA during the Great Depression on pp. 270–279.

16. Weiskotten was professor of pathology and dean at the University of Syracuse Medical School. Ireland was former United States Surgeon-General.
17. Tracy to Sheppard, 21 January 1935, Sheppard Papers, box 8, folder 113; William Cutter to Sheppard, 20 February 1935, Sheppard Papers, box 8, folder 112.
18. "Woman's Medical College of Pennsylvania. Philadelphia, Pennsylvania. Inspected by Dr. H. G. Weiskotten [and] Dr. M. W. Ireland. January 14, 15, 16, 1935," typescript report, in Liaison Commission on Medical Education, Survey Reports, box J in IM box 238, Archives of the Association of American Medical Colleges, Washington, D.C. [hereafter Weiskotten and Ireland], p. 5. Other sources used for this discussion of the 1935 inspection are: Tracy to Sheppard, 21 January 1935, Sheppard Papers, box 8, folder 113; Tracy to Sheppard, 19 February 1935, Sheppard Papers, box 8, folder 112.
19. Weiskotten and Ireland, p. 80.
20. Tracy to Wilbur, 1 March 1935, in Sheppard Papers, box 8, folder 112. Wilbur was a prominent physician-educator, former president of the AMA, former Secretary of the Interior under Herbert Hoover, and president of Stanford University.
21. During the crisis Walter L. Sheppard wrote to Mrs. Starr that "I never realized what a tremendous asset Dr. Rodman was to the institution until I became involved in these negotiations." Indeed both Rodman and his wife, who became a member of the board, served the school with uncommon devotion. Sheppard found himself also "profoundly impressed with the depth of regard and respect in which Dr. Tracy is held by the leading members of the medical profession engaged in educational work." (Sheppard to Starr, 27 March 1935, Sheppard Papers, box 8, folder 112.)
22. Walter L. Bierring to J. S. Rodman, 5 March 1935, in Sheppard Papers, box 8, folder 112.
23. Quoted in Sheppard to Starr, 7 March 1935, in Sheppard Papers, box 8, folder 112.
24. Ibid.
25. Ibid.
26. Sheppard to Starr, 27 March 1935.
27. Ibid.
28. Starr to Sheppard, 18 March 1935, Sheppard Papers, box 8, folder 112.
29. Starr to Sheppard, 30 March 1935, Sheppard Papers, box 8, folder 112.
30. See, e.g., William A. R. Chapin, ed., *History: University of Vermont College of Medicine* (Springfield, Mass.: 1951), pp. 55–59; and Edward J. Van Liere and Gideon S. Dodds, *History of Medical Education in West Virginia* (Morgantown: West Virginia University Library, 1965), pp. 42–49.
31. See Janet Tighe, "Never Knowing One's Place: Temple University School of Medicine and the Medical Education Hierarchy," *Transactions and Studies of the College of Physicians of Philadelphia*, ser. 5, 12 (1990): 311–334.
32. Sarah Evans, *Born for Liberty: A History of Women in America* (New York: Free Press, 1989), pp.197–98.
33. Margaret W. Rossiter, *Women Scientists in America: Struggles and Strategies to 1940* (Baltimore: Johns Hopkins University Press, 1982), p. xvii.
34. Cutter to Tracy, 19 March 1935, Sheppard Papers, box 8, folder 112.
35. The author has read a large body of correspondence between Cutter and WMC officials during 1935 to 1937, not all of which will be cited specifically. It is of

interest that his tone became less truculent in later letters and at times he even portrayed himself as an ally in the rebirth of the College! Perhaps he was influenced by further acquaintance with such solid representatives of the College as Tracy, Sheppard, Rodman, Jump, Francis, and Macfarlane.

36. Weiskotten and Ireland, p. 81.
37. Bickings-Thornton was a WMC graduate of 1904 and served on the College faculty from 1905 until 1935, when she became emerita. She died in 1956 at age seventy-six; "Dr. Mary Bickings-Thornton Dies; Physician 52 Years," *Philadelphia Evening Bulletin*, 8 September 1956.
38. John Henry Wyckoff and Willard C. Rappleye, "Report of Inspection of Woman's Medical College of Pennsylvania [April, 1935]," in Liaison Commission for Medical Education Survey Reports, Archives of the Association of American Medical Colleges, box 5 in IM box 238, Washington, D.C.
39. Martha Tracy, "Memorandum on Status of Graduates of the Woman's Medical College of Pennsylvania Before the National Board of Medical Examiners," in Student Affairs Collection, AMA Survey 1935, folder 2.
40. "Mrs. Starr's Remarks at Faculty Meeting May 10, 1935," typescript in Student Affairs Papers, box 1, American Medical Association Survey, folder 1.
41. MBC, 19 June 1935.
42. Ross V. Patterson, dean of Jefferson Medical College, to Tracy, 24 June 1935, in Student Affairs Collection, box 1, Survey of College, AAMC January 1935 folder.
43. Greisheimer's curriculum vitae as of 1938 is part of a "Report on the Woman's Medical College of Pennsylvania 1936–38" (hereafter "Report 1936–38") sent to Fred C. Zapffe, secretary of the Association of American Medical Colleges, dated 22 December 1937, in Student Affairs Papers, American Medical Association Survey, folder 1. For women in physiology in this period, see Toby A. Appel, "Physiology in American Women's Colleges: the Rise and Decline of a Female Subculture," *Isis* 85 (1994): 26–56.
44. A brief biographical note by a friend and student is Joachim Gerlach, "Hartwig Kuhlenbeck, 1897–1984," *Applied Neurophysiology* 48 (1985): vii–xi. A large collection of Kuhlenbeck papers, memorabilia, books, etc. is at ASCWM. Useful biographical information was found in several folders within this only partly processed collection, and in a Kuhlenbeck folder in Dean's Office Papers (accession 183, box 4). Selected biographical items have been placed in a folder in the Vertical Files. Kuhlenbeck's concern for students was described in conversations with alumnae Rachel Pape, Doris Bartuska, and Phyllis Marciano. Kuhlenbeck's last published book was *The Human Brain and Its Universe*, ed. by Joachim Gerlach (Basel and New York: Karger, 1982).
45. For information on the backgrounds of Greisheimer, Fay, Kuhlenbeck and Harned at the time of their appointments, see "Statement of Professional Personnel in the Pre-Clinical Departments of the Woman's Medical College of Pennsylvania as Re-organized 1935–1936," in Student Affairs Papers, box 1, folder "Survey of College, A.A.M.C. 1935."
46. For grants to the basic science faculty, see "Report, December, 1937," in Student Affairs Papers, box 1, AMA Survey 1935, folder 3. Martha Tracy also reported each grant at faculty meetings during the late 1930s.
47. Peckham to Maude Abbott, no date but from other evidence almost surely 1911, Maude Abbott Papers.
48. See "Report 1936–38"; Tracy to Starr, 14 December 1938, George Hay Materials, box 2.

49. Bott became chair of physiological chemistry in 1947 when Marion Fay was dean. For more on Bott's renal research, see Carl Gottschalk, "The Application of Micropuncture Techniques to Analysis of Renal Function: A Personal View," *American Journal of Kidney Disease* 16 (1990): 536–540.

50. The grant is recorded in MF, 18 March 1938. A ten-year report is Catharine Macfarlane, Margaret C. Sturgis, and Faith Fetterman, "Control of Cancer of the Uterus: Report of a Ten-Year Experiment," *JAMA* 138 (1948): 941–942.

51. "Notes from the Woman's Medical College of Pennsylvania [includes an obituary of Linda Bartels Lange]," *Medical Woman's Journal* 54 (July 1947): 33.

52. For the plight of women scientists in American higher education for the period under discussion, see Rossiter, *Women Scientists in America*, especially pp. 160–217 and table on pp. 170–171. See also Appel, "Physiology in American Women's Colleges," p. 45.

53. See Cutter to Henry Jump, 27 February 1936, Catharine Macfarlane to Council on Medical Education, 13 May 1936, Cutter to Jackson, 18 May 1936 and 19 June 1937; all in Student Affairs Papers, box 1, AMA Survey 1935, folder 3; MECBC, 16 June 1936, 3 March 1937; John Wyckoff to Tracy, 24 June 1936, William David [WMC treasurer] to Cutter, 2 June 1937 [regarding improved financial condition at WMC], Fred Zapffe to Tracy, 4 November 1936 [restoration to membership in the AAMC], all in Student Affairs Papers, box 1, Survey of College AAMC, January 1935 folder; MF, 12 March 1937.

54. Mrs. Starr learned that the new building contained 500,000 face bricks, 36,000 glazed bricks used for the interior, and about 1,500,000 common bricks in the walls (Howell Lewis Shay [architect] to Starr, 15 March 1937, in Macfarlane Papers).

55. William M. David (WMC treasurer) to Fred Zapffe, 22 December 1937, in Student Affairs Papers, AMA Survey 1935, folder 3.

56. David to Sheppard, 27 December 1938, in Student Affairs Papers, AMA Survey 1935, folder 3.

57. MF, 6 September 1940.

58. Extensive information on Craighill is lacking. There is a folder under her name in the Vertical File containing several newspaper clippings (e.g., "College Picks Woman Dean," *Philadelphia Public Ledger*, 7 September 1940, and an obituary, "Dr. Margaret D. Craighill, at 78, Former Dean of Medical College," *New York Times*, 27 July 1977).

59. MECBC, 5 March 1941.

60. "Report to the Council on Medical Education and Hospitals of the American Medical Association. Hospital of the Woman's Medical College of Pennsylvania. Inspected by A. R. Bowles, M.D., January 31, 1941," in Vida Francis Papers, "Battle" folder.

61. Craighill to Starr, 24 July 1940, Sheppard Papers, box 8, folder 116.

62. Sheppard to Craighill, 12 February 1941, Francis Papers, "Battle" folder. In this letter, Sheppard, loyal to Mrs. Starr, asked Craighill to resign.

63. Craighill to Sheppard, 18 February 1941, Francis Papers, "Battle" folder. That Craighill sought an AMA review to gain leverage over Mrs. Starr was confirmed by Marion Fay in the interview conducted with her by Regina Morantz-Sanchez, 11 July 1977, p. 17, in Oral History Project on Women in Medicine.

64. Bowles, "Report to the Council."

65. MECBC, 12 March 1941.

66. "Communication to the Board of Corporators, March 19, 1941," in Francis Papers, "Battle" folder.

67. Vida Hunt Francis to Donald G. Price, 28 April 1941, in Francis Papers, "Battle" folder. Ellen Culver Potter (WMC, 1903), former faculty member and College loyalist, served as acting president from 1941 until 1943.
68. Margaret [Majer] Kelly herself was not of Irish descent. She was college educated, highly intelligent, and like her husband, athletic. John B. Kelly Sr., one of ten children of immigrant parents, had grown up in the Falls. His major business was Kelly for Brickwork. He was both "construction and brickwork magnate," but also an Olympic rowing champion and major figure in Philadelphia politics. See David Iams, "'Guiding Light' for Kellys," *Philadelphia Inquirer*, 9 January 1990; John Lukacs, *Philadelphia: Patricians and Philistines, 1900–1950* (New York: Farrar Strauss Giroux, 1981), p. 332. An informal account of the Kelly family is Arthur H. Lewis's *Those Philadelphia Kellys . . . With a Touch of Grace* (New York: William Morrow and Co., 1977).
69. Fay interview, p. 20.
70. Ibid., pp. 20, 46.
71. Primary sources concerning the proposed merger with Jefferson Medical College include: Margaret Craighill, "Report on the State of the College and Recommendations," 10 April 1946, "Minutes of a Meeting of the Board of Corporators, Faculty and Alumnae of the Woman's Medical College of Pennsylvania held at 4:00 p.m. on Wednesday, April 10, 1946 at the College of Physicians," letter signed by Catharine Macfarlane, Winifred Bayard Stewart, Isabel M. Balph, Miriam Butler, and Emily P. Bacon to Walter H. Robinson [secretary of the board of corporators], 9 April 1946, letter signed by basic science faculty to Margaret Craighill, 7 April 1946; all in MBC, folder for special meeting of 10 April 1946; also, Catharine Macfarlane, "Report [to the Alumnae Association] on the Woman's Medical College," undated, in Board of Corporators Collection, "Charter, Statutes, Mergers," box 1. See also account of the events in Fay interview, pp. 22–25.
72. Interview with Katharine Boucot Sturgis conducted by Regina Morantz-Sanchez, 11 and 12 July 1977, p. 62, in Oral History Project on Women in Medicine.
73. Catharine Macfarlane, "Woman's Medical College of Pennsylvania, 1850–1946. The History of an Amazing Interlude. Chronologically Presented," typescript, in Board of Corporators Collection, "Charters, Statutes, Mergers," box 1. Rodman's passionate statement is recorded in "Minutes of a Meeting," pp. 4–5.
74. "Minutes of a Meeting," p. 4.
75. The telegram is in the folder for the MBC, 10 April 1946.
76. Fay interview, p. 25.
77. Catharine Macfarlane, Typescript Autobiography, p. 22, in Macfarlane Papers, and another copy at Library of the College of Physicians of Philadelphia.
78. This discussion is drawn from: Burton Clark, *The Distinctive College* (New Brunswick and London: Transactions Publishers, 1992; originally published in 1970); and idem, "Belief and Loyalty in College Organization," *Journal of Higher Education* 42 (1976): 499–515.
79. Clark, "Belief and Loyalty," p. 510.
80. Clark, *Distinctive College*, p. 252.
81. Ibid., p. 256.
82. Ibid.

Chapter 10   **The Marion Fay Years**

1. Dean Marion Fay cited figures indicating that at WMC the actual annual cost per student was $3,649.00 while the tuition was $875.00, and such a discrepancy was not considered uncommon (Marion Fay, "Dean's Report, 1943–46; 1946–56," in MBC, 28 September 1956).

2. For medicine, science, and medical education in post–World War II America, see Paul Starr, *The Social Transformation of American Medicine* (New York: Basic Books, 1982), esp. pp. 335–347; and pamphlet publications of the National Fund for Medical Education (NFME), such as *Medical Education in the United States: The Problem—The Cost—The Horizon* (1950). For the Ford Foundation program in support of medical education, see its *Annual Report* (Dearborn, Mich.) for 1956 (pp. 32–34) and 1957 (pp. 4, 5, 13). The Ford Foundation made direct grants for medical school endowments and supported the NFME.

3. Hill-Burton was Public Law 79–75, The Hospital Survey and Construction Act, passed in 1946. Federal funds for hospital expansion within this program were channeled through the states, to which applications were made. The original intent was to favor regions lacking adequate hospital facilities. See Starr, *Social Transformation*, pp. 347–351; Rosemary Stevens, *In Sickness and in Wealth: American Hospitals in the Twentieth Century* (New York: Basic Books, 1989), esp. pp. 216–223.

4. For the history of N.I.H. grants programs to medical schools, see Starr, *Social Transformation*, pp. 338–347; Richard Mandel, *A Half Century of Peer Review 1946–1996* (Bethesda, Md.: Division of Research Grants of the National Institutes of Health, 1996).

5. For the status of American women in the 1950s, see Sara M. Evans, *Born for Liberty: A History of Women in America* (New York: Free Press, 1989), pp. 243–262; William H. Chafe, *The Paradox of Change: American Women in the 20th Century* (New York and Oxford: Oxford University Press, 1991), pp. 175–193. For important revisionist essays, see Joanne Meyerowitz, ed., *Not June Cleaver: Women and Gender in Postwar America, 1945–1960* (Philadelphia: Temple University Press, 1994). I am grateful to Regina Morantz-Sanchez for suggesting this collection to me.

6. For tabular data on numbers and percentage of women medical students in the twentieth century, see Stephen Cole, "Sex Discrimination and Admission to Medical School, 1929–1984," *American Journal of Sociology* 92 (1986): 549–567.

7. *Viewpoints*, April 1950; "Centennial Events," *News Letter* [of the Alumnae Association of the Woman's Medical College of Pennsylvania] 4 (1950), 1:1–3. *Viewpoints* was a public relations newsletter issued by WMC from 1945 until 1969. Issues were not paginated; most comprised four to six pages.

8. "Centennial Events," p. 2.

9. Esther Pohl Lovejoy and Ada Chree Reid, "The Medical Women's International Association. An Historical Sketch, 1919–1950," *Journal of the American Medical Women's Association* 6 (1951): 29–38. Dr. A Charlotte Ruys, president of the Association, offered a "brief inspired address."

10. Ibid., p. 3.

11. Pearce spent almost her entire career at the Rockefeller Institute for Medical Research where her research centered on infectious and inherited diseases. She helped develop the curative drug for African Sleeping Sickness. She served as part-time WMC president from 1947 to 1951.

12. Frequently cited for their investigative work, grants, and presentations were Hartwig Kuhlenbeck in neuroanatomy and Phyllis Bott in renal physiology

(both of international reputation), Roberta Hafkesbring in physiology, Ruth E. Miller in microbiology, and later in the 1950s and into the 1960s, Sidney Ellis in pharmacology and I. Nathan Dubin in pathology.

13. *News Letter* [of the Alumnae Association of the Woman's Medical College of Pennsylvania] 10 (Spring 1957): 2.

14. "Ground Broken for Nurses' Home," *Viewpoints*, August 1950. See also fund-raising letter, "The Horseshoe Nail," arguing that a nursing building was key to growth of the College, in MBC, 28 September 1949.

15. Description from "New Nurses' Home Completed, Last Word in Comfort, Design," *Viewpoints*, December 1951. For the nursing shortage in postwar America, see Joan E. Lynaugh and Barbara L. Brush, *American Nursing: From Hospitals to Health Symbols* (Cambridge, Mass.: Blackwell Publishers and Milbank Memorial Fund, 1996).

16. Elizabeth Hirsh Fleisher (1892–1975), a Philadelphian of Jewish background, was educated at Wellesley College and Cambridge School of Architecture, and was the fourth woman architect registered in Pennsylvania.

17. This relatively early grant from the Hill-Burton program is documented in MBC, 26 October 1949, 27 January 1950, and in a letter from Ira J. Mills, Director, Bureau of Community Work of the Commonwealth of Pennsylvania Department of Welfare, to George Hay, Comptroller of WMC, 9 February 1950.

18. Another grant from Hill-Burton of $278,826 paid for additional renovations in the hospital portion of the central building (MF, 16 September 1956).

19. MF, 19 November 1952. The building plan was announced by Burgess L. Gordon, WMC's first salaried, administrative president, who served from 1951 until 1957. He was a physician with expertise in chest diseases and occupational medicine.

20. For the research wing, see MF, 21 November 1956, 15 May 1957, 26 June 1957, 19 March 1958, 17 September 1958, 21 January 1959, 29 June 1960; "$2,000,000 Research Wing Started," *Viewpoints*, January 1959; articles on dedication ceremonies in *Viewpoints*, December 1960; various folders in MCP Buildings Collection. In 1981 the wing was named the Marion Fay Research Building.

21. MF, 23 March 1960; "New Wing Construction Underway," *Viewpoints*, April 1965; "College Family Preview—New Clinical Teaching and Services Wing—March 10, 1968," Publications Collection.

22. For the training grants, see MF, e.g., 21 September 1955 and 9 September 1956; Fay, "Dean's Report," 1943–46 and 1946–56.

23. For the cervical cancer project, see MF, 21 November 1956, 18 September 1957; "$300,000 Research Project Opens. Cancer Research Project Launched at WMC," *Viewpoints*, October 1957. The intent of the study was to screen "women in industry" using cervical cytologic examination in order to explore better ways of detecting such cancer and uncovering risk factors.

24. MF, 20 January 1960. In May of 1961 Fay relayed the Board's request that faculty apply for more grants to help deal with a deficit that year (MF, 17 May 1961).

25. By the 1950s, the deans of the five Philadelphia medical schools worked together in securing the biannual stipend, which for WMC reached $362,000 by 1955–57. For state aid to WMC in this period, see Marion Fay, "Annual Report of the Dean."

26. MF, 19 September 1956, 15 May 1957. The Ford Foundation gave a total of $600,000 to WMC toward endowment.

27. For the National Board and Commonwealth Committee, see *Viewpoints*, April

1953, May 1954, August 1957. Some records of these organizations are at ASCWM.

28. MF, 20 May 1959.

29. Sidney Ellis revised the pharmacology course and I. Nathan Dubin the program in pathology.

30. MF, 19 March 1958, 21 May 1958, 18 February 1959.

31. MF, 21 April 1948.

32. Ibid.

33. MF, 19 May 1948.

34. MF, 21 March 1951, 17 October 1951, 25 June 1952.

35. MF, 23 June 1954, 19 October 1955.

36. E.g, interview with graduates of the Class of 1948, WMC, 30 May 1998, Philadelphia. I have heard such statements frequently from WMC alumnae of the period. See Interview with Marion Fay conducted by Regina Morantz-Sanchez, 11 July 1977, p. 13, in Oral History Project on Women in Medicine.

37. Marion Fay, "Annual Report of the Dean, 1948–1949," in MBC, 29 June 1949. Her summative report for the years 1943–1956 contains no reference to special educational programs for women students nor research concerning women's health. The cancer screening program would qualify as an example of the latter.

38. This section on Katharine Boucot Sturgis and the rebirth of preventive medicine at WMC is based on Bonnie Ellen Blustein, *Educating for Health and Prevention: A History of the Department of Community and Preventive Medicine of the (Woman's) Medical College of Pennsylvania* (Canton, Mass.: Science History Publications, 1993), pp. 38–58; and Interview with Katharine Sturgis, conducted by Regina Morantz-Sanchez, 11 and 12 July 1977, Oral History Project on Women in Medicine, esp. pp. 62–65, 72.

39. Sarah I. Morris applauded Boucot's initiatives and supported the reborn department financially.

40. Boucot's departmental colleagues and fellows over the years included Hildegard Rothmund, Bernard Behrend, William Weiss, Lila Stein Kroser (WMC, 1957), Dorothea Glass (WMC, 1955), and Judith Mausner. Kroser became a practitioner and teacher of family medicine and alumnae activist, Glass a respected practitioner of rehabilitative medicine.

41. Catharine Macfarlane and Rebecca Rhoads to board of corporators, 7 June 1966, Jean Gowing Papers.

42. The word "homeland" in this context was suggested to the author by June Klinghoffer, M.D. (WMC, 1945), professor of medicine.

43. Lalla Iverson, a Johns Hopkins M.D. graduate, when being recruited by WMC was chief of the Geographic and Infectious Diseases Branch of the Armed Forces Institute of Pathology. Her area of special expertise was "infectious, mycotic, and granulomatous disease"; see entry in Jacques Cattell, ed., *American Men of Science*, 10th ed. (Tempe, Ariz.: Cattell Press, 1960).

44. For recruitment of the new chair of pathology, see Minutes of Faculty Council, 15 February 1954, 10 May 1954, 13 September 1954, 15 November 1954, 17 January 1955, 7 March 1955. The assessment of Nathan Dubin is based on personal acquaintance during the 1970s and recollections of alumnae of the 1960s. Some of Dubin's papers are held at ASCWM.

45. See correspondence in "Biochemistry, Candidates for Professorship" folder, Student Affairs Collection; Minutes of Faculty Council, 14 January 1963.

46. Marshall to Glen Leymaster, 27 March 1964, "Physiology Candidates" folder,

Student Affairs Collection. Leymaster had just succeeded Fay as dean, but Fay had initiated communications with Jean Marshall. The identity of the first woman who declined an offer for the chair of physiology is not known; see Marion Fay to Armand Guarino, 17 January 1963, copy in "Biochemistry, Candidates" folder, Student Affairs Collection. Jean McElroy Marshall held a Ph.D. from the University of Rochester and was assistant professor of physiology at Johns Hopkins before holding the same title at Harvard Medical School. Her research area was the "electrical and mechanical properties of cardiac and smooth muscles." See entry in Cattell, *American Men of Science*.

47. Fay Interview, p. 39. Fay, a subtle and witty conversationalist, liked to employ the word "interesting" to stand in for a seemingly endless variety of attributes, including attractive, peculiar, difficult, etc.

48. Ibid.

49. The greater increase in the number of women faculty in American medical schools occurred in the 1970s and beyond. Even by 1984, however, the A.A.M.C found only twenty-three women chairs in basic science, and thirty-one in clinical sciences of which ten were pediatrics and five in rehabilitative medicine. See Association of American Medical Colleges, "Women in Medicine Statistics," January 1985; Janet Bickel, "A Statistical Perspective on Gender in Medicine," *Journal of the American Medical Women's Association* 48 (1993): 141–144.

50. Katharine Boucot Sturgis strongly believed that Marion Fay's fundamental fondness for men influenced the choice of WMC faculty; see Sturgis Interview, pp. 73–74.

51. Marion Fay, "Annual Report of the Dean, 1948–1949," in MBC, 29 June 1949.

52. Fay did much to build and better WMC. Although neither physician nor alumna, like the other great women deans she embraced the College's history and served the school steadfastly. In 1970 she came out of retirement at a time of near-crisis to serve for one year as acting president.

53. Voci held the M.D. from the University of Rome and earned another degree at the University of Paris. See MF, 21 March 1956. For the cardiac catheterization, see "Task Force against Heart Disease," *Viewpoints*, October 1958.

54. For the historic importance of women role models to women students, see Regina Morantz-Sanchez, *Sympathy and Science: Women Physicians in American Medicine* (New York and Oxford: Oxford University Press, 1985), pp. 255, 268–269.

55. The sources for the discussion which follows on student viewpoints where not otherwise specified include: Replies to 1938 Survey of Students' Opinions of WMC carried out by Catharine Macfarlane, in Macfarlane Deceased Alumna Files, box 1 (hereafter Macfarlane Replies); Interview with Doris Bartuska Conducted by Regina Morantz-Sanchez, 4 and 5 April 1977, Oral History Project on Women in Medicine; Interview with Boots Cooper Conducted by Janet Miller, 23–25 March 1992; interviews conducted by the author (recorded but not transcribed) with members of the class of 1947, 24 May 1997, with members of the class of 1948, 30 May 1998, with Phyllis Marciano, 22 May 1998, with Lila Stein Kroser, 28 August 1998; informal conversations with June Klinghoffer, Doris Bartuska, Rachel Pape, Jean Forrest, and other WMC alumnae of the 1940s and 1950s.

56. Cole, "Sex Discrimination and Admission to Medical School, 1929–1984."

57. Macfarlane Replies.

58. Bartuska Interview, pp. 21–22; Cooper Interview, p. 69; Marciano Interview; Kroser Interview.
59. All quotes from Macfarlane Replies.
60. Macfarlane Replies.
61. During interviews, the author has heard remarkably disparate recollections and opinions of certain faculty members, ranging literally from reverence to revulsion.
62. "Report of Survey," pp. 9, 20, Dean's Office Papers (accession 183 series), box 5.
63. *Student Handbook*, 1955–1956.
64. *Student Handbook*, 1959–60.
65. Many alumnae of the 1940s and 1950s have, at times with some discomfort, confided in the author that women faculty much more than the men were excessively hard on students. See, e.g., Bartuska Interview, p. 23; Kroser Interview.
66. See Bartuska Interview, p. 26, for a discussion of this hypothesis by Regina Morantz-Sanchez and Dr. Bartuska.
67. Staff at the newly-opened Veterans Administration Hospital in Philadelphia wishing faculty appointment at one of the city's medical school's drew lots to determine their school of affiliation (personal communication from Ralph Myerson, M.D., August 1998; MF, 21 May 1958).
68. Personal communication, A. Deborah Goldstein, M.D., (WMC, 1962).
69. Katharine Boucot Sturgis, "Catharine Macfarlane, 1877–1969. Recollections of Kitty Mac," dean's hour presentation, Medical College of Pennsylvania, April 1978, in Sturgis Papers, box 5. A succinct biography of Catharine Macfarlane is Sturgis's "First Woman Fellow of the College of Physicians of Philadelphia: Memoir of Catharine Macfarlane, 1877–1969," *Transactions and Studies of the College of Physicians of Philadelphia* ser. 4, 38 (1971): 157–160. Macfarlane was the first woman member of Philadelphia's prestigious College of Physicians. Her unpublished autobiography has been cited frequently in this work; copies are held both by ASCWM and by the Library of the College of Physicians of Philadelphia. The ASCWM holds a collection of her papers and memorabilia.
70. Renate Soulen to the author (email), 22 January 1998.
71. A "geographic full-time" clinical faculty member is not fully salaried, but maintains a private practice centered at her or his medical school rather than in an office elsewhere.
72. General statements in this section are based on: references to student activities in faculty minutes 1947–1962; minutes of the Student Government Council 1949–1960; group and individual interviews already cited; photographs in the *Iatrian* (the yearbook) beginning with 1956.
73. MF, 19 November 1947, 18 February 1948; Student Council minutes through the early 1950s also refer to a "foster parent plan" and mention a collection of books for Korea on 4 March 1954.
74. "Medical Journals, Textbooks Needed for Students Abroad," *Germantown Courier*, 20 May 1948, in College Clippings Collection, leaf 1442. Historian and activist Walter Lear discussed the origins of AIMS in his paper "The Nation's First Medical Student and House Staff Movement, 1934–1954," presented at the American Association for the History of Medicine, Toronto, May 1998.
75. Ivan H. Peterman, "Young Medics Entangled in Pinkish Group," *Philadelphia Inquirer*, 9 November 1949. A follow-up column by the same writer was "Official Quits Student Unit for Red Taint," *Philadelphia Inquirer*, 1 December 1949.

76. MBC, 25 November 1949, 27 January 1950; MF, 16 November 1949, 15 February 1950.
77. See minutes of Student Government Council, 10 November 1954, 17 November 1957.
78. MF, 16 May 1962.

Chapter 11   **Coeducation**

1. Interview with Marion Fay Conducted by Regina Morantz-Sanchez, 11 July 1977, Oral History Project on Women in Medicine, p. 41.
2. For Glen Leymaster, see "PMJ Interview: Dean Leymaster of Woman's Medical College," *Pennsylvania Medical Journal* (September 1964) p. 21.
3. During his years in office the College showed a sharp rise in the number of full-time faculty and the completion of important physical expansion. He also recruited several key departmental chairpersons.
4. Winifred D. Wandersee, *On the Move: American Women in the 1970s* (Boston: Twayne Publishers, 1988), pp. 103–106.
5. MF, 12 February 1969.
6. MF, 20 September 1967; "Admit Men, Panel Urges Woman's Medical College," *Philadelphia Evening Bulletin*, 24 May 1967; see also Albert R. Pechan's "preliminary draft" reports titled "Medical Training Facilities and Medical Practice in Pennsylvania," in the August, September, and October 1967 issues of *Pennsylvania Medicine*, the journal of the Pennsylvania State Medical Society.
7. Reported regularly in minutes of both faculty and board meetings. The deficits were worrisome but not huge.
8. Ibid.
9. MF, 15 January 1969, 25 June 1969, 21 January 1970. At the latter meeting, it was reported that during the current academic year nine students sought transfer out of WMC, five for "marital reasons," one for financial reasons, and three "dissatisfied with the College." Six of the nine ranked in the upper third of their classes.
10. MF, 25 June 1969.
11. MF, 26 June 1968.
12. Ibid.; MF, 12 February 1969. This was a special meeting Leymaster called to discuss issues of morale and governance after he realized "with force" that there had arisen in the College "a sense that we had lost momentum; that we were stalled, so to speak."
13. Stuart Brown, "Woman's Medical College to Continue All-Female Policy under New President," *The [Philadelphia] Sunday Bulletin*, 29 December 1963.
14. "Women's New Role in Medicine," *Medical World News*, 10 April 1964, p. 84.
15. Glen R. Leymaster, "An Answer: A National Center for Medical Education for Women—Forecast or Fantasy," *Journal of the American Medical Women's Association* 20 (1965): 346–348; idem., "Women in Medicine," *Philadelphia Medicine* 62 no. 1 (January 1966): 15–16; "GNP Versus Women Physicians," address at Rotary Club Luncheon, 12 April 1967, in Presidents' Collection, Leymaster folders.
16. The then-vice president for planning and development, Charles Glanville, believed that Leymaster at first was "firmly devoted" to the single-sex policy ("Summary of Interview with Charles Glanville," conducted by Regina Morantz-Sanchez, 1977?, in Oral History Project on Women in Medicine, supporting materials, Marion Fay box). Marion Fay concurred.

17. Leymaster's analysis is found in MECBC, 11 June 1968, and is reproduced as Appendix A of the "Report of the Committee on Admissions Policies" (hereafter "Report 1969") in Board of Corporators Papers, box titled "Statutes, Charters, Mergers." Another copy is in the Jean Gowing Collection.

18. Report 1969, Appendix C. See also his memorandum to Mrs. Paul Kaiser [Louise Kaiser] formally requesting appointment of the committee, with MBC, 25 September 1968.

19. "Excerpt from Letter of Alvan Feinstein" [Department of Internal Medicine, Yale University School of Medicine], undated, in Jean Gowing Papers, "Admissions Policy" folder; MECBC, 18 February 1969 (Leymaster obtained permission from the executive committee of the board to make this commitment several months before the Committee on Admissions Policy issued its report and recommendations).

20. MBC, 10 September 1968. Low salaries and lack of university status may also have affected the desirability of the institution for potential faculty and residents. See comments on lack of American house officers in MECBC, 10 September 1968.

21. Report 1969, Appendix A.

22. Report 1969, Appendix E.

23. David E. Goldman to Mrs. John T. Brugger, 24 February 1969, copy in Gowing Papers, "Co-Education" folder.

24. Conversation with Jay Roberts, Ph.D., 11 December 1998.

25. William G. Rothstein, *American Medical Schools and the Practice of Medicine: A History* (New York and Oxford: Oxford University Press, 1987), p. 290 (table).

26. In 1967 women filled only 13 percent of full-time faculty positions in American medical schools; Association of American Medical Colleges, *Women in Medicine Statistics* (Washington, D.C.: 1985).

27. The student was Susan Benes (WMC, 1975), the assistant dean Mary Ellen Hartman (Interview with Susan Benes Conducted by Regina Morantz-Sanchez, 10 March 1978, Oral History Project on Women in Medicine).

28. Report 1969, Appendix A.

29. Report 1969.

30. Mrs. Kaiser, an active member of the WMC board since 1959 and its chair since 1965, also had volunteered for other charities and educational institutions. Her husband was president of Tasty Baking Company, a large business located a few blocks from WMC. Mrs. Kaiser's work for WMC again typified its nucleus of local support.

31. Report 1969.

32. A sample copy of this letter forms Appendix B of Report 1969.

33. The Report indicates that 24 percent of the letters were against a policy change, 35 percent expressed support for a conditional policy change, and 41 percent supported an unconditional change in admissions policy (Report 1969, Appendix B).

34. MF, 15 January 1969.

35. Ibid.

36. Report 1969, Appendix B for analysis of responses; Appendix F for Dr. Cooper Bell's objections.

37. Norris to Leymaster, undated, Leymaster Papers.

38. Frances S. Norris, "Medical Womanpower," *New England Journal of Medicine* 281 (1969): 910–911.

39. Hall to Kaiser, 28 August 1969, Phyllis Marciano Papers.
40. E. Cooper Bell to Advisory Committee on Admissions Policies, 7 February 1969, copy in Phyllis Marciano Papers.
41. Petition to the Board of Corporators of the Woman's Medical College of Pennsylvania from the Delaware Valley Chapter of the Alumnae Association, 29 August 1969, Phyllis Marciano Papers.
42. "WMC Goes Coed: The Story behind the Headlines," *The Woman's Medical College of Pennsylvania Alumnae News*, November 1969, pp. 2–3.
43. Michael G. Michaelson, "Medical Students: Healers Become Activists," *Saturday Review*, 16 August 1969, p. 42.
44. MBC, 27 September 1968, 25 October 1968, 13 December 1968, and 31 January 1969.
45. "President's Report to the Board of Corporators Re Staffing and Morale, February 28, 1969," filed with MBC, 28 February 1969.
46. "An Open Letter to the Board from Concerned Students," 17 March 1969, filed with MECBC, 18 March 1969.
47. Report 1969, Appendix E.
48. Ibid.
49. "To the Committee on Admissions Policies," 24 March 1969, copy in Marciano Papers.
50. Nancy Coyne, "Editorial on the CBA Conference," *Vital Signs*, March 1969. CBA refers to the Committee on Black Admissions, previously mentioned.
51. Ibid.
52. Lourdes Corman, "Another Committee," *Vital Signs*, May 1969.
53. Corman to Mrs. John T. Brugger Jr., Chairman and Members of Advisory Committee on Admission Policies, 18 February 1969, copy in Gowing Papers, "Co-Education" folder.
54. For students' concern over educational issues, communications, and their desire for a role in policy, see "An Open Letter to the Board," "To the Committee," Corman, "Another Committee," and recording of the executive committee of the board's interview with student representatives, MECBC, 9 April 1969.
55. For alumnae insistence that men not displace women students, see responses to a postal card survey of alumnae in Marciano Papers.
56. MECBC, 9 April 1969, 21 April 1969.
57. MF, 16 April 1969.
58. MF, 25 June 1969.
59. Report, 1969, p. 2. The Report is dated 15 May 1969 and was formally proffered to the board at its meeting of 6 June 1969.
60. MBC, 26 September 1969.
61. Ibid., 5 September 1969.
62. "The Male Coeds: A New Breed," *Woman's Medical College Today*, November 1969.
63. "A Tale of 239 Girls and Three Men," *Philadelphia Inquirer Magazine*, 4 January 1970, p. 7.
64. "Reactions Mixed Over Three Men Attending Woman's Medical College," [Allentown] *Evening Chronicle*, 27 October 1969.
65. Interview with Lawrence Byrd, M.D., 23 May 1997, Philadelphia. Similar perceptions have been expressed to the author by other early male graduates such as Hardy Sorkin and Martin Schimmel (both MCP 1972).
66. MF, 15 October 1969.

67. Association of American Medical Colleges, "Women in Medicine Statistics," January 1985.

68. These statements are based on: data supplied by Linda Hiner, associate dean for student affairs; inspection of class lists in the annual catalogs, for the period noted; "MCP Student Body Data" (1993) in "WMCP/Statistics" folder in Vertical Files; and author's experience as a second-year course director (Introduction to Clinical Medicine) from 1982 until 1996. The "Mission Planning Council" appointed by Dr. Leymaster in 1970 in its 1971 report, "A Star to Steer By," stated that "a minimum of 60 places in the entering class will be reserved for qualified women," and that "as our facilities expand we anticipate a gradual increase in the percentage of men students, but their number will not be allowed to exceed the number of women students" (p. 10). When the number of men admitted exceeded the number of women in the late 1980s, it is likely that alumna and professor of medicine June Klinghoffer "eldered" members of the Admissions Committee.

69. "Dr. Leymaster Invites New Name Ideas," *Woman's Medical College Today,* December 1969, p. 5.

70. Phyllis Marciano, "Year in Review," *Alumnae News,* May 1971, p. 4. Correspondence concerning alumnae displeasure over the change of name is found in the Marciano Papers.

71. Ibid., p. 4.

72. The phrase "homeland" was used by professor of medicine and 1946 graduate June Klinghoffer in a conversation with the author, 10 February 1999. Dr. Klinghoffer through the late 1990s directed teaching programs in the Department of Medicine and increasingly represented a valuable linkage to the traditions and memories of Woman's Med. A vivid statement of alumnae feelings about the changes at WMC/MCP is Boots Cooper's "President's Statement" in the December 1972 *Alumnae News.*

73. For these antidiscrimination laws and the College's response, see Bernard Sigel, "Progress Report No. 2," 30 June 1972, and "Fact Sheet," unsigned, 7 September 1972, both in Alumnae Association and Special Trust Fund Binder, Margaret Gray Wood Papers (kindly made available by Dr. Wood); MBC, 23 June 1972; "Report to Board on Anti-sex Discrimination Legislative Efforts," with MBC, 23 February 1973 (Glanville was vice president for Planning and Development). Surgeon and researcher Bernard Sigel became dean under Leymaster in 1969 when the separate deanship was resumed, then became acting president as well, succeeding Marion Fay in 1971.

74. MBC, 23 February 1973.

75. The hoped-for amendment to other health bills actually called for a deferment of compliance until 1978.

76. For the Special Trust Fund, see Margaret Gray Wood, "Our Special Trust Fund," *Alumnae News,* February 1972, pp. 5–6; also other reports in the *Alumnae News* (e.g., December 1972, pp. 4–6; January 1974, p. 7; February 1975, p. 14). Correspondence about the formation of the fund, including animosity between its founders and officers and College leaders, is found in Margaret Gray Wood Papers, which also include minutes of meetings of the trustees of the fund.

77. Marion Fay, "Annual Report of the Dean, 1948–1949," in MBC, 29 June 1949, discussed in the previous chapter.

78. Wandersee, *On the Move.*

Chapter 12   Medical College of Pennsylvania

1. Medical College of Pennsylvania, *A Star to Steer By: Statement of Mission* (Philadelphia, 1971), p. 5.
2. Ibid.
3. *MCP Today*, September 1970. *MCP Today*, known as *Woman's Medical College Today* for its first few issues, was the official College publication through the 1970s and much of the 1980s. Its frequency of publication varied over these years.
4. *MCP Today*, November 1970, January/February 1971. The Presidents' Collection contains a small amount of material dealing with Leopold's aborted presidency but does not shed light on his reasons for withdrawing.
5. "Dr. Fay Announces Freeze on Jobs . . . Salaries . . . Budgets," *MCP Today*, Summer 1971. Information on the financial crisis of 1971–1972 is also found in MBC, 24 September 1971, 5 November 1971, 10 December 1971, 25 February 1972, 21 March 1972. The crisis grew largely out of unreimbursed hospital expenses for free emergency care and disputes with the local Blue Cross insurer.
6. MBC, 5 May 1976; Interview with Joseph Leighton [professor and chair of pathology] conducted by Sandra Chaff [archivist], 7 October 1987.
7. Leighton Interview. The author also recalls an MCP faculty member being "thanked" at a historical meeting by a faculty member at the University of Wisconsin School of Medicine for solving that school's perceived problems with Cooke. The MCP search committee had not been sufficiently astute in its inquiries.
8. For Robert Cooke's presidency, see *MCP Today*, April/May 1977, Fall 1978, Fall 1979, and a small collection of materials in the Presidents' Collection. For faculty protest, censure, and the board's deliberations, see MBC, 5 September 1979, 4 October 1979, 28 November 1979. A committee of the board investigating the allegations did not substantiate an accusation concerning diversion of funds, and chose in its report to not specifically support or refute the other charges. Cooke received four additional years of pay as "consultant."
9. "Maurice C. Clifford, M.D., Elected 17th President," *MCP Today*, Fall 1980; MBC, 29 October 1980 (includes "Recommendation and Report of the Presidential Selection Committee," 15 October 1980). Materials concerning Dr. Clifford are housed at ASCWM.
10. Information concerning Dr. Sutnick is derived from interview conducted by the author, 12 and 26 February 1999; curriculum vitae and other materials provided to the author by Dr. Sutnick; "The New Dean: Alton Sutnick, M.D.," *MCP Today*, Summer 1975. The ASCWM holds a sizeable collection of records from his deanship. His earlier research work centered on pulmonary surfactant and the "Australia Antigen," later linked to Hepatitis B.
11. Interview with Doris Bartuska conducted by Regina Morantz-Sanchez, 4 and 5 April 1977, p. 65, Oral History Project on Women in Medicine.
12. Sutnick Interview and conversation with Sandra Chaff, the first director of ASCWM.
13. "Dean Sutnick's Era: Growth and Stability," *MCP Today*, Fall 1988.
14. *Medical College of Pennsylvania 1987 Annual Report*, p. 28. The figure includes training grants.
15. "The New Dean."
16. MBC, 19 May 1972.
17. Ibid.

18. *MCP Today*, February/March 1973.
19. For addition of technologic medicine, see *MCP Today*, Fall 1978; Winter/Spring 1979; Summer 1981; Winter 1981; and *Annual Report* for 1983.
20. Plasmapheresis is a technique for removing substances such as antibodies from the blood in order to treat certain immunologic diseases. A hyperbaric chamber is a form of oxygen treatment employed for treating carbon monoxide poisoning and, experimentally, other disorders.
21. *MCP Today*, Winter 1980.
22. *MCP Today*, Special Edition, 1986; MBC, 22 June 1983; "MCP Building Project Chronology of Events," attachment to MBC, 28 March 1984. The College experienced difficulty in floating a bond with a favorable rating, and ended up paying a high rate of interest on the $32 million issue.
23. For the Retraining Program, see WMC, *President's Report 1968–1969*, p. 4; *MCP Today*, October/November 1972; "Programs of the Center for Women in Medicine," *Alumnae News*, February 1975; folder "Retrainee Program" in Public Affairs Collection. For this and other "programs for women" see Alton I. Sutnick, Susan McLeer, "Programs Developed from Concerns for Women in Medicine," *Journal of Medical Education* 54 (1979): 627–631. The Retraining Program in its early years won several large grants. It continued well into the early 1990s.
24. For the Learning Center, see Sutnick and McLeer, "Programs Developed." For its closing, see MBC, 22 June 1983.
25. Margaret Gray Wood, "Special Programs for Women," *Alumnae News*, December, 1972, p. 7; "First in the Nation: MCP Established Internship in Acute Care Medicine," *MCP Today*, December 1971/January 1972.
26. Susan McLeer, "Update: Women in Medicine at MCP," *Alumnae News*, Summer 1979, pp. 6–8.
27. Early discussions of the Office and Center for Women in Medicine are found in *Alumnae News*, December, 1972 and February 1975; *MCP Today*, February/March 1972, Summer 1973; folders on "Women's Programs at MCP," in Dean's Collection (Sutnick files).
28. The planning grant for ELAM was obtained in 1994 by former MCP president D. Walter Cohen and his associate Patricia Cormier; the program continues as this is written.
29. Woodside to Sutnick, 26 February 1976, in folder "Women's Programs at MCP, 1976–1978, Dean's Collections, Sutnick files; Charles Glanville to Jeanne Brugger, 7 October 1976, in folder "Women's Programs at MCP, 1975–1976," Dean's Collections, Sutnick files. ASCWM holds in remote storage a collection of materials from the CWIM, not examined by the author.
30. McLeer to Sutnick, 10 May 1978, in folder "Women's Programs at MCP, 1976–1978, Dean's Collections, Sutnick files.
31. *MCP Today*, Spring 1981.
32. Jan Schneider, an authority on high-risk pregnancy and obstetrical education, was recruited from the University of Michigan. There was no formal protest by alumnae surrounding this appointment but considerable unhappiness, not aimed, of course, at the individual (personal communication, June Klinghoffer, M.D.).
33. See discussion about the origins of the CWIM in *Alumnae News*, December, 1972. The entire story of the attempts to incorporate women's programs at MCP during the 1970s through the 1990s warrants a much fuller analysis than can be provided here.
34. The figures are based on a count of assistant, associate, and full professors from

the 1986–1987 *Bulletin* of MCP and the February 1987 edition of the Association of American Medical Colleges' "Women in Medicine Statistics."

35. Responses to a survey carried out by the Alumnae/i Association of the Woman's Medical College of Pennsylvania and Medical College of Pennsylvania (Alumnae/i Survey), intended to gather reminiscences and ideas for planning sesquicentennial activities; copies kindly provided to the author by the Association. These will be deposited in ASCWM. Admittedly the percentage of return for this survey was small, and no doubt those with more positive feelings about their medical school years at WMC or MCP would have been more likely to return the questionnaire, thus biasing its results.

36. Alumnae/i Survey.

37. The quotation is from the Alumnae/i Survey response of Camilla Graham (MCP, 1994). The same experience was described by Marianne Rothschild (MCP, 1991) and Alexia Gordon (MCP, 1995).

38. An abridged selection of the interviews was published as Regina Markell Morantz [Sanchez], Cynthia Stodola Pomerleau, and Carol Hansen Fenichel, *In Her Own Words: Oral Histories of Women Physicians* (Westport, Conn.: Greenwood Press, 1982). The early staff of the Archives and Special Collections included Sandra Chaff (its first director), Margaret Jerrido, Barbara Malinsky, Jill Gates Smith, and Ida Wilson. They transformed the previously little-known materials into a collection of national importance.

39. Alumnae/i Survey.

40. Author's telephone interview with Mary Ellen Hartman, M.D., 8 February 1999. The interest in students and helpfulness of Drs. Hartman and Beasley were widely acknowledged at MCP.

41. Alton Sutnick, "Update: Status of Competition for Medical Students," attachment to MBC, 18 May 1983. See also Alton Sutnick, "Achieving in the Eighties," *Alumnae/i News*, Fall 1985, pp. 18–20.

42. Maurice Clifford, excerpts from his "Inaugural Address," in *MCP Today*, Spring 1981. These words had special meaning following the discord of the Cooke affair.

43. The quotation is from the Alumnae/i Survey response of Mark Rovner (MCP, 1987).

44. Hartman interview; *Medical College of Pennsylvania 1984 Annual Report*, p. 5. In 1984, Dr. Hartman was senior associate dean for Student and Graduate Medical Affairs. The minority admissions program involved a collaboration with Bryn Mawr College.

45. *MCP Today*, Fall 1976; Susan Greenberg, "Medical Humanities: The Fine Art of Medicine," *Alumnae/i News*, Fall 1983, pp. 2–5; Bonnie Ellen Blustein, *Educating for Health and Prevention: A History of the Department of Community and Preventive Medicine of the (Woman's) Medical College of Pennsylvania* (Canton, Mass.: Science History Publications, 1993), pp. 85–87, 101–104. This program was led first by cleric and social worker John Sorenson, and later expanded by Janet Fleetwood, an ethicist and philosopher.

46. For information on the early Standardized Patient Program, see "The Vanishing Patient" in *MCP Today*, Winter/Spring 1989.

47. For some of these computer innovators, see "Hardware, Software, Studentware," *MCP Today*, Winter/Spring 1989.

48. Though it must be pointed out that throughout the MCP years the number of women chairs remained low.

49. Clifford, "Inaugural Address."

50. MBC, 26 June 1985.
51. Personal communication with Kenneth Ludmerer.
52. Lankenau Hospital, Mercy Catholic Medical Center, and Frankford Hospital; MBC, 22 June 1983.
53. MBC, 20 May 1987.
54. Ibid.

Afterword

1. "Affiliation Agreement" in bound volume "Affiliation Between Allegheny Health Services, Inc. and The Medical College of Pennsylvania, Closed April 27, 1988," in Board of Corporators Collections; *MCP Today*, Summer 1988.
2. The building, on Queen Lane, had been offices of the Lutheran Church in America. The transformation into a teaching and research facility was a triumph of architect and builder.
3. "Case Studies: Medical College of Pennsylvania" (1994), p. 21 (photocopy supplied to author by D. Walter Cohen).
4. "Hospitals Discuss a Merger," *Philadelphia Inquirer*, 13 December 1989; various memoranda concerning aborted merger with Hahnemann University, author's collection. Many MCP faculty and students opposed the merger for all or some of the following reasons: fear that the larger Hahnemann would dominate; loss of the intimate scale and milieu of MCP; a perception that MCP's science departments were superior; Hahnemann's clinical departments were highly oriented toward private practice; and in recent decades the school had been scarred by a variety of scandals (see Naomi Rogers, *An Alternative Path: The Making and Remaking of Hahnemann Medical College and Hospital of Philadelphia* (New Brunswick, N.J.: Rutgers University Press, 1998).
5. "New Names for University and Hospital System Unveiled," *University Times*, 21 June 1996 (the latter was a new internal newsletter).
6. "Absorbing Graduate Health Entails Risk," *Philadelphia Inquirer*, 11 August 1996; "Message from the President [Sherif S. Abdelhak]," 17 April 1997, announcing "integration of the former Graduate Health System" into Allegheny Health, Education and Research Foundation, author's files.
7. "Hospital Bosses Are Growing Richer," *Philadelphia Inquirer*, 19 January 1997. The reporters of the *Philadelphia Inquirer* who provided thorough coverage of the Allegheny demise included Andrea Gerlin, Josh Goldstein, and Karl Stark.
8. "Allegheny to Sell 6 Area Hospitals," *Philadelphia Inquirer*, 13 March 1998; "Allegheny CEO's Growth Strategy Proves 'Paper Thin,'" *Philadelphia Inquirer*, 7 June 1998; "Bankruptcy and Sale for Allegheny," *Philadelphia Inquirer*, 21 July 1998; "Message from the President [Anthony Sanzo, who had replaced Abdelhak]," 20 July 1998, author's files.
9. For the best existing accounts of the demise of Allegheny Health Education and Research Foundation, see *The Philadelphia Inquirer* for the following dates: 29 April 1998, 6 May 1998, 22 May 1998, 7 June 1998, 9 June 1998, 2 July 1998, 21 July 1998, 2 August 1998, 16 August 1998, 18 August 1998, 20 September 1998, 30 September 1998, 14 October 1998, 22 October 1998, 23 October 1998, 27 October 1998.
10. See Regina Morantz-Sanchez, *Sympathy and Science: Women Physicians in American Medicine* (New York and Oxford: Oxford University Press, 1985), pp. 244–249; Esther Lovejoy, *Women Doctors of the World* (New York: Macmillan, 1957), pp. 120–125.

11. Penn took its first women medical students in 1914, Hahnemann (with one exception in the 1860s) in 1941, and Jefferson in 1961.
12. *Bulletin of the Woman's Medical College of Pennsylvania* 65 (March 1915): 18.
13. Morantz-Sanchez, *Sympathy and Science*, pp. 253–254.
14. At the time of publishing his famous *Report*, Flexner did not see the continued need for separate women's medical schools, but did not single them out for closing.
15. Cited in Eliza E. Judson, *Address in Memory of Ann Preston, M.D. Delivered by Request of the Corporators and Faculty of the Woman's Medical College of Pennsylvania* (Philadelphia, 1873), p. 19.

Index

Abaza, Nabil, 234
Abdelhak, Sherif S., 252
Abbey, Charlotte, 116
Abbott, Maude, 154
Acorn Club, 59
Adams, Lida Stokes, 71
Addams, Jane, 68
Alexander, Virginia, 161, 242
Allegheny Health, Education and
    Research Foundation (AHERF),
    252
Allegheny Health Systems, Inc.
    (AHSI), 250, 251
Allison, Mary Bruins, 163
Alsop, Gulielma Fell, 63, 66; History of
    the Woman's Medical College, 188
American Chemical Society, 29
American Female Medical Education
    Society, 10–11
American Medical Association
    (AMA), 30, 31, 61; Council on
    Medical Education and Hospitals,
    122, 167, 177–178
American Medical Women's Associa-
    tion, 180
Anderson, Caroline Still Wiley, 116,
    118–119, 183
Anderson, Marian, 188
Anderson, Matthew, 118
Arey, Harriet, 205
Association of American Medical
    Colleges, 61, 73, 124, 167
Association of Internes and Medical
    Students (AIMS), 208

Audenried, Ada, 80

bacteriology, 57, 74, 76, 81
Barnes, Ann, 234, 241
Barton, Amy, 80
Barton, Isaac, 29, 40, 129
Bartuska, Doris, 198, 200, 224, 233
Bassett, James, 198, 206
Baumann, Frieda, 184, 198, 205, 242
Beasley, Andrew, 198, 234, 245
Behrens, Charles F., 188
Bell, E. Cooper, 216–217
Bell, Whitfield J., 30
Bennett, Alice, 86, 115
Berean Manual Training and Industrial
    School (Berean Institute), 118
Berman, Nancy, 241
Biemuller, Martha, 198
Bierring, Walter L., 168
Birdsell, Sylvester, 20, 21
Blackwell, Elizabeth, 7, 16, 14
Blackwell, Emily, 7, 71, 74
Bleier, Ruth, 208
Blockley, see Philadelphia [General]
    Hospital
Bodley, Rachel, 29, 31, 40, 42, 63–
    68, 79, 91; alumnae survey by, 61,
    63–65; botanical interests, 63; 1881
    address, "The College Story," 63–65
botany, 29
Bott, Phyllis, 174, 175, 195
Boucot Sturgis, Katharine R., see
    Sturgis, Katharine R. Guest Boucot
Brenner, Andrew, 223, 224

About the Author

Steven J. Peitzman, M.D., a native of Philadelphia, has taught internal medicine, nephrology, and the history of medicine at the Medical College of Pennsylvania and its successor for almost twenty-five years. He has contributed articles and chapters to both clinical and historical publications and lectured widely on the history of medicine and medical education. He has served on committees and the council of the American Association for the History of Medicine and on the editorial boards of two medical history quarterlies. He is currently working on a history of nephrology. Dr. Peitzman holds degrees from Central High School of Philadelphia, the University of Pennsylvania, and Temple University.